TRAPPED: FAMILIES AND SCHIZOPHRENIA

Lloyd H. Rogler
Albert Schweitzer University Professor
Fordham University

August B. Hollingshead
William Graham Sumner Professor Emeritus
Yale University

WATERFRONT PRESS
Maplewood, N.J.

Copyright 1985 by Lloyd H. Rogler

Originally published in 1965 by John Wiley & Sons, Inc., New York City. Reprinted 1975 by Robert E. Krieger Publishing Co., Huntington, N.Y.

This edition published by:

WATERFRONT PRESS
52 Maple Ave.
Maplewood, N.J. 07040

All rights reserved under international and Pan-American Copyright Conventions

ISBN: **0-943862-28-0**

Printed in the United States of America, 1985.

Preface to Third Edition

The preface to the reprint edition of *Trapped: Families and Schizophrenia* which follows examined the professional reactions to the book during the first decade after its publication. Now, ten years after the issuing of the reprint edition, the book's findings continue to be assimilated into the professional literature along the same lines described in the previous preface. Thus, in terms of its continuing influence, the book represents the conclusion of a successful collaborative effort between the late Professor Hollingshead and myself. Perhaps the reader will be interested in a somewhat personal but brief backward glance at some of the events associated with this collaboration.

One requirement for the Ph.D. degree in sociology at the University of Iowa during the 1950s was substantial mastery over what the graduate students, including myself, pejoratively labelled as "cloud hopping" theories. The attitude associated with the label expressed the disdain of the young, developing social scientist toward highly abstract, architectonic systems of theory then fashionable among some sociologists. We doubted the relevance of such theories to a scientific sociology. After immersion in them, it was a distinct relief to turn to the work of other sociologists who, being empirically oriented, were making observations and providing data relevant to delimited theoretical issues. Noteworthy among them was Professor August B. Hollingshead. Along with other graduate students, I was familiar with most -- if not all -- of his published research. We admired the thorough way in which he brought systematic observations to bear upon some carefully defined point of theory or public policy. The more we were exposed to the lofty machinations of the "grand" theorists, the greater became our esteem for the work of sociologists such as Hollingshead.

In the fall of 1956, when I was beginning my last year of graduate studies toward a Ph.D., I received a letter from Professor Hollingshead. In it he said that he had heard about me from a colleague who had taught at the University of Iowa, and that he understood I was born and raised in Puerto Rico and was fluent in Spanish. He explained that he had been invited by the Social Science Research Center of the University of Puerto Rico to develop research on sociocultural components of mental illness in the island. He ended the letter by inquiring as to my interest in joining this effort. The letter elated me and I immediately accepted his offer.

At that time, Hollingshead, a professor of sociology at Yale University, was completing *Social Class and Mental Illness* (John Wiley and Sons, 1958), in collaboration with Dr. Fredrick C. Redlich. Already, however, the articles which had been published from the same research were foreshadowing a major scientific contribution to issues which were little understood. The book's promise was to be amply fulfilled. To this day, *Social Class and mental Illness* remains an unsurpassed contribution to our understanding of how processes enmeshing persons in the social class system shape the emergence of mental illness, the effects of such illness upon persons and families, the efforts made to alleviate the mental distress they bring, and the differential treatment emotionally distressed clients receive when they turn to the official mental health system. These articles brought Hollingshead's name to the attention of Dr. Millard Hansen, then Director of the Social Science Research Center of the University of Puerto Rico. Under Hansen's leadership, the Center had produced a number of research-based books, now widely recognized, focusing interdisciplinary attention upon the convulsions of social change Puerto Rico was then experiencing. Emotional distress and mental illness, Hansen believed, should be the object of research in a society undergoing such change. He invited Hollingshead to Puerto Rico to explore the possibility of initiating research. Hollingshead's letter to me was the result of that visit.

Several months later I flew from Iowa to San Juan. Still a graduate student, and very much in awe of Hollingshead's research accomplishments and academic stature, I was uneasy and apprehensive as I nervously shook hands with him in Hansen's office. "Please call me Sandy," he said, referring to his nickname. I was set at ease. There followed an open discussion between seeming coequals focusing directly upon issues associated with the research initiative being planned. This started the collaborative relationship between an older, internationally renowned researcher and a young, completely unknown, but eager researcher.

It would take many more pages than what this preface allows to convey the tribulations and excitement that went into our collaborative effort to produce *Trapped*. The effort spanned contrasting environments, from the abysmally wretched slums of the San Juan Martin Pena Channel, where much of the data were collected, to the cathedral-like high-ceilinged buildings in Yale's Old Campus where the book was drafted. Not having the space to present such retrospections, I shall limit myself to one memory which remains vivid, namely, Sandy's direct attitude toward the essential task of the sociologist, the understanding of the social world. Circumlocutions were anathema to him, and so were elliptical statements and jargon. Although he was a masterful and enthusiastic storyteller, often drawing from his early life on a ranch in the west where his father raised horses, and enjoyed the storytelling talents of other persons, he was notably impatient at professional talk that rambled without direction. The culprit often would be the focus of his fixed, blue-eyed gaze, and often he would then display a surprising aptitude for getting to the point.

Sandy evidenced this attitude during his trips to Puerto Rico from New Haven, from 1957 to 1960, when the *Trapped* data were being collected. By then, I was living in San Juan and had assumed responsibility for the day to day direction of an excellent field research team we had recruited and trained. His visits, generally lasting a week or two, involved a crowded schedule of office work, team meetings, the making of decisions and plans. But a necessary part of each of his visits was going to the field to observe and interview the *Trapped* families in the slums and public housing developments of San Juan. Important as it was, office talk about the research reflected only indirectly what was occurring to the families, and it had to be balanced by visiting them. During such visits, which often involved slushing through the mud of the odiferous slums of the Martin Pena Channel, Sandy questioned me incessantly. He did not speak Spanish but was determined to know what was being said in the interviews. He pressed me to translate and explain cultural elements of Puerto Rican society. The answers to the questions rendered accessible to him the research situation in a culture different from his own and, at the same time, made me aware of features of Puerto Rican culture I had known implicitly but never before verbalized. Both of us were learning as a result of Sandy's drive to come in closer touch with the life circumstances of the study's families.

Early in the study I inadvertently became aware of the importance of spiritualism in providing care to the emotionally distressed persons in the slums and public housing developments of San Juan. (The reader will note in the preface which follows, and in the book, the therapeutic importance of this institutional pattern in Puerto Rican society.) On Sandy's next visit I told him of the work I had undertaken as a participant observer in spiritualist sessions, and why I believed the practice of spiritualism as a form of folk psychiatry was relevant to the research. He was downright enthusiastic, and no amount of office work would keep him from going to spiritualist sessions. Having anticipated his response, I had made plans. After the sessions we spent hours upon hours discussing the elaborate rituals enacted during the sessions. As substantive matters were being discussed, a point about research methods was being made. Through his own previous research, Sandy was completely familiar with the techniques of quantitative, survey-oriented sociologists. Nonetheless, he retained a fundamental conviction in the importance of methods -- more often associated with anthropological research -- in which the researcher himself is the vehicle for observations. Such methods, essential to the study of spiritualism, coincided with his own view of approaching the task of the sociologists directly.

The direct approach also was in evidence during the analysis of the data. Soon after we began the analysis at Yale, I was surprised to see Sandy spend hour after hour tediously constructing statistical tables. I suggested that a research assistant could do that work, thereby providing us with additional time to work on other facets of the analysis. He explained patiently that the construction of the tables was not an empty exercise in methodology. Rather, it represented one way in which he sought to "internalize" the study's data, in order to acquire a more direct and comprehensive understanding of the *Trapped* families. He wanted to minimize interventions which would distance him from the data and impede learning about the families. Learning occurred as each tally mark was registered. The construction of tables, however, was only a part of it. The *Trapped* data set was massive in size, the result of a three-year team effort in the field.

Much of it was qualitative, based upon open-ended interviews, observations of family and neighborhood life, participant observation in specific institutional settings, psychiatric evaluations, and other data collection procedures. In their original form, the data were in Spanish. All of it was translated into English so that it was accessible to him. The variables analyzed in the tables had to be projected against the background of the qualitative data which had been translated. Variables made no sense to him unless the human attitudes or actions they denoted could be understood or visualized. He wanted to convey the products of his research by integrating data on the relationships between variables with rich descriptions of how persons actually lived their lives from birth to death.

Writing the book was also revelatory of his attitude. *Trapped* was written over and over many times. In addition to grammatical correctness, each sentence had to designate with precision the idea being conveyed. Diction was to be obtained through repeated drafts of the manuscript. Paragraphs and chapters were organized and reorganized innumerable times. Through all of this there was one common purpose: a clear and coherent analysis and portrayal of the lives of the families rendered in simple and accurate prose. The mandate that the task of the sociologist be approached with singular directness was followed throughout, from the planning of the study to the final draft of the manuscript.

It is commonly recognized that Sandy's lifetime work represents a monumental contribution to our understanding of the human scene. A clue to how he was able to do this is to be found in what I have attempted to convey here -- his commitment to the belief that the complexity of the social world imposed upon sociologists the responsibility of rendering accounts with economy and forthrightness. I enjoyed the privilege of being his collaborator and friend.

> Lloyd H. Rogler
> Albert Schweitzer University Professor
> Fordham University

July 1985

Preface to Reprint Edition

More than a decade has now passed since the publication of *Trapped: Families and Schizophrenia* and more than a decade and a half since the data for the book were collected. The book's major findings and conclusions are still being assimilated into the professional literature. This, then, is a timely opportunity to make some observations on reactions to the book and events associated with its publication.

With few exceptions, the reactions to *Trapped* were favorable. It was acclaimed as the most important contribution yet made to our understanding of the social components of mental illness, as an interdisciplinary model of research design and execution, and as having set a new standard of excellence for research in a difficult field. It was cited as the chief modern statement of a stress theory of schizophrenia. The research team was commended for its heroism, compassion, and dedication in laboring for three years in the slums and public housing developments of San Juan, Puerto Rico to collect the data, and the authors were praised for their clear narrative style, insights, and creative interweaving of statistical presentation, case-history materials, and expository description. One reviewer, referring to it as a "monumental contribution to the analysis of Puerto Rican slum family life," concluded that "the book should be read by every civilized person." To this day, *Trapped* remains the only report of a major sociological study of mental illness in Puerto Rico.

Perhaps expectably, the findings which drew the most critical questions were those relevant to the study's first objective: the intensive examination of life-history data. The belief that all schizophrenia has its origin in childhood and adolescence is not uncommon; our findings, however, did not support such a belief, at least not with respect to the carefully diagnosed schizophrenics in the study group. Our data indicated that experiences in childhood and adolescence of schizophrenic persons do not differ noticeably from those of persons not afflicted with this illness. True, the schizophrenic persons had experienced hardships and problems during childhood and adolescence, but no more or less than had a comparable group of persons who were not schizophrenic. Had the study group been restricted to a population of sick persons, the temptation surely would have been to see the early hardships and problems of the schizophrenics as relevant to the causes of the illness—a temptation difficult to avoid in studies which deal only with clinically treated cases of schizophrenia. It is worth repeating that in this type of research carefully defined and selected control groups are needed to avoid unsound conclusions.

Some reviewers questioned the presentation of findings which led repeatedly to the acceptance of the null hypothesis that "sick" and "well" persons did not differ significantly in childhood and adolescent experiences. It is not unusual for researchers to publish only those findings which affirm true differences between the groups being studied. To be confronted with page after page reporting the absence of true differences, as the first part of *Trapped* does, makes unusual reading. The reader, accustomed to the usual publications, begins to yearn—perhaps impatiently—for the "positive" findings of the study. One reviewer, apparently annoyed at the lack of "positive" results, dismissed the findings altogether, alleging that we were victims of the sociologists' bias of minimizing the importance of childhood experiences. The exact opposite was true. In-depth life-history data were collected because we felt that such data could provide clues to schizophrenia; also, in the next-to-last chapter, data are presented on the deleterious impact upon the children of a schizophrenic mother. Findings, of course, cannot be foreordained. We believe that, if an hypothesis is worthy of testing theoretically, the results—no matter what they may be—are worthy of serious attention.

Some reviewers correctly called attention to the retrospective character of the data on childhood and adolescence. The persons studied were asked to look back upon their own life histories. Our concern for reliance upon memory is stated in the book. But after a systematic and thorough examination of the data, life-history experiences—the credibility of which could reasonably be assumed, such as whether the person's family of orientation was intact or ruptured—did not reveal differences between schizophrenic and nonschizophrenic persons. Retrospective accounts, nonetheless, must give way to carefully designed, prospective, longitudinal studies based upon direct observations and measurements.

Most of the reviewers found the data on the year preceding the perceived onset of the illness to be of compelling importance to a stress theory of schizophrenia: during that year, the schizophrenic persons experienced a relentless and ever-increasing bombardment of problems which exceeded by far the nonschizophrenic persons' experiences during a comparable year. For the person decompensating into schizophrenic reactions there was no escape from his difficulties. His increasing idiosyncratic and bizarre behavior, in turn, involuntarily drove him into the stigmatized role of the *loco*, causing him to suffer further cruel punishment and social ostracism (thus, the title *Trapped*). Scholars interested in a labeling theory of mental illness have found such data to confirm the importance of the dialectical interplay between the person's emerging symptoms and society's harsh, punitive reactions to the deviant acts he commits. Society's reactions are conceived to reinforce and direct the deviance leading to illness. Thus, the schizophrenic's withdrawal from customary social relations results from the interaction between the deviant acts attached to the emerging illness and the punishment society inflicts upon the afflicted person.

The absence of differences between schizophrenics and nonschizophrenics during childhood and adolescence, considered in relation to the data relevant to the stress theory, led competent researchers to the inference that *Trapped* is a study of "reactive" schizophrenia, as distinguished from "process" schizophrenia. Process schizophrenia usually makes its appearance in childhood and develops incrementally over time, whereas reactive schizophrenia is a comparatively sudden reaction to massive stresses. By definition, this formulation fits *Trapped's* schizophrenics. The choice of married schizophrenics in the study group could have tended to exclude persons afflicted with a long-developing process schizophrenia and to have included those with reactive schizophrenia, but in no way is it correct to conclude that stress factors do not play a role in the schizophrenias which may originate earlier in life. The *Trapped* data on the next generation (Chapter 20) demonstrate how the children of schizophrenic mothers, enmeshed as they are in structurally chaotic and punitive family environment, show evidence of serious emotional disturbances. From the viewpoint of social psychiatry, the distinction between reactive and process schizophrenia may well reduce itself to the time at which and the way in which stress impinges upon the person's life arc to initiate, shape, and stabilize the developing illness.

The reviewers of *Trapped* expressed unqualified enthusiasm with the findings on the impact of schizophrenia on the family. In families free of schizophrenia, conjugal solidarity is based upon sex role complementarities associated with the cultural division of labor. We thought at first that the impact of schizophrenia would be pervasively disorganizing, that the presence of schizophrenia among the spouses would rupture the family's unity, envelop the husbands and wives in conflict, mutual recriminations, and bitter disillusionment. This hypothesis applies to families in which the wife is schizophrenic, regardless of the husband's mental health status, but families with schizophrenic husbands only exhibit a strikingly different pattern: in the husband-schizophrenic families, customary marital roles are reversed. Role relationships between the spouses are reorganized as the husbands and wives cope with problems stemming from the illness, and sick husbands and well wives develop unifying bonds as a result of their mutual efforts to preserve the family by coping with the husband's illness. *Trapped* meticulously delineates this process of change which progressively relegates the sick husband to a dependency role while enlarging the scope of the wife's role to that of breadwinner and family therapist. *Trapped* followed the classic sociological model of explanation by reaching outward to identify influences stemming from broader sociocultural parameters: it identified the dimensions of sex-role differences as root, cultural elements of Puerto Rican society and examined them in the larger context of the extended family, the overarching system of cultural norms, and the external social structures impinging upon the family as an institution.

Students of the family, of Puerto Rican society, and of Latin American culture patterns have seen in such findings the possibility of developing general theoretical propositions about family dynamics in response to stress. In turn, clinically oriented scholars saw in the findings a need for modifying and refining therapeutic interventions according to the sex role of the afflicted person and the social consequences in the family which derive from the illness. The reorganization of family roles, they believe, could be conceived as a therapeutic objective, thus making use of socially supportive patterns of help in the family and the community. The "well" wife's heroic efforts to cope with the problems associated with her husband's illness provide one model of therapy *in* the family to be used as a source of learning by clinicians *of* the family.

Of all the findings reported in *Trapped*, the material on spiritualism stirred the greatest interest, if not downright enthusiasm, in Puerto Rico, Latin America, and the United States. The therapy practiced by spiritualist mediums in small group sessions (Chapter 12) was cited as a significant contribution to our understanding of folk psychiatry. Energetic researchers have pursued the leads in the material, and, so far, their observations and data substantially confirm what we reported. Looking back, it seems curious—perhaps even strange—that when the research plans for the study were first made we did not set out to study spiritualism, although we did have an explicit interest in uncovering patterns of social support in the community. The discovery of the importance of spiritualism was the serendipitous result of incidental observations made during the early pretesting of the study. When we became aware of the importance of spiritualism in the care of emotionally disturbed persons, it became a focal point of the research effort. The public's interest in the findings, however, was aroused while we were still collecting data. The Social Science Research Center of the University of Puerto Rico organized a series of lectures to be given by the Center's research staff who were conducting a variety of studies. Small groups of interested professional researchers on the Island were expected to attend the lectures. When preliminary findings on mental illness and spiritualism were presented at the first lecture in the series, the auditorium was filled with about 300 students, professors, social and behavioral scientists, government officials, administrators from public and private agencies, psychiatrists and other medical doctors, and lay persons, and last but not least spiritualist mediums and their followers from San Juan and outlying towns—a standing-room only crowd. Planned for sixty minutes, the presentation went on for almost three hours, prolonged by questions and answers, persons making their own speeches, and an occasional medium invoking the spirits for guidance. In the days which followed, the lecture was cited in numerous letters to the editors of local newspapers, and there were letters and telegrams to the authors themselves. San Juan-based organizations invited us to speak on spiritualism. A Puerto Rican millionaire commissioned his attorney to secure a copy of the lecture at any cost; brandishing a checkbook, the attorney was incrédulous that a copy of the lecture was available at no cost. A wealthy Brazilian proposed that the University of Puerto Rico establish an institute for the study of spiritualism. Local mediums visited our research offices to bring us literature on spiritualism while expounding their views on religion. The responsive chord the topic of spiritualism struck was indicative of the character of this institution in Puerto Rican society. Striving for recognition, public acceptance, and legitimacy, the leaders of spiritualism took the University of Puerto Rico's sponsorship of such a lecture as a sign that spiritualism had earned full academic credentials. They saw no distinction between the presentation of research findings and advocacy in behalf of spiritualism's ideology.

Alas! Some of our psychiatrist friends—without whose cooperation the study could not have been carried out—failed, too, to make this distinction and accused us of championing primitive beliefs over medically based psychiatry. To them, the research findings were invalid, and the researchers misguided. Friendships were strained. One psychiatrist argued that therapy was uniquely and exclusively tied to the services rendered by psychiatrists; thus, by definition, mediums could not administer therapy. But the therapeutic importance of spiritualism—carefully studied and systematically documented through field observations—was not to be ruled out by definitional fiat. In response to such criticism, we actively sought to present the *Trapped* findings in lectures and informal conferences, both on the Island and on the mainland, to psychiatrists and allied health professionals, mental health workers, social and behavioral scientists, in brief to any group of persons willing to discuss with us the significance of the research findings. Clinically oriented reviewers of *Trapped*, in turn, argued pointedly that much could be learned about therapy from the medium's skillful treatment of persons with socio-emotional problems.

Psychiatrists in Puerto Rico are now much more accepting of spiritualism, some embracing its therapeutic doctrines and practices with a suspicious degree of enthusiasm, but the authors can claim only modest credit for this change. The change was due much more to the rise and impact in the decade of the '60s of the community mental health movement, with its central premise that patterns of therapeutic support can be found in the structure of society at large and are not restricted to the efforts of particular professional specialties.

Convulsive social changes, affecting Puerto Rico since World War II and through the years when the *Trapped* data were collected, continue on to the present. During the past 30 years, Puerto Rico has been transformed into an urban society. The number of registered motor vehicles has increased sevenfold since the study's data were collected. Along with increasing per capita income, the traditional occupations are still giving way to occupations based upon manufacturing, commerce, government, and professional services.

There is an increase in the number of physicians relative to the increasing population size, and Puerto Rico exhibits the mortality pattern of an industrializing society. Mortality rates attributable to infectious and parasitical diseases are decreasing as mortality attributable to degenerative diseases increases.

This portrait of a society's progress, however, quickly can turn into a caricature if it beclouds the evident fact that a significant proportion of the Island's population still lives in wretched, abysmal poverty, with the accompanying misery and agony documented in the pages of *Trapped.* In 1970, 49 percent of the Island's families lived on an annual income of less than $3,000 while 10 percent had incomes of $10,000 or more. Most of the San Juan slums described in the book remain comparatively intact, although cosmetic efforts at "urban redevelopment" have removed shacks bordering some of the new thoroughfares—shacks offensive to the eyes of the passing suburban commuters. Desperately poor families still struggle to find their niche in the urban community, but now some of them do it with new organizational knowhow: along with the individualized efforts of particular families to stake out lots to build their homes, as described in the pages of *Trapped*, families now collectively band together in organized attempts at slum invasion, thus recreating land-settlement patterns long established in the Latin American republics.

The most notorious slum in San Juan in the early '50s, *El Fanguito*, was bulldozed out of existence, and the area was leveled and filled. As we were collecting data in the late '50s, squatters had begun to erect shacks on the same land which was becoming known as *Tokio*. Mr. Ubarri, whose family was the last one studied, had built a shack out of miscellaneous scraps of lumber on the other side of the Martin Peña Channel. He was inordinately proud of his home and of the leaky, handmade rowboat docked at the door which he had baptized with the name of a local politician because the boat, like the politician, had a bulging stern. Soon after Mr. Ubarri returned from serving eight months in La Princesa Jail for bootlegging rum, urban redevelopment reached the area and the Ubarri shack disappeared. So did the boat! But across the channel the *Tokio* slum grew; now it has over twelve hundred inhabitants, all living very much in the same poverty as the Ubarris did a decade-and-a-half ago.

LLOYD H. ROGLER
Albert Schweitzer University Professor
Fordham University

AUGUST B. HOLLINGSHEAD
William Graham Sumner Professor Emeritus
Yale University

June 1975

Preface

This book examines the intimate, detailed life histories of a series of families who live in the slums and public housing projects of San Juan, Puerto Rico. The life stories of these people were gathered in the course of a research study. The purposes of the study were threefold: to identify the distinctive experiences of persons who are nonschizophrenic in comparison with those who are afflicted with schizophrenia; to determine the circumstances associated with the onset of the mental illness; and to assess the impact of mental illness on family life. Briefly stated, the findings indicate that experiences in childhood and adolescence of schizophrenic persons do not differ noticeably from those of persons who are not afflicted with this illness. At an identifiable period in the life of the schizophrenic person, however, a set of interwoven, mutually reinforcing problems produces an onrush of symptoms which overwhelm the victim and prevent him from fulfilling the obligations associated with his accustomed social roles. The impact of schizophrenia on the family depends on the sex of the person afflicted.

We begin the story of our research with the families of orientation in which the sick and well persons were born, then turn to the families of procreation in which they are spouses, and finally focus on their children. We hope our findings, based on the study of a sequence of three generations, contribute to an understanding of schizophrenia as well as to the culture of poverty in an emerging society.

The study was initiated in 1956 when Millard Hansen, Director of the Social Science Research Center of the University of Puerto Rico, invited August B. Hollingshead, a sociologist, and Manuel Augusto Torres Aguiar, M.D., a psychiatrist, to direct an epidemiological study of mental illness on the Island. The prospect of a sociological study of mental illness in a rapidly changing society, such as Puerto Rico, was a challenging opportunity to Hollingshead who for several years had been involved in community studies of mental illness in the greater New Haven area. Shortly after the first plans were made, Lloyd H. Rogler, a sociologist who was born and raised in Puerto Rico, was brought into the collaborative effort to serve as resident field director of the project.

In the summer of 1957 plans for the large-scale epidemiological study of mental illness had to be abandoned because we were unable to secure adequate financial support. The pressing need remained, however, to uncover personal and family dimensions of schizophrenia. Consequently, we proceeded to design and carry out an intensive, controlled case study of families in half of which at least one spouse is afflicted with schizophrenia; the spouses in the other families are free of schizophrenia. The families were studied in great detail with a variety of methods by successive visits to the home and the neighborhood in which the families live.

From mid-1957 to the summer of 1960, Rogler lived in Puerto Rico, directing the day-by-day activities of the research staff. He exchanged numerous letters relevant to field problems with Hollingshead, whose frequent visits to the Island enabled the authors to share in the major decisions of the project. After the field work was completed in early 1960, Rogler brought all the data to Yale University where the project was housed until its completion. From the analysis of the data to the drafting of this manuscript, the authors have written and rewritten every paragraph as a team. The book is a joint effort.

The study was carried out through the Social Science Research Center, College of the Social Sciences, University of Puerto Rico. It was supported, in part, by a research grant from the National Institute of Mental Health, United States Public Health Service, the University of Puerto Rico, and Yale University.

We have been careful to present the findings in straightforward prose; whenever possible we have avoided the use of unnecessary, technical terms. Although it is a report of scientific research, the text is directed toward both professional and lay readers. The data and conclusions should excite psychiatrists, psychologists, sociologists, educators, anthropologists, social workers, and nurses as well as the questing layman. It should be of interest to all persons who are concerned with the effects of poverty and mental illness on the individual and the family.

LLOYD H. ROGLER
AUGUST B. HOLLINGSHEAD

New Haven, Connecticut
December 1964

Acknowledgments

The initial stimulus for a study of mental illness in Puerto Rico was provided by Millard Hansen, Director of the Social Science Research Center. He also recruited the first members of the professional staff and participated in many conferences through the field phase of the project. Without his sustained support, counsel, and cooperation, this study would not have been possible.

Dr. Manuel Augusto Torres Aguiar became Sub-Secretary of Health in the Department of Health of the Commonwealth of Puerto Rico before the field work was completed and, consequently, was unable to continue on the project. While on the staff, he helped plan the study, conducted the Survey Sample of households, assisted in the development of the Mental Status Examination Schedule, and reviewed the mental health evaluations made by the psychiatrists. We thank Dr. Torres Aguiar for his thoughtful and enthusiastic contribution to our work.

Dr. Fernando Canino, Dr. Manuel Rodríguez Pérez, and Dr. Leopoldo Gárcia, all psychiatrists, conducted the mental health examinations of the persons whom we studied; we thank them for the diligence with which they made the evaluations.

We are indebted to Dr. Juan A. Rosselló, psychiatrist and Head of the Department of Psychiatry, School of Medicine, University of Puerto Rico, for permitting us to screen persons who were referrals to his clinics. We are grateful to our companion and friend, Dr. Juan Enrique Morales, psychiatrist and professor in the Department of Psychiatry, who was at all times a source of encouragement, stimulus, and assistance.

E. Seda Bonilla, anthropologist, was our associate during the early phase of planning and pretesting the study. We thank him for his contributions to the Life History and Family Life Schedules.

The interviews and field observations on which this study is based were carried out by a group of skilled workers who gave their time unstintingly, night and day, weekends, and holidays. We express our deepest gratitude to Francisca Santos de Limardo who worked on the project from the planning phase to the preliminary tabulation of the data. Her enthusiasm, boundless energy, and field-tested experience, gained through participation in social science studies on the Island, proved to be indispensable during the field phase of the study. Eugenia D'Acosta de Ruíz also worked through the entire field phase of the project. In addition to interviewing, she maintained the administrative records of the project and coordinated the complex arrangements that had to be made between the respondents and the psychiatrists to carry out the mental status examinations. We thank her for the efficiency and diligence with which she performed her work.

It has been an incalculable pleasure and learning experience to have had as associates: Esperanza Acosta, who worked in the screening phase to specify the study group, interviewed, and carried out valuable studies on the structure of spiritualistic sessions; Elsa Torres de Dávila, who performed valuable services in interviewing during the period we studied the families free of schizophrenia; Ricardo Márquez Rivera, who conducted many interviews with sick and well heads of households and provided us with excellent reports of his field observations; Juan Muños Valentín, who interviewed sick and well husbands; and Rosa Elena Martínez de Vega and Ana Teresa Fábregas, who worked during a portion of the field phase. All together these persons composed a cohesive, motivated, and congenial field staff.

At one time or another, the following persons were research assistants: Alejandro Rodríguez Fortis, Celia Elisa Fernández, Servando Echandía Valentín, and Héctor Jiménez Juarbe. We received valuable secretarial and administrative help from Carmen Herenia López, Conchita Torruellas Correa, Esmérida Tirado de Santos, Carmen Lydia Benítez, Isabel Rodríguez Mundo de Barbosa, Esmérita Fiol de Moreno, and Eleonora Arana Castro.

The sample design for the survey of households carried out in the early stages of the study was constructed by Miguel A. Valencia. Many of the items in our schedules were drawn from studies conducted by Reuben Hill, J. Mayone Stycos, Kurt W. Back, Melvin Tumin, and Howard Stanton in the Social Science Research Center. We thank them for the use of the items.

We thank especially Chancellor Jaime Benítez of the University of Puerto Rico for both his encouragement during this study and his dedication to the development of the social sciences on the Island. Adriana Ramu de Guzmán, Dean of the College of Social Sciences, University of

Puerto Rico, maintained a close connection with the study, participated in staff discussions of the families studied, and facilitated the progress of the study.

The discussions we have had with Charles Rogler and Carmen Canino on Puerto Rican culture patterns and family structure have been most helpful. Robert Wilson, Franco Ferracuti, and Howard Stanton gave us advice at the beginning of the study. The photographs in the book are by Donald W. Keillor.

In New Haven, we have been assisted in the analysis of the data by: Marcia Derfner, Marjorie Koski, Florence Guerra, Julia Limbert, George N. Clements, Edward L. Smick, and Alan Mallach. We have received secretarial assistance from Blossom Segaloff, Dorothy Thompson, Carol Cofrancesco, Margaret Paugas, Eda Calechman, Nora Quiocho, Alice Venable, Karen Slater, and Lillian Smith. Dr. Raymond S. Duff gave us advice in classifying physical diseases.

Janet Turk has edited this book with professional competence and skill. To her fell the responsibility of preparing the index. We owe her a special debt of gratitude for the enthusiasm and consistent effort which she brought to the preparation of our manuscript.

Finally, we acknowledge with gratitude the unmeasured obligations to our families. Elaine Rogler was faced with caring for a young family in a strange cultural setting for three years. Carol Hollingshead was often left in New Haven for weeks at a time while her husband worked in Puerto Rico. Those who wait behind have to solve the problems at home without an awareness of what is going on in the field. They too contribute to the search for new knowledge.

L. H. R.
A. B. H.

Mental Health Evaluation of the Families Studied

Fictitious Family Names	Mental Health Status	
	Husband	Wife
Aparicio	no mental illness	no mental illness
Aponte	schizophrenic	schizophrenic
Badillo	no mental illness	psychoneurotic
Berríos	schizophrenic	no mental illness
Cardona	schizophrenic	no mental illness
Cortés	no mental illness	personality disorder
Dávila	schizophrenic	borderline mental deficiency
Domínguez	no mental illness	mental deficiency
Escudero	no mental illness	personality disorder
Espinosa	schizophrenic	psychophysiological disorder
Feliciano	no mental illness	schizophrenic
Fuentes	no mental illness	no mental illness
Gallardo	schizophrenic	schizophrenic
Guerrero	no mental illness	no mental illness
Herrero	schizophrenic	no mental illness
Hidalgo	no mental illness	psychoneurotic
Iglesias	no mental illness	schizophrenic
Iriarte	psychoneurotic	no mental illness
Janer	no mental illness	schizophrenic
Julía	personality disorder	no mental illness
Lebrón	no mental illness	schizophrenic
Lugo	no mental illness	no mental illness
Medina	psychoneurotic	schizophrenic
Molína	no mental illness	psychoneurotic
Nieves	no mental illness	schizophrenic
Núñez	no mental illness	no mental illness
Oliver	psychoneurotic	no mental illness
Oliveras	no mental illness	schizophrenic
Padilla	no mental illness	schizophrenic
Porrata	no mental illness	no mental illness
Quintero	personality disorder	no mental illness
Quiromo	schizophrenic	schizophrenic
Ramos	schizophrenic	no mental illness
Rosado	no mental illness	no mental illness
Santano	schizophrenic	schizophrenic
Soltero	no mental illness	psychoneurotic
Tirado	schizophrenic	psychophysiological disorder
Toro	no mental illness	no mental illness
Ubarri	personality disorder	psychoneurotic
Urrutia	no mental illness	schizophrenic

Contents

Part I. The Problem and the Method ... 1
   Chapter 1. The Research Problem, 3
   Chapter 2. Methodological Procedures, 10
   Chapter 3. The Social Setting, 44

Part II. The Childhood Years ... 67
   Chapter 4. Families of Orientation, 69
   Chapter 5. Parent-Child Relations, 85
   Chapter 6. Socialization, 98

Part III. Becoming an Adult ... 117
   Chapter 7. Jobs, Geographic Mobility, and Illness, 119
   Chapter 8. Courtship and Marriage, 133

Part IV. Becoming a Schizophrenic ... 151
   Chapter 9. Illness and Death, 153
   Chapter 10. The Problematic Year, 173
   Chapter 11. Mental Illness, 215
   Chapter 12. Coping Behaviors, 243

Part V. The Impact of Schizophrenia on the Family ... 261
   Chapter 13. Family Structure and Process, 263
   Chapter 14. Economic Dimensions of Family Life, 276
   Chapter 15. Social Control in Marriage. I, 293
   Chapter 16. Social Control in Marriage. II, 314
   Chapter 17. Sexual Conflicts, 332
   Chapter 18. Nuclear and Extended Families. I, 347
   Chapter 19. Nuclear and Extended Families. II, 360

Part VI. The Future ... 379
   Chapter 20. The Next Generation, 381
   Chapter 21. Summary and Conclusions, 401

Appendix 1 ... 419
Appendix 2 ... 421
Appendix 4 ... 425
Appendix 3 ... 429
Index ... 431

PART I THE PROBLEM AND THE METHOD

1
The Research Problem

This book is the report of an exploratory study of interrelations between the performance of social roles in families and schizophrenia. The family has been linked to schizophrenia in medical literature for over a century. In 1857 Morel announced his theory of degeneration.[1] Briefly, he thought that physical and mental illnesses are progressive over several generations: The first generation is characterized by nervous temperaments in the parents. The children are subject to neuroses, epilepsy, hemorrhages of the brain, and general physical weaknesses. The third generation is prone to insanity, evil acts, and disorderly conduct. The fourth generation is degenerate; dementia praecox (schizophrenia), sterility, ficklemindedness, idiocy, and cretinism afflict its members. Morel's theory indiscriminately mixes physical pathologies, social behaviors, and moral values. It assumes that the deleterious conditions he described are transmitted through the germ plasm. This theory was compatible with the heavy emphasis placed on organic explanations of behavior in the nineteenth century. Morel did not prove his theory, but it had a profound influence on medical and lay thinking about schizophrenia, other mental illnesses, and disorganized social behavior. Although some researchers continue to look for a genetic base to explain functional mental illnesses,[2] others

---

[1] B. A. Morel, *Traité des dégénérescences physiques, morales, intellectuels de l'espèce humaine*, J. B. Ballière, Paris, 1857.
[2] E. Inouye, "Similarity and Dissimilarity of Schizophrenia in Twins." Paper read before the Meeting of the American Psychiatric Association, Montreal, May 1961. F. J. Kallman, "The Genetic Theory of Schizophrenia," in C. Kluckhohn and H. A. Murray (eds.), *Personality in Nature, Society, and Culture*, Alfred A. Knopf, New York, 1948. F. J. Kallman and B. Roth, "Genetic Aspects of Preadolescent Schizophrenia," *Am. J. Psychiat.*, 112 (1956), 599–606. H. Luxenburger, "Untersuchungen an schizophrenen Zwillengen und ihren Geschwistern zur prüfung

believe that the tangled skein of human misery psychiatrists label schizophrenia can be unraveled by careful studies of the family as a social group.[3] For the sociologically oriented researcher, the family continues to be the focal point of studies aimed at discovering the causes of schizophrenia.

We studied mental illness in the family and the community rather

---

Realität von Manifestationsschwankungen," *Z. ges Neurol. Psychiat.*, **154** (1935), 351–394. David Rosenthal (ed.), *The Genain Quadruplets*, Basic Books, New York, 1963. This recent study is concerned with both the hereditary and environmental aspects of the etiology of schizophrenia. The book is a must for anyone desiring to look at the literature and to explore both sides of the problem. The bibliography is excellent.

[3] P. G. S. Beckett, et al., "Studies in Schizophrenia at the Mayo Clinic: I. The Significance of Exogenous Traumata in the Genesis of Schizophrenia," *Psychiatry*, **19** (1956), 137–142. M. Bowen, et al., "Study and Treatment of Five Hospitalized Family Groups Each with a Psychotic Member." Paper read before the Meeting of the American Orthopsychiatric Association, Chicago, March 1957. Stephen Fleck, et al., "The Intrafamilial Environment of the Schizophrenic Patient. II. Interaction between Hospital Staff and Families," *Psychiatry*, **20** (1957), 343–350. Fleck, et al., "The Intrafamilial Environment of the Schizophrenic Patient. V. The Understanding of Symptomatology Through the Study of Family Interaction." Paper read before the Meeting of the American Psychiatric Association, May 1957 (mimeographed). D. L. Gerard and L. G. Houston, "Family Setting and the Social Ecology of Schizophrenia," *Psychiat. Quart.*, **27** (1953), 90–101. Donald D. Jackson (ed.), *The Etiology of Schizophrenia*, Basic Books, New York, 1960. This volume critically examines theories regarding schizophrenia from the viewpoints of genetics, biochemistry, physiology, psychology, and sociology. D. W. K. Kay and M. Roth, "Environmental and Hereditary Factors in the Schizophrenias of Old Age (Late Paraphrenia) and Their Bearing on the General Problem of Causation in Schizophrenia," *J. Ment. Sci.*, **107** (1961), 649–686. Melvin L. Kohn and John A. Clausen, "Social Isolation and Schizophrenia," *Am. Sociol. Rev.*, **20** (1955), 265–273. E. Gartly Jaco, "The Social Isolation Hypothesis and Schizophrenia," *Am. Sociol. Rev.*, **19** (1954), 567–577. Theodore Lidz, et al., "The Intrafamilial Environment of Schizophrenic Patients. I. The Father," *Psychiatry*, **20** (1957), 329–342. Lidz, et al., "The Intrafamilial Environment of Schizophrenic Patients. II. Marital Schism and Marital Skew," *Am. J. Psychiat.*, **114** (1957), 241–248. Lidz, et al., "The Intrafamilial Environment of the Schizophrenic Patient. IV. Parental Personalities and Family Interaction," *Am. J. Orthopsychiat.*, **28** (1958), 764–776. Lidz, et al., "Intrafamilial Environment of the Schizophrenic Patient. VI. The Transmission of Irrationality," *Arch. Neurol. and Psychiat.*, **79** (1958), 305–316. T. Lidz., "Schizophrenia and the Family," *Psychiatry*, **21** (1958), 21–27. S. Reichard and C. Tillman, "Patterns of Parent-Child Relationships in Schizophrenia," *Psychiatry*, **13** (1950), 247–257. Victor D. Sanua, "Sociocultural Factors in Families of Schizophrenics," *Psychiatry*, **24** (1961), 246–265. L. C. Wynne, et al., "Pseudomutuality in the Family Relations of Schizophrenics," *Psychiatry*, **21** (1958), 205–220.

than in the hospital and the clinic. This procedure is in accord with a trend that has developed in the study of mental illnesses during the last twenty years. Speaking broadly, the shift has been away from the examination of patients in clinics and hospitals toward the study of persons and groups in nonmedical settings. Studies of patients in medical institutions have continued, but clinical and laboratory researches have been supplemented by field studies of nonpatient populations. In field studies the "healthy" as well as the "sick" are of interest to the researcher. He asks such questions as: How many persons of a given age, sex, race, and socioeconomic stratum are mentally ill in a given population? What is the extent of the sick person's impairment? How is the mental illness related to the sociocultural environment? Field studies have added substantially to our knowledge of the distribution, onset, and course of mental illnesses in specified population groups.[4]

The research reported in this book grew out of experience gained in the study of mental illnesses in New Haven in the early 1950's.[5] The New Haven study indicated a need for more detailed knowledge of the sociocultural settings in which mentally ill persons live. The specific need was for the careful investigation of interrelations within families and between the members of family groups and (a) the development of clinical symptoms and (b) the ways in which disturbed individuals affect other persons and groups who live with them. In the summer of 1956 the opportunity was presented to Hollingshead to organize a field study of mental illness in Puerto Rico. Two years were devoted to the formulation of the research plan, the pretesting of

---

[4] August B. Hollingshead and Fredrick C. Redlich, *Social Class and Mental Illness*, John Wiley and Sons, New York, 1958. Charles C. Hughes, Marc-Adelard Tremblay, Robert N. Rapaport, and Alexander H. Leighton, *People of Love and Woodlot*, Basic Books, New York, 1960. E. Gartly Jaco, *The Social Epidemiology of Mental Disorders*, Russell Sage Foundation, New York, 1960. A. H. Leighton, *My Name Is Legion*, Basic Books, New York, 1959. D. C. Leighton, J. S. Harding, D. B. Macklin, A. M. Macmillan, and A. H. Leighton, *The Character of Danger*, Basic Books, New York, 1963. A. H. Leighton, T. A. Lambo, C. C. Hughes, D. C. Leighton, J. M. Murphy, and D. B. Macklin, *Psychiatric Disorder Among the Yoruba*, Cornell University Press, Ithaca, 1963. Jerome K. Myers and Bertram H. Roberts, *Family and Class Dynamics in Mental Illness*, John Wiley and Sons, New York, 1959. Leo Srole, T. S. Langner, S. T. Michael, M. K. Opler, and T. A. C. Rennie, *Mental Health in the Metropolis*, McGraw-Hill, New York, 1962.
[5] Hollingshead and Redlich, *op. cit.* Myers and Roberts, *op. cit.* A. B. Hollingshead, "Some Issues in the Epidemiology of Schizophrenia," *Am. Sociol. Rev.*, 26 (1961), 5–13.

research procedures and techniques, and the recruitment of a research team. The details incident to the development of the project are told in the next chapter. Here, we wish merely to record that we focused this research on one type of mental illness in a single social class, rather than attempted to gather data on all kinds of mental illnesses in the social structure.

We selected schizophrenia for a number of reasons. First, it is the most frequently occurring psychosis in the public mental hospital in Puerto Rico. Second, the etiology of schizophrenia is largely a matter of speculation. Third, schizophrenia is a disabling illness. We limited our attention to the lowest class because earlier studies reported that schizophrenia is concentrated unduly among persons of low socioeconomic status.[6]

Schizophrenia is the most persistent and disabling mental illness in our society, but knowledge about its etiology, onset, and course of development is limited. Approximately one-fourth of the hospital beds in the United States are occupied by persons suffering from schizophrenia. These patients are confined in mental hospitals for months, years, and, in many instances, for the remainder of their lives. In the United States we probably care for most schizophrenics in publicly supported mental hospitals. In Puerto Rico, coping with the illness is almost exclusively the responsibility of the family. The Commonwealth of Puerto Rico had one public mental hospital, housing some 1500 patients, at the time we assembled the data for this study. Conservative estimates indicate there are at least 10,000 psychotic individuals in the population of the Island. These individuals are living with their families.

The organizing frame of reference of our research postulates that a person's experiences in his effective social environment condition the development and onset of schizophrenia. In turn, schizophrenia influences the social environment, modifying old arrangements or creating new ones. The key ideas in this frame of reference—schizophrenia and effective social environment—had to be defined before we could use

---

[6] R. E. Clark, "Psychoses, Income, and Occupational Prestige," *Am. J. Sociol.*, 54 (1949), 433–440. R. E. L. Faris and H. W. Dunham, *Mental Disorders in Urban Areas*, The University of Chicago Press, Chicago, 1939. Hollingshead and Redlich, *op. cit.* Clarence W. Schroeder, "Mental Disorders in Cities," *Am. J. Sociol.*, 48 (1942), 40–48. Two recent large-scale field studies have reported a strong inverse relationship between mental illnesses and socioeconomic status, but neither one analyzed the data in terms of a schizophrenic diagnosis. This relationship is found in D. C. Leighton, et al., *op. cit.* and Leo Srole, et al., *op. cit.*

them in our research. For purposes of the study, we assumed that a fully trained psychiatrist possesses the knowledge and skills to diagnose schizophrenia. The reliability and validity of the psychiatric diagnoses are reported in the next chapter.

The effective social environment is conceived as being encompassed primarily by the family. The family is the most persistent group in which a person is enmeshed throughout his life. He is born into a family, he is reared in a family, and he enters into a new type of family relationship upon marriage. Each person, in the course of his life, is usually a member of both a family of orientation—the family group into which he is born—and a family of procreation—the family group that is created through marriage and the birth of children.

The effective social environment also includes members of the kinship group outside the immediate family, work associates, friends, neighbors, and other persons in the life space who are meaningful to a particular person. Persons who are in interaction with one another are continually in the process of reciprocally defining and evaluating one another within a framework of culturally defined role expectations. Role expectations are premised on a person's position in the family as well as on his age, sex, and class status. Each person customarily plays a number of roles in daily life and may, or may not, satisfactorily fulfill the norms associated with the roles he is expected or required to play.

Other dimensions of the effective environment include such diverse things as the physical aspects of the home and neighborhood in which persons live and opportunities open to them, as well as limitations imposed by their class status, abilities, motivations, aspirations, and state of health.

We believed an extensive examination of sociocultural factors in carefully specified family groups, which permit a maintenance of well-being and adequate social and psychological functions in some persons but which result in a personal decompensation in others, would enable us to determine if schizophrenia is linked in meaningful ways to the experiences individuals have in the course of their lives. The objectives of the research required that the families to be studied be divided into two categories—families with a schizophrenic member and families without a schizophrenic member—and that the families be as similar as possible in all other control variables. In other words, they were to be as similar as possible on the biosocial criteria but diagnostically different in mental status. The inclusion of persons suffering from schizophrenia in one series of families, and the exclusion of psychotics in the other series of families, was planned so that the two types of families could be compared after the data had been assembled.

The study group is composed of twenty families, each containing a schizophrenic husband, wife, or both; the other group of twenty families is composed of spouses who are mentally healthy or have neurotic traits. These families may be viewed as either psychiatrically "sick" or "well." In the language of research methodology, the sick families are the experimental group, the well families are the control group. However, we did not perform any experiments on either the well or the sick families. We simply studied them in their homes and in the neighborhoods where they live.

The 40 husbands and 40 wives who united in marriage to form families of procreation before we began the study are the central focus of interest. We collected detailed data, however, on three generations in each family. We systematically gathered retrospective information on each of the 80 spouses, the 160 parents of their families of orientation, and the brothers and sisters of the spouses. The information accumulated about the family of orientation enabled us to reconstruct the life history of each person from his birth to the present. In addition, very detailed data were gathered on the family of procreation, as a social group, subsequent to marriage. These individual and family data are supplemented by extensive observations of each spouse and the family of procreation. Finally, we systematically gathered data on the children in the families we studied; there were 136 children in these families when we ended the field work.

By comparing the detailed information on three generations of family members and family groups, we are able to answer the three basic questions underlying this research:

1. Is the life history of a person who develops schizophrenia markedly different from one who does not?

2. When and under what conditions do symptoms become evident to the afflicted person, his family, and his associates?

3. What are the effects of schizophrenia on the family of procreation?

During the presentation of the data we will learn whether our frame of reference is viable or whether it should be abandoned. The realization of this objective should enable us to throw new light on the assumed interrelations between the performance of social roles and the presence or absence of schizophrenia. Our emphasis is on the social structure of families, the sociocultural environment in which these families live, the interpersonal relations of their members, and the adequacy with which they fulfill the demands contingent on the social roles they are expected to play in their position in the family and the society.

We embarked on this study imbued with the conviction that a field study of schizophrenia among families in the lowest socioeconomic stratum of a well-defined population would be an intellectually challenging enterprise. This book is the product of our commitment to this venture.

2
Methodological Procedures

This chapter describes the detailed research procedures used to achieve the goals of the study. By research procedures, we mean the formal or logical design of the study as well as the informal, usually unwritten, strategies designed to cope with a variety of problems in the field. Field studies involve cooperative efforts between persons who are doing the study and those who are being studied. As researchers endeavor to penetrate the sociocultural milieu being studied, difficulties sometimes arise. We relate the ways we coped with such problems without sacrificing the goals embodied in the design of the study.

The professionals on a research team determine what data are collected, how carefully the work is done, and how the materials are utilized in drawing up the report of the group's activities. In this instance, sociologists, psychiatrists, an anthropologist, and psychiatric social workers were engaged in some phase of the study from its conception to its conclusion. The authors, who are sociologists, designed the study and worked on it through every vicissitude, from the selection of the staff to the completion of the manuscript. Four psychiatrists were involved in the early phases. One, a full-time member of the staff for approximately two years, was primarily responsible for the design, development, and pretests of the Mental Status Examination Schedule. He also checked the psychiatric evaluations of the three psychiatrists who examined the spouses in the study. The anthropologist worked on the project for about six months, devoting his efforts primarily to the development of the Life History Schedule. Five psychiatric social workers and two social science researchers were engaged either in the planning or during the field phases. When the field director (Rogler) was appointed, the staff consisted of the study director (Hollingshead), the psychiatrist, and two women who remained with the project until all the field work was completed. One is an experienced and professionally trained psychiatric social worker; the other is an experienced professional research worker in the Social Science Research Center of the University of Puerto Rico where she has been a key figure in several studies carried out by the Center in the last decade.

We assumed that a strong fear of the mentally ill would create serious problems in the establishment and maintenance of a close relationship with individuals and families, so candidates for the position of fieldworker who expressed strong fears of mentally ill persons were not considered further. On the other hand, candidates who had an excessively solicitous attitude toward the mentally ill, who would tend to give advice in the field, also were eliminated on the assumption that a strong help-giving orientation would influence the replies to the questions in the interviews. The field director searched educational institutions, psychiatric hospitals, general hospitals, and public welfare agencies in the government for persons qualified to work with us. During a 5-month period over 100 candidates were considered, but only five were selected.

Each person was trained before being allowed to interview the families selected for study. Readings in social psychiatry and in interviewing were assigned; then staff discussions were held on the assignments, with special emphasis given to the applicability of selected interviewing techniques in the sociocultural setting in which we were to work. Simulated interviews were held before the other members of the staff. Performances in these interviews were discussed and criticized. The new members of the staff went out with the more experienced fieldworker to observe actual interviews. Gradually, the new members came to assume the role of interviewer. We did not send to the field a member of the staff whom we did not consider to be fully prepared. With one exception, the training of the staff was completed before the actual field work was begun. All members of the field staff and the examining psychiatrists are Puerto Rican. All the questions were asked in Spanish and the replies recorded in Spanish.

After we had settled on the frame of reference sketched in the preceding chapter, the next step was to develop questions that would provide the information we needed to answer our three basic questions. Specific questions were phrased to throw light on possible connections between interpersonal supports, the structure of family roles, diverse aspects of the social environment, and the mental status of each person. For 15 months we framed questions and tested them on individuals and families. Gradually, our questions were brought together into eight schedules in anticipation of the yet-to-be-done field work. The questions on each schedule were designed to penetrate in depth the life space of the families to be studied. We now describe each schedule in some detail.

1. *The Screening Schedule.* This schedule is a series of questions about age, education, occupation, illness experience, marital status, and psychiatric history. It was used to identify persons who fulfilled the prerequisites of the study.

2. *Mental Status Examination Schedule.* This schedule provides the outline for the psychiatric examination. It is divided into eight sections, each of which focuses on an area of psychiatric interest. The first division is concerned with the general appearance and manner of the person being examined. The second division encompasses his sensorium and intellectual resources. The third is concerned with thought patterns—their content and processes—and with powers of abstract and rational thinking. The fourth division deals with the emotions, the prevailing mood and its intensity, and the stimuli that affect the emotions. Each individual was queried on inappropriate emotional responses, and his mood changes were noted and described.

The fifth division involves motor responses; subsections of it deal with the quantity, expressiveness, deficiency, quality, and inappropriateness of the action. The sixth division focuses on the examinee's relationships with other people; a descriptive statement of how other people affect the examinee was requested from the psychiatrist in each case. The seventh division is concerned with attitudes, in particular relationship to self, to other people, to social situations, to play, to recreation, and to self-expression and emotions. Section 8 is a summary statement in which the psychiatrist describes the mental traits, signs, and symptoms of the examinee. After the mental status evaluation, the psychiatrist was required to state, in psychiatric terms, the diagnosis of the patient and to justify why he placed this diagnosis on the patient.

3. *The Health Opinion Survey.* This schedule was developed in the Stirling County study by the late Allister Macmillan, who provided us with a copy and gave us permission to use it. In translating it into Spanish we were as faithful as possible to the literal meaning of each question in English but adapted the phrasing to the vernacular of the lower class. The translation was pretested on a number of lower-class persons during the planning and the schedule development phase

of our research. The Health Opinion Survey Schedule is composed of 72 questions which cover the interviewee's opinions about his health and about the availability of medical facilities and services in the community where he lives.

4. *The Life History.* This schedule collected information on a person's experience through time. Its questions cover five areas of interest: (a) composition of the family of orientation and its sociobiographical characteristics; (b) early childhood experiences and socialization patterns to which the person was exposed; (c) educational experiences and relationships with peer associates; (d) attitudes toward sex and sexual experiences; and (e) medical history and that of the members of the family of procreation, that is the spouse and the children.

5. *Family Life.* This schedule focuses on the following social and cultural aspects of family life: (a) composition of the family of procreation and the sociobiographical characteristics of its members; (b) current and past marital experiences of the spouses; (c) occupational history of the spouses; (d) geographic mobility of the spouses since they were born; (e) intergenerational social mobility between the family of procreation and its corresponding families of orientation; (f) aspirational levels for the spouses and their children; (g) perceptions and definitions of the class structure—a number of items collected information about a respondent's opinions of his location in the class structure as well as of the class identifications of his friends, neighbors, and relatives; (h) social participation, including frequency of visits to friends, neighbors, religious organizations, and community institutions—information was collected also on the frequency and kinds of mass media of communication to which an individual is exposed; (i) job satisfaction; (j) social values such as dignity, respect, and marital faithfulness; (k) patterns of family activities including entertainment, shopping, household work, and training of the children; and (l) expectations about the roles of husband, wife, father, mother, and child— information was collected also about the performance of these roles from the point of view of the spouses.

6. *Conceptions of Mental Health.* This schedule gathers information on the ideas that each person has about mental illness, his conceptions of the *loco* (the crazy person), what psychiatrists do, and how psychiatric treatment is administered.

7. *Spiritualism in Everyday Life.* This schedule gathers information on the extent to which the respondents were integrated into the

religious system of spiritualism and their use of this system to solve everyday problems.

8. *Problematic Areas.* This schedule probes the problems the nuclear and extended family experienced during a 1-year period. It is organized into the following areas: (a) health problems; (b) economic problems; (c) matrimonial problems; (d) relations between nuclear and extended families; (e) relations with neighbors; (f) frustrated aspirations; and (g) loss of personal prestige.

Specific items in each schedule were either of the fixed-choice or open-ended variety. Fixed choices were specified for items only when our experience in pretesting indicated that the choices meaningfully and comprehensively covered the replies respondents were likely to make. Open-ended items required further probing by the interviewer or the examining psychiatrist.

The Screening Schedule, the first one used on a family, enabled us tentatively to include or exclude families. If a family met the sociobiographical criteria, the husband and the wife were invited to submit themselves to a mental status examination. A fully trained psychiatrist then administered the Mental Status Examination Schedule. Persons who met our criteria with respect to psychiatric diagnosis were included in the study group; those who did not were excluded. The details pertinent to the inclusion or the exclusion of a family are discussed in the next section of this chapter.

The other schedules were not administered in a set order. The overall order in which the schedules were used depended upon our understanding of the rapport that would be required between the interviewer and respondent in gathering certain kinds of information. For this reason, schedules calling for intimate information were used toward the end of the interviewing sequence.

Items within the schedules were organized into the areas of inquiry we have listed in preceding paragraphs. Within an area of inquiry some items had to be presented to the respondent in a certain sequence. For example, in the Family Life Schedule, after the interviewer had established that the respondent had a conception of the class structure, a set of items was presented in the following order: (a) How many social classes do you think there are in Puerto Rico? (b) In what way or ways do the persons in these social classes differ from one another? (c) To which one of these social classes do you belong? (d) To which one of these social classes would you like to belong? (e) To which of these social classes did your parents belong? (f) To which one of these social classes would you like your children to belong? and (g) To which one of these social classes do your best friends belong? Such a sequence allows one item to be premised on the replies to a former item, enabling the interviewer to operate within the respondent's frame of reference.

In other sequences fixed-reply questions were followed by open-ended items so as to identify the reasons for the choice of alternatives. As an example, we asked the question, "If you had to live your life again, would you marry the same person, a different person, or would you not get married?" After the respondent had made a choice, he was then asked why he had made that choice. The "why" question almost always led to a "spill-out" of information bearing on marital satisfaction or dissatisfaction.

A sequence of two items, the second with a provocative intent, was used to probe for information. We were interested in uncovering a respondent's attitudes toward *locos*. Therefore, we asked him to describe what came to his mind when he thought about *locos*. When he had exhausted his powers of description, the interviewer then asked, "Would you marry a person such as the one you have described?" Typically, the respondent would add new information which revealed deeper psychological layers of his stereotype of the *loco*.

In asking questions, we adopted the assumption that the effective stimulus to which the respondent reacted was the meaning of the question rather than its precise and specific phrasing. For this reason, the fieldworkers were permitted *when necessary* to rephrase during the interview if they thought that rephrasing would more successfully convey the meaning of the question to the respondent. The other alternative would have bound the interviewer to the exact phrasing of the item, a procedure which would have allowed the respondent to assign varied and idiosyncratic meanings to the items presented. Admittedly, this decision placed a great responsibility on the interviewer. It assumed that the interviewer both possessed the verbal skills required for such rephrasing and was sensitive to nuances in the speech habits of the respondent. Finally, it assumed that the interviewer had a clear idea of the meaning of the items. We made these assumptions and rested our confidence on the competence of the interviewers because they had been carefully selected and trained, and they were knowledgeable about the purpose of each question.

The research design required that the families be as similar as possible on a number of sociocultural characteristics but that they differ on mental status. We established five criteria of similarity for families to be included in the study:

1. Residence in the San Juan metropolitan area.
2. An age range from 20 through 39 years.
3. Spouses living in the same household.
4. Low socioeconomic status.
5. No contact with a psychiatric agency prior to May 1, 1958.

We imposed residence in the San Juan metropolitan area as a criterion for two reasons: first, we needed ready access to the families to carry out the interview program, and, second, access to psychiatric agencies in the San Juan area is important in order to determine relationships between families and psychiatric agencies. No family in the study lives more than a 50-minute automobile drive from the psychiatric hospital and clinics; a network of public and private transportation covers the area.

An age range from 20 through 39 years ensured that we would be working with a relatively young, but mature, group in the period of the life cycle in which schizophrenia is encountered most frequently in a patient population. In this age range the problems of adolescence and childhood would be behind the husbands and the wives, and the problems of aging would be ahead of them.

Only spouses living in the same household are included because our primary interest is centered on the intimate interpersonal relations that take place in a family. We selected couples who are recognized as marital partners in a neighborhood. Low socioeconomic status is a criterion of selection because we desired that all the families live under similar sociocultural conditions. Furthermore, field studies indicate that the highest prevalence of schizophrenia occurs in the lowest socioeconomic stratum of a population.

Socioeconomic status is measured by Hollingshead's *Two Factor Index of Social Position*.[1] This index relies on the occupation of and the years of school completed by the head of the household as indicators of socioeconomic position. To calculate the social position score for the head of a household, we measure his occupation and education on a seven-point scale. Then the scale values of his education and occupation are multiplied by their respective weights: occupation is given a weight of 7 and education a weight of 4. The results are then

---

[1] August B. Hollingshead, *Two Factor Index of Social Position*, New Haven, Connecticut, 1957, privately printed.

totaled. Scores may range from 11 to 77 points. The lowest socioeconomic positions are represented by scores that fall between 62 and 77 points, the class V group. The score for every family in this study falls within the 62–77 range.

No previous contact with a psychiatric agency was a criterion because we did not want the subject matter of the study to show residues of psychiatric intervention. Although the families are similar with respect to these five criteria, the further specification of schizophrenia in at least one spouse in one series of families or no psychotic illness in the spouses of the other series divides the families into a "sick" group and a "well" group.

The actual finding of couples who met our criteria for inclusion in the study was a crucial step. We decided to locate schizophrenic individuals before we tried to find families to be included in the well series. To obtain a preliminary estimate of the difficulties involved in assembling the sick group, we analyzed the records of 375 individuals who were receiving out-patient care at the psychiatric hospital during December 1957 and January and February 1958. Only five of these patients fulfilled the criteria of the sick group. Statistical analysis of another group of 500 patients receiving ambulatory care in a psychiatric clinic indicated that less than 3 per cent would fulfill our requirements. These results indicated that a screening program would have to be instituted which would guarantee a maximum coverage of persons who solicited psychiatric aid.

Interviews with responsible officials, records clerks, and secretaries as well as our own informal observations demonstrated that a central list of individuals who had asked for or were soliciting psychiatric aid was not available. Therefore, a record system was established to enumerate all individuals who were seeking psychiatric help or had been referred to a psychiatric clinic in the area. Referrals were made by local officials in public health units, the police, physicians, and, sometimes, family members. Daily visits were made to psychiatric agencies, and all of the appointments which had been given were listed. All letters requesting or recommending psychiatric aid were read. After this procedure was firmly established, three visits each week were required. This inventory of solicitants was maintained from May 1958 through April 1959, during which time 2805 requests for aid were registered in our inventory. This inventory listed the name, sex, age, source of referral, and address of the solicitant or referred person.

The second step in the search for schizophrenic persons was a home visit. Home visits were made to every solicitant who might fulfill the criteria of the sick group as far as this could be determined by the limited information collected in the inventory.

To administer the Screening Schedule, 319 visits were made to the homes of solicitants. Questions bearing on the criteria of the study group, with the exception of the diagnostic one, were asked. We collected information also on the main complaint of the solicitant and an abbreviated life history and made a judgment as to whether or not the solicitant could be interviewed for a prolonged period of time. This latter information was to serve as an orientation toward the person, should he be selected for the sick group. Solicitants who fulfilled the sociobiographical criteria were taken to a psychiatrist for a diagnosis. If the psychiatric diagnosis indicated schizophrenia, the solicitant became a member of the sick group.

The well families were selected after all of the sick families had been diagnosed and interviewed. From the interview data we knew the neighbors with whom the sick families had social relations. Each sick family was matched by a family living in a contiguous residential area but outside the radius of neighbors who were friends of the sick family. We chose households outside the life space of the sick families because we wanted to avoid communication about the study between a sick family and a well family. Owing to the arrangement of dwellings, there was seldom any doubt about the segment of a residential area to be selected for the well family.

All the households in a selected segment were interviewed with a schedule that contained approximately 25 sociobiographical questions. A random sample of 1 was taken from the families in each segment that fulfilled the criteria of the study group. Of the 468 families living in the segments we enumerated, 118 families fulfilled the sociobiographical criteria of the study. The 20 well families are drawn from these 118.

This method of selecting the well families enables us to introduce an additional control beyond the criteria common to the sick and the well groups, namely area of residence. For every slum family in the sick group, there is a slum family in the well group; public-housing dwellers are also evenly distributed in both groups. More specific, unknown, residential variables also may have been controlled.

Persons who fulfilled our criteria were asked to cooperate with us. The study was explained to the members of the family, and they were invited to participate in it. Husbands and wives were told that they would be taken to a psychiatrist and given a mental health examination. They were told also that we would visit them many times to gather information about the family. After their consent to be studied was obtained, the husband and wife were taken separately to the office of a project psychiatrist. The psychiatrist gave the same mental status examination to each spouse in the well series as to those in the schizophrenic series. Ideally, every spouse in the well group would have had a diagnosis of no mental illness, but persons with some neurotic symptoms were included. Before a family could be included in the well group, both spouses had to show a diagnosis of *no psychotic illness*. In brief, a psychiatric diagnosis of schizophrenia in one spouse placed a family in the sick series; a diagnosis of no mental illness or of neurotic symptoms in both spouses placed a family in the well series.

An intensive field study designed to make heavy demands on time and to probe into intimate, delicate areas of personal and family life might be expected to gather a large number of refusals. Ours did not! Of all the persons who were asked to cooperate only three, all from the control segments, refused to participate in the study *before* they were taken to a psychiatrist. After the families accepted our invitation to be taken to a psychiatrist there were no refusals to participate further in the study. We attribute the fact that we had few refusals to the quality and perseverance of the field staff and the hospitality accorded the fieldworkers by these families. We may add that hospitality to comparative strangers is an important value in Puerto Rico.

The question of representativeness bothered us from the beginning. Did the criteria imposed on the study group result in a biased cluster of families different from other families that could have been included but, for unknown reasons, were not? If the study group is biased, any generalizations beyond the 40 families is hazardous. However, if the study group is representative of other families living in the area who fulfill our sociobiographical criteria, then generalizations from the studied to similar, unstudied groups are possible.

We were able to answer this important question by comparing the 40 families in the Intensive Study with 104 families in the Probability Sample we interviewed in an earlier phase of this project. The earlier phase involved the collection of information on a representative sample of individuals living in households in the urbanized area of the San Juan community. This sample was based on the sampling frame the Department of Labor of Puerto Rico has for the entire Island. Its quarterly Labor Force Survey uses this frame. In general terms, it is a rotating sample of households in clusters of ten in urban areas and clusters of twenty in rural areas.[2]

All clusters are subdivided into four parts so that each part constitutes a probability sample; that is, the probability of selection for every household in Puerto Rico is the same and equal. In any quarterly sample, the sampling ratio is 1 in 140 households. Each quarter, one-fourth of the households is eliminated so that a different sample is used each year. The Department of Labor furnished us with the list of households dropped from its labor force sample in the quarter before we began our survey. These sampling lists were checked against the most up-to-date maps of the Planning Board and the Housing Authority. In addition, we checked the latest changes in new developments with the contractors by visits to the construction sites. A total of 1144 households were included in the Survey Sample that was constructed from the lists provided us by the Department of Labor, the Planning Board, and the Housing Authority.

Personal face-to-face interviews were held by a member of the field team with one or more adults in each household in the sample. Data were gathered on the age and sex of every person who lived in the household, the relationship of each person to the head of the household, the highest grade of school completed by each one, the occupation of gainfully employed members, the type of dwelling, and the family's tenure in it. In addition, the schedule contained a series of questions on the illnesses each person in the household had experienced.

The survey was made to obtain vital statistics on a current sample of the population. Another objective was to make first approximations on the amount of geographic mobility and the prevalence of recognized illnesses in the population. We planned originally to follow up this phase of the study with systematic psychiatric examinations on all persons 15 years of age and older in the sample.[3] We were unable to realize this plan.

For present purposes we selected from the Survey Sample all households in which the head of the household is living with a spouse, the

---

[2] A. C. de Irizarry, "Sampling Procedures Used for the Labor Force and Other Surveys in Puerto Rico," 3400b (IASC), Department of Labor, San Juan, Puerto Rico, March 1956 (mimeographed).

[3] The representativeness of this sample is demonstrated by comparisons with the United States Census on three crucial items: number of persons in the household, age, and sex of the two populations. The detailed data for these comparisons are in Appendix 1, Tables 1 and 2.

husband and wife are between 20 and 39 years of age, the household is located in a *caserío* or slum, and the family is lower class. The criteria were met by 104 out of a total of 708 lower-class households in the Survey Sample. We were able to compare persons in these 104 households, whom we know are representative of a selected segment of the community's population, with persons in the 40 families in our study to determine if the two series of families are similar and if the 40 families are also representative. The 104 families from the Probability Sample are compared with the 40 families in the Intensive Study on a series of items. The results are presented in Table 1.

Each comparison shows that the 40 families in the Intensive Study are very similar to the 104 families in the Probability Sample. The families in the Intensive Study do not differ statistically from the families in the Probability Sample on any item. The two series clearly come out of the same population. These comparisons demonstrate that the 40 families in the Intensive Study are representative of lower-class families in their age group who are married and live in either a *caserío* or a slum. Therefore, we may generalize from the families selected for the Intensive Study to the larger segment of similar families who live in the San Juan urbanized area.

TABLE 1 Comparison of 104 Families in the Probability Sample with 40 Families in the Intensive Study

	PROBABILITY SAMPLE	INTENSIVE STUDY
Mean number of persons in household	5.0	5.5
Mean age of husbands	31.9	32.1
Mean age of wives	28.3	28.4
Years of school completed by		
Husbands	5.2	5.5
Wives	4.2	4.4
Mean *Index of Social Position* score	70.0	68.0
Mean years lived in present residence	3.5	3.6
Per cent of residences owned	45.0	40.0
Median value of residences owned	$990.00	$975.00
Per cent of residences rented	55.0	60.0
Median monthly rental	$16.40	$16.90
Per cent of residences in slums	71.0	65.0
Per cent of residences in *caseríos*	29.0	35.0
Per cent of husbands semiskilled workers	40.0	35.0
Per cent of wives gainfully employed	19.2	17.5
Per cent of legal marital unions	61.5	67.5

22 Problem and Method

The examinations for mental status were conducted by fully trained psychiatrists in the privacy of their air-conditioned offices. The examining psychiatrist made his diagnosis of each individual from the clinical evidence he gathered during the course of the mental health examination which lasted about two and one-half hours. The evidence elicited from the examinee was recorded on the Mental Status Examination Schedule. After the diagnosing psychiatrist filled out the schedule, it was checked for completeness by the team psychiatrist who also wanted to see if the diagnosis was supported by the symptoms and main pathological trends of the examinee. This procedure provided professional supervision over the mental status evaluation. There were no disagreements between the team psychiatrist and the examining psychiatrist.

Each husband was taken to a psychiatrist at a different time from his wife. Usually the spouses were taken to different psychiatrists, the time and place depending on both the convenience of the respondent and the hours at which the psychiatrist was available. To locate the sick group, 35 of the 42 persons who met the sociobiographical criteria we established were taken to a psychiatrist for a mental status evaluation; the other 7 persons were not taken because they were found toward the end of the screening operation when we had already secured the sick group. The diagnoses of the 35 persons who were examined were: schizophrenic, 26; manic depressive, 1; psychoneurotic, 6; and personality disorder, 2.

Of the 26 schizophrenics, 20 became members of the sick group. Two of the remaining 6 were not studied; one because the husband abandoned his wife to migrate to the United States, the other because the husband and wife were not living together and did not plan to be reunited. Four were held in reserve to be used should some families be lost.

The 20 spouses of the schizophrenics in the sick series were diagnosed as follows: schizophrenic, 4; psychoneurotic, 1; mentally deficient, 1; psychophysiological disorder, 2; and no mental illness, 12.

Mental status examinations were given to 53 individuals belonging to families living in the control residential segments. The psychiatrists diagnosed them as follows: schizophrenic, 3; psychoneurotic, 9; personality disorder, 8; psychophysiological disorder, 1; chronic brain syndrome, 1; mentally deficient, 1; and no mental illness, 30. Of these individuals, 40 are the husbands and wives in the well series. Seven of the 53 psychiatrically diagnosed persons were eliminated from further study because of their or their spouses' diagnoses. (The 3 schizophrenics and the chronic brain syndrome were in this category.) Two husband-wife pairs had to be dropped after the psychiatric examination because they gave false information during the screening interview. One husband-wife pair was lost when the family moved to a town outside of San Juan.

In sum, 73 individuals who had not solicited or been referred for psychiatric care were given the mental status examination; 20 of these persons are the spouses of the 20 schizophrenics in the sick group; 53 individuals were from the control residential segments. When the 53 individuals from the control segments are combined with the 20 spouses of schizophrenics in the sick series, their psychiatric diagnoses are: schizophrenic, 7; psychoneurotic, 10; personality disorder, 8; psychophysiological disorder, 3; chronic brain syndrome, 1; mentally deficient, 2; no mental illness, 42. We draw no conclusions from these figures, but it is of some interest to note that only 57.5 per cent are free of mental disability of some kind.

This project assumes that the psychiatrists who worked with us possess the knowledge and required skills to make a valid and reliable distinction between schizophrenic and nonpsychotic symptomatology. We were aware that among professionals who study mental illness there is controversy about the diagnoses of functional mental disorders. To ensure comparability between the examinations given by the different psychiatrists to different persons we developed the Mental Status Examination Schedule and used it as the basis for the psychiatric evaluation. In addition, the examining psychiatrist stated explicitly the main pathological characteristics and trends, if any, on which he based his diagnosis. The completed schedule was examined in detail by another fully trained psychiatrist who decided whether the evidence warranted the diagnosis.

After all the field work was completed, two types of statistical tests were made to assess the acuity of the psychiatric diagnoses. One involved an item analysis of the Mental Status Examination Schedule; the other compared the diagnosis placed upon each individual by the psychiatrists with the same individual's answers on the Health Opinion Survey Schedule. We tested 113 items on the Mental Status Examination Schedule to see if the individuals diagnosed as schizophrenic differed from individuals diagnosed as nonschizophrenic. In 95 out of the 113 items, schizophrenic males differed significantly from nonschizophrenic males; female schizophrenics differed from nonschizophrenic females on 103 items out of the 113. The item analysis indicates that the psychiatrists made meaningful discriminations between the schizophrenics and nonschizophrenics.[4]

The comparison of the psychiatrists' diagnoses with the Health Opinion Survey (hereafter referred to as the H.O.S.) was made in three different ways. First, we made a direct application of Allister Macmillan's procedure to our data. Second, we compared the psychiatric diagnoses and the H.O.S. scores, using our own analytical scheme. Third, we tested the reliability of the psychiatrists' diagnosis against the H.O.S. scores.

The 20-Item H.O.S. Allister Macmillan selected 20 questions indicative of mental disorder from the Health Opinion Survey Schedule and analyzed his data by discriminate function analysis. This enabled him to assign numerical weights to each response to the 20 questions he believed to be universally symptomatic of the presence or absence of mental disorders.[5] The questions are structured, usually, so that a respondent may answer them in one of three ways: "often," "sometimes," or "never." An individual's mental status may be computed from his answers to these 20 questions. A low score indicates that the individual is "sick"; a high score indicates he is "well." The range of theoretically possible scores is from -30.2 to 117.0. A person with a score of -30 would be really "sick," whereas a person with a score approaching 117 would be "mentally healthy" indeed.

We compared the diagnoses of the psychiatrists with the item scores of each individual, using the same 20 items Macmillan did and the same weights. The psychiatrists made their diagnoses, independently of the H.O.S. items, on the basis of the individual's behavior, verbal and gestural, during the psychiatric interview. The psychiatrists did not know we were using the H.O.S. Schedule. With this brief explanation we turn to the question: Is there a significant difference between the persons diagnosed as schizophrenic and those diagnosed as nonschizophrenic in their answers to Macmillan's 20 H.O.S. questions? In other words, are the psychiatric diagnoses valid according to Macmillan's items?

---

[4] The summary of the data from the Mental Status Examination Schedules is presented in Appendix 2, pp. 421–424.

[5] The rationale, the procedures followed, the items used, and the weighing of each response are discussed in Allister M. Macmillan, "The Health Opinion Survey: Technique for Estimating Prevalence of Psychoneurotic and Related Types of Disorder in Communities," *Psychological Reports*, No. 3, 1957, pp. 325–339.

TABLE 2 Mean Scores on 20 Universal Items of H.O.S. by Sex and Diagnostic Group

	MALES	FEMALES
Schizophrenics	32.4	24.8
Nonschizophrenics	65.7	60.7

$p < .001$

The mean scores of the schizophrenics, males and females, are less than one-half of the mean scores for the nonschizophrenics. The range of scores for the males is -9 to $+89$. The range for the females is -1 to $+91$. A test of the significance of difference between means reveals that the schizophrenics have scores that are significantly lower than those for the nonschizophrenics. The data are summarized in Table 2. The results of this test substantiate the diagnoses made by the psychiatrists. The schizophrenics are mentally "sick"; the nonschizophrenics are far "healthier" by the criteria of the 20-item H.O.S.

The 17-Item H.O.S. We made an item analysis of each question on the H.O.S. to see which questions discriminate between the schizophrenics and the nonschizophrenics; 17 items were found to discriminate between schizophrenics and nonschizophrenics in both males and females.[6] To determine the mental status score for each individual we arbitrarily assigned weights to the replies of the 17 items. The alternatives to each item were given weights of 0, 1, or 2. For example, the item—"Do you wake up during the night?"—had three alternatives: "often," "sometimes," and "never." If the person answered "often," he received a score of 0 for that particular item; if he answered "sometimes," he received a score of 1; if he answered "never," he was given a score of 2. The mental status score for each person was calculated by the simple summation of his scores on the 17 items. The theoretical range is from 0 to 34, the observed range from 1 to 34. The lower scores are toward the mental illness end of the range, and the higher scores are toward the mental health end of the continuum.

To gain more precise information on the relationship between the psychiatric diagnoses of individuals and their mental status scores on the 17-item H.O.S., we classified individuals into three groups: schizo-

---

[6] Fisher's Exact Probability Test was used to determine the statistically relevant differences. The 5 per cent level of confidence was set as the criterion of difference.

phrenics, individuals with neurotic symptoms, and individuals who had no mental illness. We analyzed the data from the males and females separately. An analysis of variance, single classification of these three groups, yields an F ratio of 34.71 for the females and 30.25 for the males—with 2 and 37 degrees of freedom in each sex group. Both of the F ratios are significant.

Tests of the significance of difference between the means of the 17-item H.O.S. scores of persons in the three diagnostic groups were then made. The following results were found for the males: (1) The mean score of the schizophrenics, 10 ($n = 11$), is significantly smaller than the mean score of those with neurotic symptoms, 22 ($n = 6$). (2) The mean score of those with neurotic symptoms, 22 ($n = 6$), is significantly smaller than the mean score of those who had no mental illness, 27 ($n = 16$). All other possible comparisons between means yield statistically significant differences in the predicted direction.

The results of tests on the significance of differences between the three groups of females follow: (1) The mean score of the schizophrenics, 10 ($n = 13$), is significantly smaller than the mean score of those with neurotic symptoms, 22 ($n = 11$). (2) The mean score of those with neurotic symptoms, 22 ($n = 11$), is significantly smaller than the mean score of those who have no mental illness, 27 ($n = 16$). All other possible comparisons between means yield statistically significant differences in the predicted direction. Because the sample sizes are all small, the T test was used.

It is interesting that males and females in each diagnostic group have the same mean scores. More important, however, is the fact that, even though the 17 items were selected because they differentiated between schizophrenics and nonschizophrenics, the scores enable one to make more refined differentiations of mental disorders.

As mentioned before, each psychiatrist was required to fill out the Mental Status Examination Schedule which was then checked by the team psychiatrist. This procedure was designed to ensure relative uniformity in examination and diagnosis from person to person and among the three examining psychiatrists. A two-way analysis of variance was made to determine if there were significant differences in the judgments the psychiatrists made of the examinees' symptoms or lack of them. Each psychiatrist's diagnostic judgments were compared with the score the diagnosed persons made on the 17-item H.O.S. The responses each person made to the different questions were scored in the manner discussed earlier: 0, 1, and 2. The score of each individual was grouped by diagnosis for each examining psychiatrist. Sex was ignored. The unadjusted mean scores by examining psychiatrist and diagnostic group are shown in Table 3.

The scores for the three diagnostic groups are significantly different from one to another. However, the scores do not vary significantly from one psychiatrist to another. Finally, there is no significant difference for interaction. The psychiatric diagnoses *are* reliable. Persons diagnosed as schizophrenic have low scores, and persons suffering from neurotic symptoms have scores more than twice as high as the schizophrenics but lower than those who were diagnosed as having no mental illness.

TABLE 3 Analysis of Variance of the 17-Item H.O.S. by Diagnostic Group and Psychiatrist

		MEAN SCORES		
PSYCHIATRIST	NUMBER EXAMINED	SCHIZOPHRENIC	NEUROTIC SYMPTOMS	NO MENTAL ILLNESS
A	33	9.0	20.6	27.2
B	27	9.8	22.9	26.6
C	20	11.5	25.5	28.5
N = 80	Mean scores	10.4	22.3	27.2

The necessary adjustment of these scores for disproportionality yields the following:

SOURCES OF VARIATION	DEGREES OF FREEDOM	MEAN SQUARE
Diagnosis	2	1986.4296
Psychiatrist	2	31.3279
Interaction	4	13.2858
Within	71	32.4122

For diagnosis	1986.4296	$F = 61.2865$
	32.4122	$p < .01$
For psychiatrists	31.3279	$F = .9665$
	32.4122	$p > .05$
For interaction	13.2858	$F = .4099$
	32.4122	$p > .05$

Before we began the field phase of the study three issues faced us: the deeply rooted fear of mentally ill people, the danger of interviewing in impoverished neighborhoods both day and night for many hours, and the anxiety which resulted from serious doubts that husbands and wives selected for the study would allow members of our staff to take them to a psychiatrist for a mental health evaluation. These issues were the object of lengthy discussions and animated interchanges between the members of the staff. Fears began to crystallize around these issues as the date approached for the beginning of the field work. The fears, however, coexisted with the understandable enthusiasm of facing a challenging task we all considered to be important. The questions were real but the answers were not available; simply put, we did not know what would happen in the field.

Although candidates for the job of fieldworker who had expressed a strong fear of the mentally ill were not recruited, it soon became evident that among those who had been selected the deeply ingrained fears of the *loco* and the widespread unfavorable attitude toward mental illness in the culture had been internalized before they became members of the staff, and even those who had had frequent contact with the mentally ill openly expressed fears as the field work came closer. The more experienced members of the staff rationalized their fears by arguing that their contacts with mentally ill persons had always been in hospital and clinical settings where help could be summoned immediately should the mentally ill person become hostile and aggressive. Those who had had less experience with the mentally ill took their cues from their more experienced colleagues. In point of fact, to talk with a schizophrenic in the comfort and safety of an office or hospital where one is surrounded by doctors, nurses, and guards is different from the task our workers faced. To walk into the depths of a vast slum seeking a schizophrenic person, to talk with him, to persuade him to cooperate in interviews, and to return to visit him time and again for several months *is* a different work experience. Our prospective fieldworkers were keenly aware of this difference. The men were as uneasy as the women, and, as the time came to start the home visits, the anxiety level mounted to the point where it threatened to paralyze the project.

The field director urged the psychiatrists who had agreed to make the mental status examinations to talk with the members of the staff. This was done in the hope that expert advice would alleviate anxieties, but the "pep" talks did little to still fears. Psychiatric advice was discounted immediately because the fieldworkers knew that psychiatrists, themselves, had had little experience with or knowledge about the ways lower-class schizophrenics would act outside the walls of hospitals, clinics, or private offices. Direct and personal experience in the field proved to be the only effective antidote to the stereotype of the hostile and aggressive schizophrenic. Despite our fears, the schizophrenics did not harm us. They were visited and interviewed in their homes without incident.

Closely linked to the fear of the mentally ill was the fear of failure. Would the persons who had been found suitable submit to an examination by a psychiatrist? An implicit correlative to this question was another one: If a person is asked to go to a psychiatrist for a mental health examination, will he or she interpret this as an indirect way of telling him that we think he may be a *loco*? If the answer to this question was positive, cooperation would be difficult, if not impossible, to secure. These questions had to be faced squarely. Each person selected for a psychiatric examination was told honestly and clearly the kind of medical doctor he was being asked to see. Experience proved that the anticipatory fears of failure were groundless. Had the mental health examinations been carried out at the insane asylum instead of at the private offices of the psychiatrists, we are convinced the individuals would not have cooperated. But, to see a doctor, even a psychiatrist, in a private office was, for lower-class persons, a personally gratifying experience which conferred prestige on them.

The personal danger involved in being in a slum area for hours during the day and night was anticipated, but, unlike the other fears which proved to be groundless, this fear had some basis in fact. The local press describes criminal acts occurring in precisely the residential areas we proposed to study. Almost daily, thefts, fights, and killings are described in the newspapers. To alleviate the fears of the staff, we decided that female interviewers would be accompanied by male interviewers, which not only would provide some protection but also would enable us to interview husbands and wives simultaneously. If husbands and wives could be interviewed with the same schedule at the same time, the possibility of interspouse communication leading to the contamination of responses would be controlled.

Although the staff's anxieties about the personal dangers in repeated and long exposure to lower-class areas were exaggerated prior to the field work, our experiences in the field indicate that there was some danger. An interviewer, who by dress, manner, and speech was not a member of the subculture, was conspicuous in the desperate poverty of the congested slums. To reach a family's home, the interviewer often had to walk several hundred yards through a labyrinth of alleys, narrow passageways, and on wooden planks placed over the mud and soaked by the incoming tides of the lagoons. Our interviewers were often tracked by observant eyes as they went to and from the homes. They came upon men playing dice or waiting their turn at the entrance of a prostitute's quarters. Such encounters elicited mumbled threats of violence from men who thought our interviewers were *chotas* (agents of the government who spy and report infractions of law to the police; they are the objects of profound hatred). On one occasion the misidentification of an interviewer as a *chota* created a dangerous situation; the fieldworker writes:

> When I arrived at the house I greeted the lady of the house and made the usual introduction. When I started to interview her, someone shouted through the window that she should not answer the questions. The one who had shouted was calling someone else. Soon a man about six feet tall, naked from the waist up and perspiring freely, came running into the house. He looked very mad. He demanded angrily that I leave the house. He said he hated people like me who work for the government spying on what people in the slums did for a living. He said he was not afraid to go to jail if it was for killing a *chota!* He would not listen to my explanation of why I was there. Then he blocked the door and would not let me out. He had his right hand hidden behind his back and I thought he probably had a rope or a knife. I tried to disguise my fears by smiling and thanking him for having let me rest at his home. He replied that he had seen me in the neighborhood with a man [Rogler] early in the morning asking questions. Then he turned around to see if anybody else was spying. I ran out of the house. As I was interviewing in the house next door, I saw through the window that this man was distilling rum clandestinely in his back yard.

The husbands of the female interviewers often accompanied their spouses into the slum areas and returned to get them after the interview was over. Several times male respondents accompanied female interviewers through the slums with the admonition, "Mrs., you are not safe here." Lest such precautionary measures conjure up images of slum life as extraordinarily dangerous, we must say that in 3 years of day and night field work *the staff had only one incident of actual personal harm*—an interviewer was bitten by a dog. The precautions decreased opportunities for harm, but they were relatively low.

The home interviews for each family stretched over a period of 4 to 7 months. On the average, 40 visits were necessary to gather the data required of the families with a schizophrenic member, and 35 with the well families. The interviewers spent from 110 to 125 hours in face-to-face interviewing with the members of a family.

The field work was a give-and-take process. We interviewed where we could and when we could. Most of the interviews were carried out in the homes, but some were conducted in small, street-corner coffee shops, bars, barber shops, beauty parlors, the interviewers' cars, parks, and jails. The male fieldworkers bought rum for some of the men, and the women fieldworkers carried food to starving wives and children. Clothing was given to several families to cover the nakedness of the children. The interviewers were drenched by unexpected tropical storms, sat on the floor when there was no other place to sit, walked thigh-deep in polluted water, and felt the homes on stilts sway precariously when high tides rolled in. One interviewer received a friendly invitation to help castrate vicious dogs impounded in the yard of one of the respondents. With minor and infrequent exceptions, the persons interviewed were cordial and cooperative.

Throughout the field phase, staff meetings were held at least once a week; some weeks we met three or four times. In these meetings we discussed problems, scheduled interviews, and developed interviewing strategy to meet the problems encountered in the field. When we completed work on a family, a staff conference was held to discuss the concepts of social support and social cohesion in the family, with particular attention given to interpersonal relationships between the husband and wife. Minutes were taken during the conferences. On other occasions, special staff meetings were held to solve outstanding problems of interviewing. One such problem was information from a wife that was contradicted by replies the husband gave. Mrs. Dávila told us she did not believe in or practise spiritualism. Mr. Dávila, a schizophrenic, claimed that the main source of domestic arguments in the family was the enthusiastic participation of his wife and mother-in-law in spiritualistic practices. As we studied the details of this couple's replies and weighed the fieldworkers' judgments, we decided that the husband was telling the truth. We inferred that Mrs. Dávila was denying her religious beliefs in fear that the interviewer was forming an implicit coalition with her husband against her and that she perceived herself as an "outsider" with reference to her religious beliefs.

We developed a plan to solve the problem. The wife was told that we were interested in religious beliefs (this was true). We told her that in interviewing other people we had found many persons who believed in and practiced spiritualism (also true). The interviewer elaborated on this theme and assumed an attitude of respect toward the subject's possible religious convictions until gradually Mrs. Dávila relaxed and began to describe in great detail her enthusiasm for spiritualism and her frequent participation in it. Her reports then coincided with those of her husband.

During the course of our work with the Feliciano family, the fieldworker interviewing the wife gained the impression that Mrs. Feliciano was not expressing the problems she had had and was having at that time with her husband. Despite the fact that this woman had formed a close attachment to the female interviewer, liked her, and welcomed her to her home enthusiastically, we felt that she was not confiding in her. At the same time, we were not having any success with the husband in our efforts to probe into his difficulties. We decided that since Mrs. Feliciano was more receptive to the female fieldworker than Mr. Feliciano was to the male fieldworker, special efforts should be made to gain her complete confidence. Our interviewer formed a friendship with Mrs. Feliciano far beyond the requirements of rapport for interviewing. She took Mrs. Feliciano for pleasant drives, shopping, to visit relatives, even to the hospital. Gradually, the details came out and the fieldworker learned what she needed to know.

Through staff conferences and discussions the field director became conversant with the experiences the interviewers had in the field. Private conferences with the interviewers provided an opportunity to discuss the field problems. The fieldworkers often described vividly and dramatically their experiences in the field, frequently providing background information which made answers to questions in the schedules more meaningful.

When a fieldworker finished an interview, the field director checked its contents. The material collected on each person was read carefully. Notes were taken on the completeness with which each question had been answered, the relevance of the answer to the question, the legibility of the interviewer's handwriting, the meaning of phrases and words in the vernacular of the subjects, and inconsistencies from one response to another. The interviewer responsible for the person and the field director then discussed the flaws and deficiencies noted and defined further questions to be made during call-backs to remedy observed deficiencies. Often it was necessary to call the interviewer's attention to the possibility of a probe that could be made during a call-back that would sharpen the meaning of the material or would provide additional richness to the case. Probes were often suggested which were based on knowledge of how the spouse of the subject had answered the same question.

Upon returning to their offices each day, the interviewers recorded their experiences on a dictaphone. These reports constitute a day-by-day chronicle of field experiences which supplements the material from the eight schedules. As soon as the interviews were completed, each fieldworker was required to write a descriptive and analytical paper on the field experiences with the families in the study. Staff conferences, private conferences between the field director and the interviewers, the interviewers' daily notes, and the summary papers provide a comprehensive account of the field phase of the project as it was seen by the staff at that time. These documents reveal the difficulties we encountered.

Four recurrent problems were experienced throughout the field work. First, the interviewers had to locate the family and identify himself or herself to the husband and the wife. Second, rapport with each spouse had to be established and maintained over time. Third, the interviews had to be carried out in privacy which was not easy to obtain. Fourth, we had to cope with the emotions engendered in the fieldworkers by the physical and emotional hardships they endured. Each problem is discussed in some detail below.

LOCATING THE FAMILY AND IDENTIFYING THE INTERVIEWER SOCIALLY

The population of the San Juan metropolitan area has increased very rapidly during recent decades, and its growth has not been orderly. Slums have sprung up in a haphazard way; streets in the slums are oftentimes unnamed, or if they have names they are known only by the local residents. Consequently, considerable energy was expended in locating the residence of the study group, in particular of the sick families.

Beyond the use of maps, the most common technique employed for locating a residence was that of simply inquiring. The fieldworker went to the general locality of the selected family's dwelling and then asked questions. One fieldworker, upon finding that the map was of no help, went from person to person asking about the residence of the family she was trying to locate. The people she spoke to were reluctant to answer; as one person hesitated over the reply, a young boy broke into the conversation and laughingly told her that the family lived in Black Ass (the local name for one slum area).

During the pretests of the schedules we discussed the manner in which an interviewer should identify himself to a respondent. We decided that interviewers would carry an official letter of identification on the letterhead of the Social Science Research Center. The letter contained a brief statement of the research and thanked the reader for the cooperation he surely would extend. After the pretests the decision was made that the interviewers should use the letter if they thought it was necessary to elicit the respondent's cooperation; it was used infrequently.

After the usual greetings, the interviewer identified himself. Slowly, as the conversation allowed, the study was described in general terms, and the fieldworker invited the cooperation of the individual selected. It was more important to satisfy the person's curiosity as to our identification than to give a long, detailed explanation of the objectives of the study which would have been confusing, if not detrimental to the development of interest of the potential respondent; a statement that we were studying the mental health of families was sufficient. On a number of occasions, the fieldworkers were identified as *chotas*, or more frequently as government welfare workers. Some persons persisted in identifying us in this manner despite the many efforts we made to dissociate ourselves from a help-giving role. We considered it extremely important not to arouse false expectations.

An important identification of the interviewers was in class terms. From the point of view of the families in the study and their neighbors, we were advantageously located in the class structure. Frequent references were made to the interviewers as "professionals" and "doctors." The prestige labels were the result of the clothing and comportment of the interviewers, as well as the common knowledge that they were on the staff of the University of Puerto Rico, an institution that enjoys a favorable reputation in the community. Class identification created social distance between respondent and interviewer. Therefore, procedures were developed to gain rapport and lessen the social gulf between the interviewer and the respondent. Our experience indicates that the prestige enjoyed by the interviewer had motivational significance for the behavior of the respondent. Interaction with higher status persons was, per se, a rewarding experience. Possible status gains were of paramount importance in sustaining the interest of family members.

ESTABLISHING AND MAINTAINING RAPPORT

Many efforts had to be made to establish a bond of identification between the interviewer and interviewee and sustain interest over several months. A newly contacted person, we decided, was not to be hurried into the interview situation. The interviewer was to assume a relaxed, undemanding attitude toward the respondent. A number of casual "get acquainted" visits were made to some homes before the interviews were attempted. During the interviews when the respondent expressed a desire to go on an errand or to visit someone, the interviewer, if asked, willingly accompanied the respondent; if necessary, he provided the transportation. Interviewers accompanied respondents to visit friends, relatives, churches, spiritualistic sessions, and public health clinics. Interviewers accepted invitations to stay for lunch or dinner, and, if the family was in serious economic distress, food and clothing were brought to the home.

This relaxed, casual, and helpful approach impressed upon each person that his cooperation was not exclusively a means toward our ends. Implicit recognition of the worth of the individual in his own right enabled us to visit each family as many times as we needed for our purposes. Our interviewers were able to establish bonds of identification with each family. Husbands and wives frequently asserted that the interviewer knew them better than anybody else. Family secrets, which would not have been mentioned in the presence of nonmembers of a family, were discussed openly in our presence. Many pieces of information were divulged to interviewers that were unknown to the other spouse. After the field work was over it was necessary to continue to visit some families in order to ease ourselves out of the relationship we had established.

This approach allowed the fieldworker to expose himself to the social life of the respondent and provided opportunities to make relevant observations of the family's intimate practices and values. Personal observations of interactions between husbands and wives, parents and children, and family members with neighbors and extended kin, which threw new light upon the data collected in the interviews, were recorded by the interviewers upon returning to the office.

As the field work progressed, the interviewers noticed differences in their experiences with schizophrenics and nonschizophrenics. Less strain was involved in interviewing the nonschizophrenics. To some extent this is related to the anxiety of interviewing a seriously deranged person; nonetheless, the interviewers' subjective feelings were linked also to the objective characteristics of schizophrenics. From the beginning, the nonschizophrenics had a clearer impression of our expectations, whereas schizophrenic individuals tended to view us as help-givers despite the numerous efforts we made to correct this impression and avoid this identity. At the same time, the staff unanimously concurred in the opinion that schizophrenics were less defensive and more spontaneous in their replies than well persons. Schizophrenics replied quickly and showed less reluctance to discuss openly the more private areas of their lives. Well persons were more concerned about the divulgence of private information.

As schizophrenics discussed the problems they had been experiencing, they looked and acted more relaxed. Frequently, they volunteered the information that by speaking to a person who had a sympathetic ear they were being unburdened; as one person put it, "A heavy weight is being lifted from my shoulders." Catharsis was probably related both to the sick person's view of us as help-givers and to his greater tendency to be spontaneous and less defensive in replies to questions. Undoubtedly, catharsis was a pleasant experience or at least a psychological relief central to his motivation to cooperate.

Although catharsis occurred among the well persons, it did not appear to be as important in motivating them to participate in the study as among the schizophrenics. Often well persons proudly introduced the interviewer to friends and relatives and loudly announced the professional identification, showing great concern for the amenities of cross-class contacts. The respondents were delighted that a person of the social status of the fieldworkers should trouble himself to make such frequent visits.

Sick persons had more difficulty keeping appointments than well persons. On any given visit an interviewer was likely to find that the sick person had forgotten about the appointment or that unexpected demands made the appointment impossible. Well persons were more skillful than schizophrenics in disentangling themselves from social obligations in anticipation of an interview. Schizophrenics had more difficulty in focusing on the question being asked and were slightly more prone to take the question as a point of departure for a lengthy, desultory discourse. By and large, the answers given by the schizophrenics were as sensible and reasonable as those given by the nonschizophrenics, but the efforts required to channel thoughts and actions of a schizophrenic person into the role of a cooperative respondent required patience and a greater expenditure of self-conscious effort. In sum, schizophrenic persons had more difficulty in learning the role of respondent than well persons; however, all persons did learn the role.

THE PRIVACY REQUIRED FOR THE INTERVIEWS

The lack of privacy in the homes was the most serious problem in the field work for two reasons. First, the families live in dwellings that are open to the noises of a congested neighborhood. In some dwellings when a window is opened it opens into a neighbor's house, and these households are subject to an incessant flow of relatives and friends. The second condition that made privacy important yet difficult to secure was our desire to keep the spouses separate during an interview to prevent one spouse from influencing the replies given by the other. It was also desirable to coordinate the interviews in the family so that neither husband nor wife would have an opportunity to discuss questions in the interview which his mate had not yet been asked. The fieldworkers sought to talk with the respondent alone, and, if this was not possible, arrangements were made to return when the respondent was free of obligations. The respondent, after having been casually and diplomatically but clearly informed that privacy was important, was asked to specify a time that would be convenient. Once a husband or wife learned the role of respondent, privacy was attained despite the many disturbances. Respondents soon learned that they should strive to disentangle themselves from friends and relatives who were visiting while the interviewer was present.

When interviewers were faced with children frequently bothering parents during the interviews, pencils and small writing pads became additional items of equipment for the field work. These items were given to the children who, in turn, often proceeded to enact the roles of interviewer and interviewee. Toys were brought for small children who could not read and write. We gave money to children to buy ice cream and fruit from peddlers who wander through these areas.

Many efforts were made to have a male fieldworker interview the husband while a female fieldworker was interviewing the wife over the same set of items, but, in fact, it was often not possible to pair the male and female interviewers in field visits. Interviewers asked probing questions at casual moments to find out whether the respondent had spoken to his or her spouse about prior interviews. After the initial curiosity of the spouses had been satisfied there was very little, if any, discussion between them about the interviews. We discovered that the lack of interspouse communication is part of a more general patterning of marital relationships in which few experiences are shared verbally. Seldom do husbands and wives establish a coequal companionship. On one occasion, however, a wife told the interviewer that she and her husband had discussed the questions on sexual activity after they had answered them. This woman was curious to learn whether a woman could initiate love play prior to sexual intercourse.

PHYSICAL AND EMOTIONAL HARDSHIPS OF THE INTERVIEWERS

The families are all poor, some are destitute, and one-half are afflicted with a psychotic illness. The many hardships they suffered were shared with the fieldworkers who reacted with sensitivity. The emotional state of the interviewers was exacerbated by the dangers and inconveniences they faced day after day as they strove to meet professional standards of field work. Tropical storms inundated the slum areas making it difficult, and sometimes impossible, to keep appointments in the field. They waded through mud, lost shoes, and threw away an unknown number of stockings soaked with sewage affluent. Cars, stuck in the mud, had to be abandoned until the weather cleared. Water, heat, mud, filth, and the ever-present hazard of an assault added to the anxieties.

The meagerly furnished, overcrowded homes complicated the work. A complete lack of chairs and tables in some homes meant that the interviews had to be conducted on the floor or on beds. During evening interviews writing was difficult because of the lack of light. Droves of mosquitos descended periodically, making it so uncomfortable that interviews had to be delayed momentarily.

Several families were plainly starving. They were subsisting on handouts from neighbors, and evidences of malnourishment were apparent in the children. Members of the staff contributed money to two families to keep the wife and children nourished to the point where we could complete the interviews. The effect of such contributions on the interviews, more specifically whether or not it contaminated the information, is unknown. We do know, however, that it is difficult to sustain a respondent's interest when he is starving.

The emotional stress experienced by the fieldworkers was a by-product of their perception of the many trials and tribulations the respondents suffered because of their abject poverty. Also, it was a by-product of their role as researcher insofar as this role did not allow them to give help in the form of orientation and information. Policy required the interviewers to hold their humanitarian impulses in check.

To sustain this role, we held numerous get-togethers as the field work progressed and discussed in great detail the problems the fieldworkers were experiencing. The boundaries of the role of the researcher as distinct from that of the help-giver were discussed repeatedly. The fieldworkers came to realize that their feelings of discomfort were common to all. Gradually, they understood that their feelings arose from the divergence of the two roles of help-giver and interviewer. To avoid the possibility that this conflict between roles would lead to the accumulation of stress through the field phase, the interviewers were allowed to give help once the whole sequence of interviews with a particular family had been completed and call-backs had been made. After a particularly difficult series of interviews with a family, the fieldworkers were encouraged to take a few days to rest and recuperate.

On at least two occasions an interviewer stepped beyond the research role and gave the respondents advice. One male interviewer, listening to the anguished complaints a husband was making about the many idiosyncrasies of his wife (a schizophrenic), explained to the husband how he could cope with his sick wife. This advice fell upon receptive ears. Fortunately, it was given during a call-back interview when practically all the information had been collected. On another occasion, a female interviewer made a number of suggestions as to how a schizophrenic mother might deal with a daughter who was suspected of having sexual relations with her boy friend. This advice may have affected some of the mother's responses to a number of questions, since several hours of interviewing remained. We have no information on its effects on the mother or the girl.

The data we collected are analyzed at two levels: the individual and the family. At the individual level the focus of analysis is the psychiatric status of the person. Which social experiences influenced the development of schizophrenia in a person? Which social conditions are related to the presence or absence of this psychiatric condition in a person? Parts II, III, and IV of the book present the findings relevant to these questions which require comparisons between schizophrenic and nonschizophrenic persons, either husbands or wives. Among the women, 13 are schizophrenic and 27 are not; among the men, 11 are schizophrenic and 29 are not. To avoid excessive repetition of the term schizophrenia, we sometimes refer to persons who are afflicted with this illness as *sick* and to those who are not afflicted with schizophrenia as *well*.

Part V and Chapter 20 of Part VI trace the impact of schizophrenia upon the family of which a person is either a husband or a wife. At the level of the family, comparisons are made between families in which neither spouse is sick (20 families), the husband but not the wife is sick (7 families), the wife but not the husband is sick (9 families), and the families in which both spouses are schizophrenic (4 families). Through comparisons among the four diagnostic family groups, the effects of the sick person's sex role on his relationships to blood and affinal relatives, to his spouse, and to his children are identified and reported. The use of the individual and the family level of analysis corresponds respectively to the period before and after marriage of the persons in the study.

Chi square, the T test, and the F ratio, which analysis of variance yields, are used for statistically significant differences at the individual or family level of analysis. In most cases, however, the data are classified into four-cell tables, and Fisher's Exact Probability Test is applied.[7] The degree of relationship between quantitative measures is ascertained by the use of the Pearson product moment correlation coefficient; the correlation coefficient is then tested for its statistical significance. In all the statistical tests the null hypothesis is rejected when differences are observed at the .05 level of significance or less. One-tailed tests are used as the direction of difference is assumed.

Some findings in Parts V and VI are presented as important even though the differences between groups do not fulfill the .05 criterion of statistical significance. Two reasons underlie this departure from the standard. First, the items in the schedules which are relevant to the solidarity or cohesion of the family yield differences which are uniformly in the same direction. Second, the pattern of differences is clearly and demonstrably supported by the material; to demonstrate this, numerous references are made both to field observations and to the personal accounts of the husbands and wives. Families and individuals who are exceptions to the patterns are identified and described and, when possible, hypotheses are advanced to explain the deviation.

Much of this report is based on case studies of persons and families. Each family is identified by a pseudonym to ensure its anonymity. The pseudonyms are common names in Puerto Rico, but none is the

---

[7] P. Armsen, "Tables for Significance Tests 2 × 2 Contingency Tables," *Biometrika*, 42 (1955), 494–511.

real name of a family in our study. The pseudonyms follow an alphabetical arrangement that goes from A through U. (No pseudonym begins with K because real names that start with this letter are rare in Puerto Rico.)

Six months were devoted to translating all the original data from Spanish into English. The translations were recorded on tapes and in written reports. Then, an assessment schedule consisting of 48 questions was used to extract inferences from the translated material. Which are the main tension points in the family? How, if at all, are the tension points in the family resolved? Questions of this type were brought to bear on the data from each family and discussed jointly by the authors; the answers were registered in typewritten reports which range from twenty to thirty pages in length for each family.

The assessment schedule served as a point of departure for the case studies. Many times, however, it was necessary to revert to the original schedules to clarify ambiguities, check inferences, and find relevant quotations. Often, additional reports were written which focused on new questions not contained in the assessment schedule. Special techniques were often used to integrate the data from each family which were relevant to a specific topic. For example, to examine the relationship of each person to his blood and affinal relatives in the four diagnostic family groups, we drew kinship maps to identify the affinal and blood relatives of the spouses, describe the quality of relationships between the persons (harmonious, neutral, or conflict-ridden), and trace the exchange of assistance between the members of the family. (Chapters 18 and 19 present some of the findings which resulted from this analysis.) The qualitative analysis, broadly based at the beginning, became progressively refined into final reports from which the chapters were first drafted.

SUMMARY

The staff of fieldworkers assembled consisted of persons experienced in interviewing who had had professional contact with mental disorders. They were trained for the project through reading assignments, staff discussions, simulated interviews, and by going into the field with the more experienced members of the staff. Three major anxieties arose prior to the field work: the danger of interviewing schizophrenics, the concern that persons might not cooperate in going to a psychiatrist for a diagnosis, and the fear of working day and night in slum and *caserío* areas. Experience demonstrated that only the last fear was realistic. Persons cooperated in going to the psychiatrist, and the schizophrenics did not harm us. There was, however, some danger in working in slum and *caserío* areas, although our fears tended to exaggerate this.

To administer the eight interview schedules to each husband and wife, a fieldworker had to locate the family, identify himself, and proceed to establish rapport. Every person in the study learned the role of the interviewee, but schizophrenics had more difficulty in doing this than did nonschizophrenics. The lack of privacy for the interviews was the most serious field problem we had to confront. Of importance, too, were the physical hardships and the emotional wear and tear experienced by the fieldworkers in gathering the data.

The study group consists of forty families. The husbands and wives in these families are of the lower class, live in San Juan, and had no contact with psychiatric agencies prior to May 1, 1958. At least one spouse is schizophrenic in 20 of the families; the other 20 families do not have a spouse afflicted with a psychotic disorder. To select the sick group, we began with an inventory that registered all persons who had sought or been referred for aid at two psychiatric agencies. Over 300 home visits were made to locate families who fulfilled the sociobiographical criteria of the study group. As the final step in locating the sick group, 55 persons were taken to our staff psychiatrists for diagnosis. The well group was sampled randomly from residential segments contiguous with those in which the sick persons live. Before we arrived at a group of 20 families in which neither spouse is psychotic, 53 persons were psychiatrically diagnosed. A series of fifteen comparisons between the 40 families in our study and the 104 Probability Sample families of equivalent age, marital status, and class status show no statistically significant differences. The study group is representative of an identifiable larger group of slum and *caserío* families in San Juan.

Three psychiatrists used the Mental Status Examination Schedule to diagnose the husbands and wives. The diagnoses had to be substantiated by specific references to psychopathologies in the person. The project psychiatrist checked this point. An item analysis of the mental health examination indicates an overwhelming number of statistically significant differences between the schizophrenic and nonschizophrenic persons. The psychiatric diagnosis is related to Macmillan's 20 universal H.O.S. items weighted and combined as he postulates. Finally, through our own analysis of H.O.S. items, we demonstrate that these scores do not vary from psychiatrist to psychiatrist and that there is no interactional effect between psychiatrist and diagnoses on the scores, but that there are significant differences between diagnostic categories.

The analysis of the data was carried out at the individual and family level. A variety of statistical tests was employed. The .05 level of statistical significance, one-tailed, is taken as the criterion of difference with an exception being made only under specifiable circumstances. The procedures involved in the case studies are outlined.

3

The Social Setting

Columbus discovered the island of Puerto Rico and claimed it for the King of Spain on his second voyage to the New World. San Antonio Bay, the only good harbor on the north side of the Island, is protected from the Atlantic Ocean by a rocky promontory on which the Spanish built their citadel, El Morro. The walled city of San Juan, with its cluster of colonial offices, grew under the protection of this fortress.

The native Indian population was decimated early in the sixteenth century by war, slavery, and disease. The new inhabitants were predominantly from Spain, but Negro slaves were introduced early in the colony's history. During the four centuries of colonial rule the racial strains became intermixed into a population that varies from predominantly Spanish to almost African in origin. The Spanish component was augmented by some settlers from Portugal, Italy, France, the British Isles, the Low Countries, and Denmark.

The political revolutions that engulfed the Americas after 1775 did not shake the Spanish loose from Puerto Rico. Political disasters in Mexico and Central and South America gave new importance to the Spanish possessions in the Caribbean. During the nineteenth century, the Spanish made efforts to tie their remaining islands to the motherland by cultural identification and force, but political unrest increased as the century neared its end. The Spanish-American War marked the end of the Spanish rule in 1898. An American army mounted an invasion, but the population did not actively oppose its march across the Island. At the end of the war, Puerto Rico became a dependency of the United States.

A relatively homogeneous culture developed on the Island between 1500 and 1898. Since 1900 the society has experienced a series of social changes. Its transition from the colony of a European state to a militarily strategic possession of the United States has been of prime importance. It retained this status until after World War II. In the postwar years, it achieved a new political status, and today it is an autonomous commonwealth associated with the United States.

A new culture is emerging from the old. A predominantly rural, agricultural, village-centered community is becoming an urban-centered, highly industrialized society. Two colonial centers have become the leading cities of the new society: San Juan on the north coast and Ponce on the south coast. San Juan is the more important of the two. It has grown much faster than Ponce, and the influences stemming from the United States are more apparent. The San Juan metropolitan area is subject particularly to the invasion of practices and values from New York City and Miami.

Culturally, the center of gravity has shifted from Madrid to New York. American leadership and know-how have been exported to the Island. American capital has been invested in sugar and pineapple plantations, urban real estate, factories, highways, docks, and ships. Technological changes introduced by American business leaders have been accompanied by the introduction of American laws, customs, and values. As the years have passed, selected American culture patterns have become interwoven with traditional Hispanic ones.

The impact of changes brought about by sociocultural forces characteristic of our time is visible throughout the Island. New opportunities are being presented to persons in all segments of the social structure. Socially, the new society is developing classes that lie between the historic, very small, aristocratic segment of wealthy families and the vast majority of poverty-stricken families concentrated in the slums and public housing projects that are being built on the Island. In differing degree, all socioeconomic groups are affected by the admixture of the new cultural complexes with the old. The impact of the new, juxtaposed with the old, has created a confused social scene. Some aspects of the culture are changing rapidly; others are resistant to change. Possible interrelations between sociocultural factors and mental health and mental illness attracted us to this natural laboratory of a society in transition.

The San Juan metropolitan area spreads out from the historic citadel of old San Juan to the flatlands around Bayamón on the west, to the newly stirring old colonial town of Río Grande on the east, and to the hill country beyond the city of Río Piedras on the south. The metropolitan area, as defined, covers fifteen *municipios* (administrative districts). It may be divided into two parts: (1) the urbanized complex revolving around the city of San Juan and (2) the outlying districts. In

1960 the population of the metropolitan area was 862,443 individuals, of which 75 per cent lived in the urbanized area and 25 per cent were spread out over the remaining rural districts and clustered in the towns. The outlying *municipios* still present many aspects of the period when the population was predominantly rural.

The population of the urbanized central area has grown much faster in the last 30 years than the population of the outlying districts. Between 1930 and 1960, the population of the city of San Juan and adjacent suburbs increased 175 per cent, whereas the population of the outer area increased only 38 per cent. The central area is congested with business buildings and homes. Modern high-speed highways have been constructed from San Juan to the outlying suburbs, along the coastal routes to the east and west, and into the interior of the Island. The new highways speed up traffic, but they add to the congestion because they consume many acres of scarce land. Likewise, the construction of new offices, factories, apartments, and public housing projects cuts into the amount of available land and also adds to the congestion in the San Juan area.

The Survey Sample encompassed the entire San Juan metropolitan area. Every household had an equal probability of being drawn in the sample. The 1144 households interviewed are representative of the metropolitan population. A total of 5326 individuals were enumerated in the Survey Sample. When these persons are stratified into classes, the resulting distribution is pyramidal. The percentage in each class increases from class I through class V, but the middle classes, II and III, represent only one-eighth of the total. From the perspective of this study, the salient point about the class structure is the large percentage of class V persons in the population: two persons out of three are in class V. The number of individuals in the Survey Sample and the proportion by class are given in Table 4.

The *Two Factor Index of Social Position* relates occupation to education to calculate class position, but, for present purposes, we discuss data on the occupation of the head of the household separately from those of education. Speaking broadly, the heads of households in each class are engaged in a relatively small group of occupations. The heads of households in classes I and II are concentrated in the major professions and the administration of large enterprises.

The owners of businesses are spread across the class structure, but there are real differences between classes in the kind of business the men operate. The class I man is a manufacturer, banker, or owner of a warehouse or some other enterprise involving large amounts of capital.

TABLE 4 Distribution of Survey Sample Population by Class

CLASS	NUMBER OF INDIVIDUALS	PER CENT OF POPULATION
I	58	1
II	259	5
III	361	7
IV	1093	20
V	3555	67
Total	5326	100

A class II man owns an insurance agency or a wholesale franchise from an American company. A class III man operates a furniture or shoe store in San Juan. The class IV man owns a café, a garage, a filling station, or a grocery store.

The class V man who is in business is generally a peddler. Although his entire capital may not exceed $10, he views himself as a businessman. He tells you he owns a business, and he is correct; he buys wholesale and sells for a profit, managing in this way to eke out a meager living for himself and his family. He may own a pushcart and sell his merchandise from its deck. For example, a pushcart peddler who specializes in oranges buys a load of oranges each morning; usually a young son, or sometimes a daughter, pushes the cart and calls the wares. The merchant peels the oranges, one by one, and sells them in the street. Other common pushcart specialties are soft drinks, household sundries, and cotton piece goods. An even more modest merchant purchases his supplies as they are needed and sells them from a tray balanced on his head. He cries his wares and makes bargains as he threads his way through the narrow streets. Ambulatory merchants frequent older residential areas, but they are seen most often in the slums. Some lower-class businessmen open a shop on their front porches by constructing a display platform of old crates on which they place a few tropical fruits and vegetables.

White-collar management positions, sales work, and clerical pursuits are concentrated in the three middle classes. The center of the skilled occupations is class IV, but there is a goodly representation of class V's. Semiskilled workers are found largely in class V. The distribution of semiskilled workers almost directly reverses that of the skilled workers. The modal skilled worker is in class IV; the modal semiskilled worker is in class V. Unskilled workers are found almost exclusively in class V. The percentage distribution of each class by socioeconomic group is given in Table 5.

The percentage distribution of educational experience by class is similar to that of the socioeconomic group of the heads of households. The higher the class, the larger the percentage of heads of households who have achieved some measure of education beyond high school. Every class I head of a household graduated from a college or university with a baccalaureate or professional degree, and 10 per cent completed graduate professional training. Among the class II's, 96 per cent completed at least 1 year of college, and 20 per cent received at least 1 year of training beyond the baccalaureate. In class III, three out of five completed high school, and about one in four completed at least 1 year of college. Elementary education is the modal achievement level in class IV, but one person out of three received at least 1 year of secondary education. Class V's have had the least education; almost two out of three have not gone beyond the fourth grade. Only 8 per cent have received any educational training beyond the eighth grade.

The percentage distribution of socioeconomic groups in each class, given in Table 5, and the years of school completed by class, recorded in Table 6, are products of the scales used in the *Two Factor Index of Social Position*. The social reality embodied in the class system as defined here is related to the perception of occupation and education, which is demonstrated when data from the Survey Sample, other than occupation and education, are presented in subsequent paragraphs.

The ecological area in which a family lives is associated with its class position. Class I families are concentrated in relatively exclusive, older

TABLE 5 Percentage Distribution of Heads of Households by Socioeconomic Group and Class

	CLASS				
	I, %	II, %	III, %	IV, %	V, %
Professions and management	100	79	15	1	—
Owners of businesses	—	5	12	11	6
Clerical and sales	—	16	58	40	1
Skilled workers	—	—	9	31	16
Semiskilled workers	—	—	6	16	37
Unskilled workers	—	—	—	1	40
N =	11	72	90	249	722

TABLE 6 Percentage Distribution of Years in School Completed by Heads of Households in Each Class

	CLASS				
	I, %	II, %	III, %	IV, %	V, %
Years of school completed					
Over 16	10	20	2	—	—
13–16	90	76	27	1	—
9–12	—	4	60	34	8
5–8	—	—	11	56	28
0–4	—	—	—	9	64
Median years of school completed	16	14	12	8	3
N =	11	72	90	249	722

residential sections, such as the Condado which overlooks the sea in Santurce, or in an expensive new area, such as San Francisco in the outskirts of Río Piedras. Class II families are divided between the better-established residential areas of Santurce and Río Piedras and high-cost new homes in planned developments. Class II and III families tend to live in the same types of residential areas. There is also about the same proportionate division between older areas and new developments. Classes II and III, like class I, are concentrated in the urbanized area centered in and around San Juan. Relatively few families in these classes live in the smaller cities and towns of the outer zone of the metropolitan area.

Class IV families live in more widely dispersed areas than the higher-class families. One class IV family out of eleven lives in a semirural area, mainly in the outer zone of the metropolitan area. Approximately one class IV family out of five lives in an urban slum, and one family in ten lives in a public housing project. New developments are attracting families at this socioeconomic level in considerable numbers. The largest proportion of class IV families, however, live in deteriorated sections of the regularly established, old residential areas. The houses are small, close together, and in need of repairs, especially paint. In the quality of housing they are close to slums, the principal characteristics distinguishing them from slums being surveyed streets, houses on regular-sized lots, sewers, and electricity and water in the houses.

Class V families are found in the same types of residential sections as many class IV families. There are marked differences, however, in the proportions of families in the two classes in the different residential areas. Almost twice as many class V as class IV families live in

TABLE 7 Percentage Distribution of Households in Different Residential Areas by Class

	CLASS				
	I, %	II, %	III, %	IV, %	V, %
Semirural area	—	1	2	9	22
Urban area					
Old residential	55	45	42	43	17
New development	45	54	55	17	2
Public housing	—	—	1	10	21
Slum	—	—	—	21	38
N =	11	72	90	249	722

slums. Likewise, more than twice as many, proportionately, live in public housing projects and in semirural areas. Many of the families in the semirural areas actually live in publicly planned and owned projects. Others live in developments laid out by the government in which the family builds its own home. The vast majority of semirural dwellers live in residential areas that are little, if any, better than the urban slums, the major difference being that the houses are not crowded so closely together in semirural neighborhoods. In the outlying towns and smaller cities, the housing conditions are very similar to the urban slum conditions described in the next section. One class V family out of six lives in a deteriorated older residential area, and one out of fifty has managed to move into a modest new development.

The percentage of distribution of the 1144 households in the Survey Sample by class position and residential area is given in Table 7. Examination of this table shows that every residential area, old or new, is occupied predominantly by families who have similar positions in the social structure.

Tenure in a residence is not related to class, nor is ownership or rental of dwellings. In class I, 55 per cent own their homes, in class IV, 50 per cent, and in class V, 62 per cent. The value of the home one owns or the rent one pays in a rental unit, however, is related very strongly to class position. This relationship is shown in the following summary:

	CLASS				
	I	II	III	IV	V
Median value of owned homes	$25,000	$16,500	$15,000	$2,020	$950
Median rental paid	$125	$81	$68	$25	$14

The dollar income of families is linked closely with class position. The higher the class, the higher the income as shown in the following tabulation:

CLASS	MEDIAN WEEKLY INCOME
I	$215
II	125
III	102
IV	49
V	26

The median income of the class I families is distinctly higher than that for any other class. Actually, the class I families have a median weekly income almost twice as high as the class II families. The dollar gap between the II's and III's is not as great, but it is significant. There are two more sharp breaks in the income distribution: class IV has less than one-half as much as class III, and the class V family has approximately one-half as much income per week as the median class IV family.

When the weekly income figures for each class are converted to a per capita basis, the distribution shifts slightly. This results from the differences in the size of families in the several classes. The median per capita weekly income by family is as follows:

CLASS	MEDIAN PER CAPITA WEEKLY INCOME
I	$40
II	35
II	26
IV	11
V	5

On a per capita basis, the largest difference is between classes III and IV. The next largest gap is between class IV and class V. Class V has the lowest income by family or individual. The weekly per capita income may be converted to a daily per capita income by dividing the median weekly figure by 7. When this is done, we find that the median daily per capita income for class V is 71 cents. It may be of interest to repeat that two out of three individuals in the San Juan metropolitan area are in class V. One-half of these lower class individuals live on less than 71 cents a day; the other half has more income, but not much more.

The marital status of the head of the household is connected with class. The spouses in classes I through III are united in civil or religious ceremonies. In class IV, about one in ten are common-law marriages, and in class V one in five is a consensual union. Although 53 per cent of the household heads in class V report they are legally married, the probability is very high that in the beginning of their marriage the relationship between the spouses was a consensual one. This generalization is documented in Chapter 8 in which courtship and marriage are discussed. The distribution of the marital status of the heads of the households is summarized in Table 8.

The data from the Survey Sample summarized in the foregoing tables indicate that the population of the San Juan metropolitan area may be divided meaningfully into classes. Each class follows relatively distinct occupational pursuits. It participates differentially in the educational system and it lives in different residential areas. The classes exhibit a gradient dollar value of homes owned or rent paid. The weekly income of each class is distinctly different from that of adjacent classes. Finally, marital status varies from one class to another.

On all characteristics presented, class V occupies a singular position in the social system: numerically, it is the largest portion of the population; economically, it is the poorest; culturally and socially, it is the most deprived.

We now focus attention on class V families living in the slums and the public housing projects in the urbanized central portion of the metropolitan area. The 40 families in the Intensive Study all live in the slums or in public housing projects known locally as *caseríos*. The slums and public housing projects are described here for the purpose

TABLE 8 Percentage Distribution of Marital Status of Heads of Households by Class

	CLASS				
	I, %	II, %	III, %	IV, %	V, %
Married, civil or religious ceremony	90	85	90	74	53
Married, common-law union	—	—	1	9	20
Single	10	7	—	6	4
Divorced	—	5	2	4	3
Widowed	—	3	4	4	12
Separated	—	—	3	3	8
N =	11	72	90	249	722

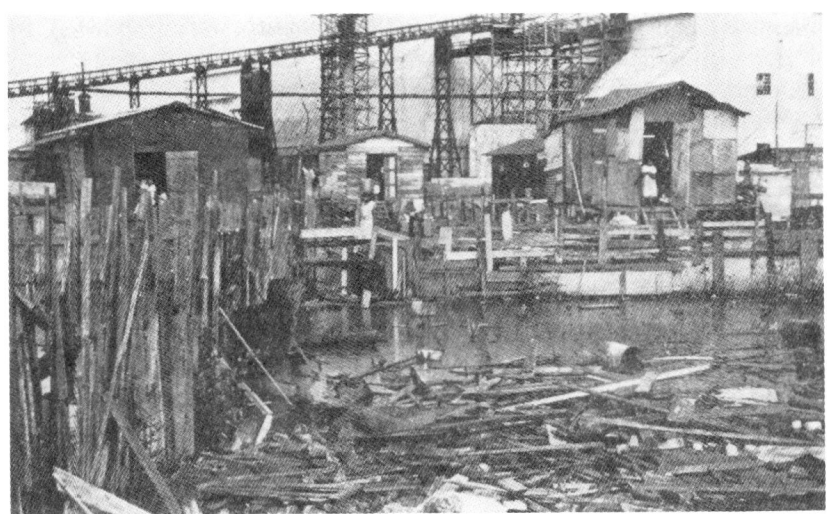

of communicating an understanding of the physical and social environments in which these people spend their lives.

The slums have been built through the efforts of individuals and their families in search of a niche where they may meet the necessities of life and death and store their meager possessions. Any place where people can build a shelter from the rain and the sun may become a slum. Slums have grown on land too swampy to support commercial buildings and on hillsides so steep they have not been attractive for other uses. The largest slums are built on low ground on both sides of the Martín Peña Channel. These slums stretch for several miles along the margins of the lagoons and backwaters of the meandering channel.

The demand for a place to build is so great that many homes are built on piles over tidal waters. The farther into the water a house is built, the longer the piles; as one moves away from the channel to higher ground, the piles become shorter. In the low-lying areas, when the wind blows and the tides run high, the houses vibrate; the longer the piles, the greater the amount of movement from tidal action. (Several fieldworkers reported getting seasick while interviewing in these homes.) Even on the hillsides the houses are built on piles to ensure circulation of air, minimize damage from termites, and provide protection from water running down the hill.

Each neighborhood within a slum has a name. One of the most

dilapidated and pestiferous is known as *Buenos Aires* (good air); another, surrounded by slightly higher ground but whose center is an odiferous pool of mud, is called Black Ass. The most infamous slum, *La Perla* (the pearl), is anchored on a steep hillside that descends to the Atlantic Ocean. The names of the slums are indicative, in a sardonic way, of the inhabitants' attitude toward them.

Slums are adjacent to regularly established streets. Entrances from these streets enable the inhabitants to come and go. The "main street" or walkway of a slum is interconnected with a network of narrow side alleys which branch into paths that end at someone's front door. In the main, the walkways meander from the entrance downhill to the edge of the lagoon or uphill from a road. In hill slums, the walkways may be downhill from a highway.

Some walkways are covered with crushed rock dumped by the city on the edge of the area. Each householder hauls the rock to the spot where his house is located so that the walk in front of the house will not be a morass during the rains. Some householders carry to their homes pieces of discarded linoleum gathered from a dump, lay them on the stones, and pound them down; others use pieces of tar paper or discarded gunny sacks to smooth the walkway. In low-lying slums, as the paths descend toward the water, the walkways are built out of wooden planks placed upon piles. These walkways are often washed away during storms and high tides.

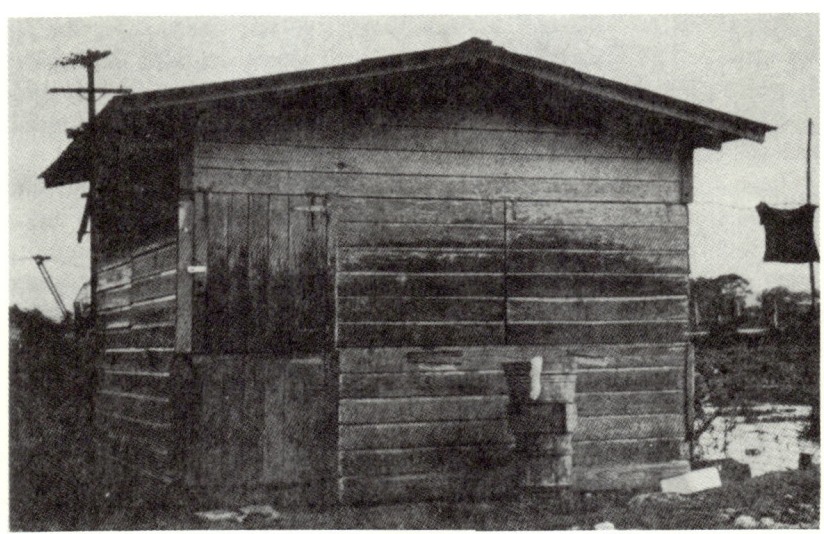

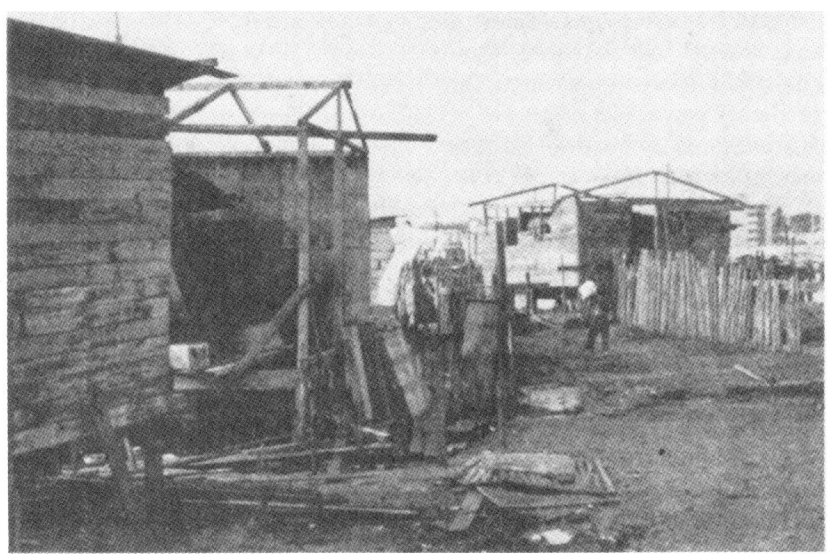

Each house is likely to be very close to another because of the scarcity of space and the desire to have the house facing a street, alley, path, or walkway. Frequently not more than a foot or two separates one house from another. The houses are not built at a uniform height above the ground or the water; each builder sets the floor level of his house to suit his fancy and needs. The floors of homes built over the channel and lagoons may be only a few inches above the water during high tide, and when storms sweep over the area these houses are flooded. The lack of uniformity in the height of houses above the water line presents a step-stair effect from the walkways or the channel.

Each house is built by a man who expects to live there as soon as possible, often while it is under construction. The builder is generally an unskilled worker who has a few simple tools. He selects a site and squats on it; he may assign his wife or child to guard "his" property so that someone else does not claim it. He scans the incoming tide for floating lumber, and after, or before, regular working hours he visits buildings being demolished. Lumber, hardware, sheet iron, and other items are carted to the building site. New construction sites are checked for possible materials, and the watchman may be bribed to look the other way while the builder clandestinely selects something he needs. Gradually, the essential pieces are brought together and the house takes shape.

These homes are rectangular; the walls are made of wood, corrugated iron, opened and flattened 5-gallon kerosene tins, and old metal signs. The gable roofs are covered usually with corrugated iron. Apertures for the windows and doors are rough and often untrimmed. The doors and windows are made of rough boards, generally hinged to swing outward, which saves inside space but which causes difficulty unless the neighbors in adjacent houses cooperate in opening and closing them. When the family is at home during the day the doors and windows are open. Otherwise, the heat is suffocating. At night, the windows and doors are closed to keep out the night air, which is believed to be unhealthy. When the family is away, the windows are secured from the inside and the door is locked from the outside with a steel hasp and a padlock.

Nearly every house has a small front porch covered with a shed roof for protection from the sun's piercing rays; the more elaborate ones may have a back porch. Inside the house the living space may be divided into rooms by partitions which may or may not extend to the roof. Only the better slum homes have ceilings since ceilings are expensive and impede the circulation of air.

Sanitation is provided by open ditches that run from the houses to the alleys and the walkways. Feces, urine, used water, coffee grounds, and other wastes are carried to the lagoon in ditches. Toilet facilities vary from commercial earthenware stools to a hole cut in the floor. The toilet empties into the sewage trench. A person walking by a home, on occasion, may see someone urinating or defecating and hear the excrement hit the waters of the trench or the lagoon. Houses on high ground have outside latrines. The yard is usually so small that the latrine is immediately beside the house and may block passage to the adjacent house.

The city has piped water into each slum by laying the water pipes on top of the walks. Some homes are connected legitimately to the city's water main. Other householders come for their water supply to the public spigots placed at intervals alongside the walkway. The water is drawn into cans or jars that were formerly containers for kerosene, vegetables, fruit, or lard. To avoid going to the public spigot, some householders run water lines to their houses by boring a hole into the main; a copper tube is then thrust into the hole and bound in place with an iron strap that encircles the main. The tube is run, in some instances, to a sink in the house and a spigot attached. More commonly, the spigot is placed at the corner of the house. Periodically, officials from the Water Authority tear out these illicit private lines.

A bathtub or shower in the home is a rare luxury, and bathing is accomplished in a wash tub, basin, or gasoline can. Some men have built showers beside their houses. A common sight is the neighborhood shower made by tapping into the water main; a pipe is run to a small vacant area, raised five or six feet above the ground, and a shower head is attached; a slat footrest is built to lay on the ground and a board wall with a door is built around the shower head, although cracks from three-quarters to more than an inch wide separate one board from another.

Some homes are either legitimately or surreptitiously connected to the city's electrical system. Electricity is brought into the house on wires fastened to insulators in one or two places so that the family can have light, a radio, and, desirably, a television set.

The slums in which most of the families live are subject to the twice-daily flow and ebb of the tides. The incoming tides bring debris from the harbor (untreated sewage from the city as well as the accumulation of sewage from the slums) into the network of house piles and walkways. To this accumulation is added the garbage from slum homes. Thrown under the houses and along the walkways is rubbish of many kinds: bottles, cans, coconut husks, grapefruit and orange rinds, gunny bags, old automobile tires, rusted pieces of iron, paper boxes, newspa-

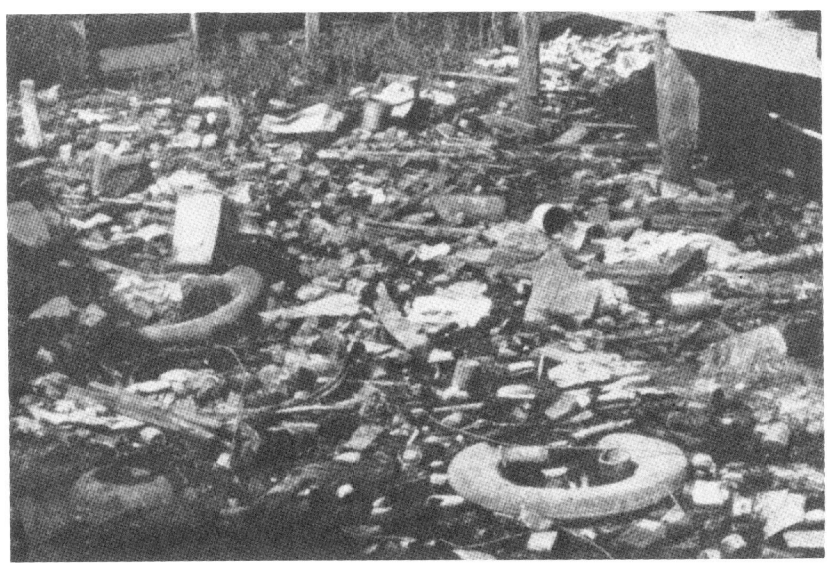

pers, IBM cards, bones of chickens and pigs, old shoes, playing cards, condoms, and so on. This mulch of garbage and rubbish is soaked periodically by the sudden rains which pass over the area. The hot, tropical sun helps decompose and dry the sodden debris and also adds to the all-pervasive stench. Gradually, the debris settles into the mud. The incoming tidal flow stirs up the sediment and washes the lower-lying areas with malodorous waters. As the tide ebbs, scum covers the lower portions of the walkways and the ground under the houses.

The public housing projects, *caseríos*, which are planned, erected, and maintained by the Puerto Rican government are a sharp contrast to the slums. The *caseríos* embody established principles of good housing for low-income families. *Caseríos* are built on solid, relatively dry land, surrounded by surveyed and paved streets. Each building is set apart from adjacent buildings. The foundations, walls, floors, stairs, and roofs are made of concrete. Sidewalks lead from the street to each building which is two, three, or four floors high. There are no high-rise buildings.

Residential buildings in *caseríos* are subdivided into 1-family apartments, each with electricity, water, and sanitary facilities. The internal space is divided into a kitchen, bath, dining-living area, and 1 or more bedrooms. The more desirable apartments have a balcony with a wall approximately 3 feet high around it. In the older *caseríos* windows are sometimes fitted with iron bars to keep thieves out of the apartments. The newer *caseríos* have jalousie windows which pro-

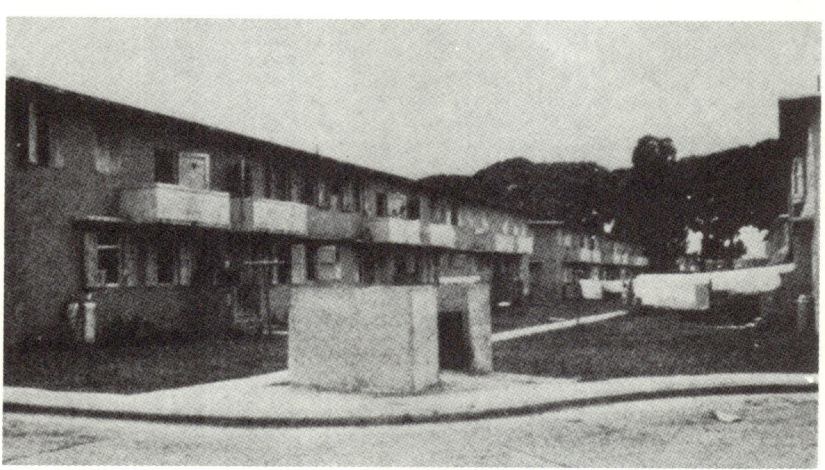

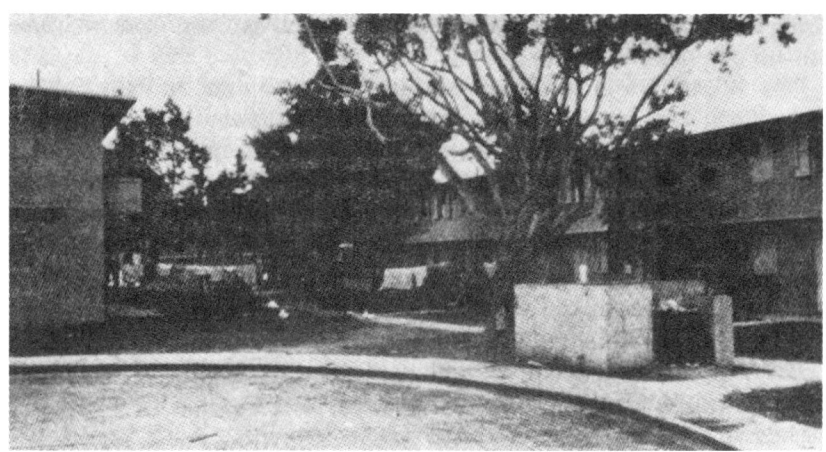

vide protection and have the advantage of being easy to open and shut.

The construction of *caseríos* to replace the slums is a major governmental objective. As the Housing Authority is able to carry out its program of building public apartments, the worst slums are demolished, but before the debris can be hauled away individuals in search of building materials carry off usable pieces. Since there is a chronic shortage of housing of any kind, slum dwellings are replaced while the Housing Authority builds new projects. Building goes on day and night—officially by day, unofficially by night. This situation can be traced to the attraction that the San Juan area has for Puerto Ricans throughout the Island. The vast majority of migrants are unskilled, poorly educated, and without financial resources. The newly arrived migrant from another part of the Island ordinarily drifts to the slums or to a *caserío* apartment of some member of his kin group. Gradually, as conditions become better for him, he moves from a room or sleeping space to a house or apartment of his own. Although the government is building public housing as rapidly as possible, slums that were once demolished are being rebuilt by migrants to San Juan.

In our study of social stratification we followed two different approaches—direct and indirect. We utilized an indirect approach in the analyses of the data on the 1144 households interviewed in the Survey Sample. Each household was stratified by the use of the *Two Factor Index of Social Position* which we assumed was a meaningful measure of social stratification in the society. The figures we have presented from the Survey Sample indicate that this indirect approach is useful on the population studied.

The 40 families in the Intensive Study were studied by both indirect and direct approaches to the phenomena of social stratification in Puerto Rico. Each family was screened originally by the *Two Factor Index of Social Position* to ensure that it met the objective criterion of low socioeconomic status. Later, we approached the subject directly by systematically querying each spouse. Each husband and wife was asked seven questions about his and her perceptions of social class. This direct approach enables us to demonstrate the existence of classes in the society.

Every person responded without hesitation, avoidance, or embarrassment to the seven questions regarding class. The answers reveal that classes in the society are accepted as a fact of life. They tell us how many classes the respondents think there are in Puerto Rico, their criteria for placing persons in a class, where they think they personally belong in the class structure, where their parents belonged, where their friends belong, and the class in which eventually they would like to see their children.

There is unanimity on the existence of classes, but the number of classes named shows some variation. A few persons think there are only two classes; more persons will name four or five; the modal number is three. Persons who believe there are three classes name them without hesitation as the rich, the mediocrity or middle class, and the poor. Persons who delineate four or five classes refer to them as the very rich (the multimillionaires or near-millionaires), the government workers in offices, the poor, and the poor-poor. Some will add the beggars as a separate class. The number of classes a person perceives and how he labels them are not as important as the fact that he knows that there are classes in the society.

We have selected the replies of one couple to illustrate the modal response to our questions. Mr. and Mrs. Ubarri believe there are three classss: rich people, middle class, and poor people, described in the following ways:

Rich people have no compassion for the poor. They have lots of money, they travel, they go to society dances, and they entertain a lot at home. Their guests are invited by formal invitations sent through the mail. They are society people. All of the members of families of society have cars. Even pet dogs and cats often have cars that are used to take them on rides.

Middle-class people are not as rich as the society people. They are salaried and have regular employment. They can afford to have nice homes and they dress well. Middle-class people work for rich people.

Poor people do not have regular employment. Their irregular employment is provided by the middle class. When they do not have jobs, they make money by gambling with cards and dice. Some of them bootleg rum for a living. There is stealing and fighting among the poor. They live in the mud in the cities or scratch a living off the hillsides in the country.

Mrs. Ubarri says she can classify anyone immediately into one of these three social classes. Even *jíbaros* (poor country folk) who go to New York City and come back with fancy coats that hang down to their knees cannot fool her about where they belong in the social system. She comments: "Any bird can be recognized by its droppings." Mr. and Mrs. Ubarri believe they are members of the poor class. Their friends and neighbors also are perceived to be in the poor class, and their children are in the poor class although they hope they will not remain there.

In the following discussion of how the husbands and wives view the class structure of their society, we confine ourselves to the modal conception of the three classes. To repeat, every adult has a good working knowledge of what determines a family's or an individual's class. Economic values are the most ubiquitous criteria associated with class position. The following is a summary of the views the husbands and wives have of the class system which enmeshes them.

The rich conspicuously display their wealth with patterns of expenditure visible to all. They live in large houses and own large automobiles. They have many clothes made of fine materials. They belong to private clubs. They go to the best hotels and order so much food they cannot eat it. They travel over the Island in big, shiny cars and stay at one another's houses. The men have secretaries and their wives have servants.

The middle class live in nice concrete homes. They own a car, but a smaller one. They dress well, but they do not have as many fine clothes as the rich. They own good furniture. They have stoves, refrigerators, and television sets. They eat regular meals and they are never hungry. Sometimes they can afford to go to the Hilton (the Caribe-Hilton Hotel) for a fine meal.

The poor do not have the things they would like to have. They have no money; they live in poverty. They eat anything and they are often hungry. They live in bad places, in shacks or a *caserío*. They have no conveniences and no hope for anything but food for the day. They have no shoes; they have poor furniture and no cars. They travel by foot or bus. The poor are lucky to live. They make sacrifices to live. Debts eat up their earnings. Only the night and the day are theirs.

The following excerpts from the remarks of family members reveal that a person's function in the economic system is identified with class. Members of each class are viewed as being engaged in a limited range of economic activities.

The rich own the businesses, the banks, and the industries. They are in the big professions (law and medicine). They live on property and rents. They own the great *fincas* (farms). They are in the money business. The middle class work all the time in government offices, banks, and stores. They wear white shirts and earn everything they need. They are the salaried ones. They sell their services for about $300, $400, or $500 a month. They have a regular life. The poor work in the cane, do odd jobs, and wander in the streets. They rent themselves to others, and they work hard to live. Their work is hard. They work with their hands in the hot sun. They are the picture of pain; they are malnourished. They have no clothes. The pain of the parents is thrown onto the children. Some have no interest in getting a job, and many cannot find the work they need in order to eat.

The relationship of a family to the monetary system is equated with class. The rich, we are told, can borrow from the Americans or the banks. The middle class obtain loans to buy things they need and pay them back out of their salaries. They receive credit at the stores. They buy homes and cars on installment. The government will loan them money. The poor have no access to money through loans or mortgages. They are constantly faced with debts as they struggle to keep a roof over their heads, food in their stomachs, and clothes for themselves and their children. They say: "Borrowing is hard. One should do without it." "When you work and need some money you borrow from your employer and you pay it back in short wages." "One cannot rely upon anyone." "When you need money and you are not working, you beg for it." One man says, "We live off what I earn. I have $5 for an emergency." A wife remarks, "With what he [her husband] makes, there is food only for the day. Poverty today, poverty tomorrow."

Noneconomic factors, however, are also essential elements in the perceptions of class. Skin color is mentioned frequently. The rich are believed to be lighter skinned than the middle or poor classes. They are referred to as "the whites," or "They are white, so they say." The middle class are called the "little whites." The poor are symbolized as the "darker ones." Qualitatively different interpersonal relations are attributed to each class. The rich are delicate in their relations with one another. Middle-class persons are affectionate to one another; they are trustful. The poor have bad relations in the family and with neighbors. Out in the deep slums no one trusts anyone; no one helps anyone. "The poor despise the poor."

Unequal personal abilities are ascribed to the different classes. The rich confront any situation and manage it. The middle class are intelligent and clever; they have struggled to gain their position. The poor have no pride; they are stupid and shy; they are physically weaker.

The power dimension of stratification is seen clearly. The rich demand privileges in public places. They intimidate officials in the offices. They are the real political leaders. The middle class are corrupted by money. The poor are timid and humble. They are helped by the government.

The ideas of religious affiliation are stereotyped. The rich are the true Catholics; they go to church and support the Church. The middle class are mostly Catholics, or claim they are, but there are other religions there too. The poor are said to be Catholic, but many are members of other religions. They turn to spiritualism for help; spiritualists help the poor.

Education is categorized by class. The rich go to private schools and they are educated. The middle class emphasize education; they strive to put their children through high school and the university. The poor attend the public schools. If one is lucky, he finishes the sixth grade.

Illness is an area of great concern, and is symbolized in simple terms. The rich purchase health; they can afford to go to private physicians and private hospitals. The middle class go to private doctors for treatment. If necessary, they go to private clinics and hospitals. The poor are sick; they are weak. They cannot afford health. They are dependent on the public clinics and the city hospital.

Interclass relations are defined in vivid language. The rich receive most of the attention: "The rich are nice people," is one pole of a judgmental axis; "The rich hate the poor," is the other. Between these extremes many values are uttered. Mr. Molína supports the position that the rich are proud but some treat the poor well. He says: "Don

64 *Problem and Method*

Luis ——— is a gentleman with all his workers. He gives life to the poor." To offset this unusual case, the other men and women aver:

> The rich do not really care about the poor. They treat their servants badly.
> The rich should give to the poor, but they do not.
> They treat the poor as inferiors.
> They humiliate the poor. They humiliate their servants.
> The rich are superior.
> The rich are egoists.
> They are refined only because they have money. They dream about money.
> The rich do not go to heaven. They live only for themselves.
> They do not like our gossip.
> They are self-willed. They do not like to be humbled.

The middle class are viewed in differing terms: They are of a different temperament. They are good people; they are simple people. The middle class rub elbows with the rich but not with the poor. They put on a front. They live by the grace of the rich. The middle class have worked for their aspirations; they live for tomorrow. They live near the rich and look to the rich. They look down on the poor. They struggle to improve themselves and get into the high class. They live beyond their means. They are strivers. They have struggled to gain their position. The middle class think they are better than the poor. The middle class is considerate; they help the poor most.

Mrs. Molína gives an account of how she was humiliated by a woman she identifies as middle class:

> I remember one day I was thirsty, and I went to the house of a nurse. The mother-in-law of this nurse came to the door. I asked for a drink of water. This woman got an old jar and gave me water in that jar. I did not want that water given to me in a jar. She was treating me as if I were going to contaminate her in some way.

They say about themselves: The poor are damned by the rich and by their own vices. They are humiliated and suffer injustices. The poor speak badly about the rich and the middle class. They disparage themselves. They are the damned ones. The true poor are proud; they will not beg or take relief. The poor live off the rich. They go to the rich for money. There are some decent people in the poor class, but there are also killings, fights, and knifings. The poor are squeezed; life is water.

The Social Setting 65

Resignation is prominent in lower-class values. "One blind man cannot help another blind man." "The poor take life as God gives it." Yet in the midst of this series of self-denigrating proverbs, one encounters now and again a faint protest: "Everyone has an equal right in life to life. People in high classes have no more right to be better than anyone else."

Few lower-class persons are bitter about their position in the social system. Their reference group is within this stratum. They are poor, their relatives and friends are poor, and their ancestors were poor.

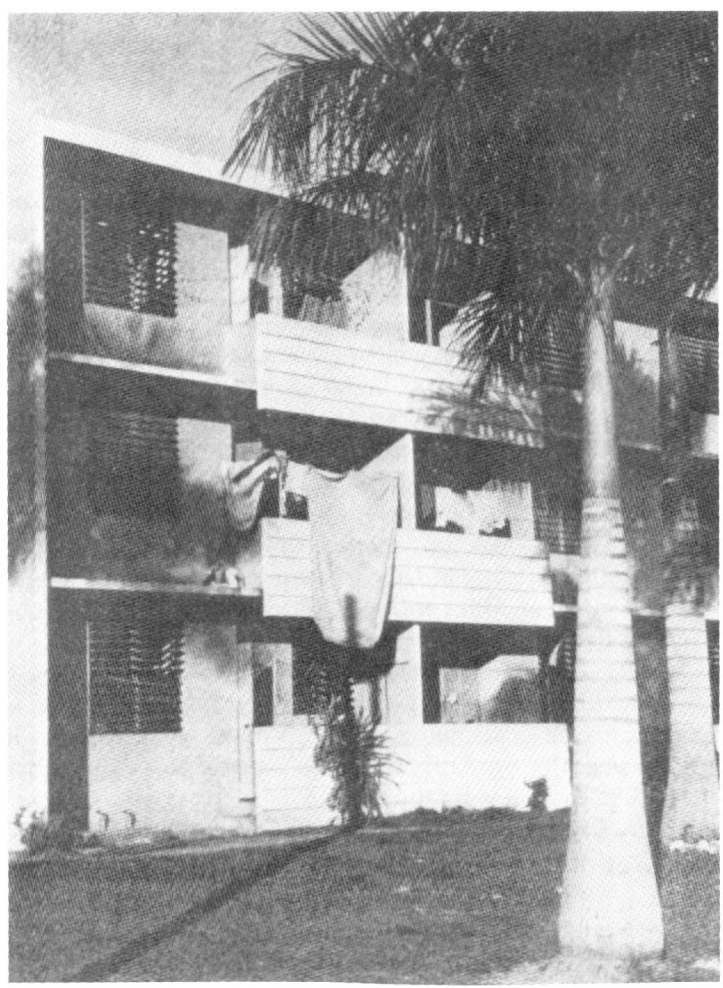

They associate with people like themselves who are struggling, also, to keep a roof over their heads, to have enough to eat each day, and to meet the burdens of illness as they arise. They are isolated from the higher reaches of the society. They know the rich class exists, but the gulf between the poor and the rich appears to be insurmountable. One woman voices this finality when she says, "One does not swim the Mona Channel."

Lower-class individuals are accustomed to a social system in which there is little equality. Throughout the colonial era the man lowest down was kept down from one generation to another. The ideology of social equality is a new ideal—one which has not been blended into the historical culture patterns.

SUMMARY

The city of San Juan has been the center of the Island's government for over 450 years. Today, the city has grown far beyond its historic boundaries. The automobile has enabled the population to spread into an extended metropolitan area, but in the last half-century population in the central zone of the metropolitan area has increased far faster than in the outlying areas, engendering extreme congestion. The competition for land upon which to build roads, factories, and office and apartment buildings has given rise to the utilization of all available space, even to the point where those least able to compete are forced to build their homes on steep hillsides, on swampy ground, and over estuaries. Culturally, the traditional is juxtaposed to the new. Socially, the population is divided into clearly delineated classes. Data from the Survey Sample highlight the differences between the classes as we have defined them. Our interests focus on the two-thirds of the population in class V.

Class V persons, who live predominantly in slums and public housing, are aware of their position in the social system that enmeshes their lives. They view themselves as poor people, struggling for a living in a society where the desirable things are controlled largely by persons and families who occupy positions higher in the social system than they do. The class V adults in our study are resigned for the most part to a life of want; only a few look forward to a better day. The prevailing judgment of their position is: "We are drowning in poverty."

PART II THE CHILDHOOD YEARS

The life history of each individual is divided into three periods. The first extends from birth to the fifteenth birthday. The second begins at 15 years of age and lasts until the individual married his present spouse. The third encompasses the years from the beginning of the current marriage to the present.

Two strategic objectives guide our examination of the life histories. First, we describe the conditions under which the 40 men and 40 women in the study were reared while they were members of families of orientation. Second, we compare individuals who are now suffering from schizophrenia with individuals who are not, to determine if the two groups differ from one another in specific areas of their life histories. We hope that a careful examination of the data will throw new light on the issue of whether individuals who have developed schizophrenia have experienced conditions in their lives that are markedly different from those who have not.

Each period of the life history receives detailed analysis in succeeding chapters. The chapters in Part II are focused on three different, but related, facets of life in the childhood years. Chapter 4 is concerned with the parents who procreated and reared these individuals. Chapter 5 examines the relations that are reported to have existed between the parents and the children in each group of families. Chapter 6 traces selected life experiences each individual faced as he became socialized into the family and the community.

In each chapter attention is focused on two principal questions: (1) What were the family settings in which they spent these formative years? (2) Are childhood experiences which are recalled related to mental status in the present? Both questions are of interest. The first enables us to describe life conditions in the families of orientation. The second represents an effort to test the widely asserted proposition that experiences in childhood mold one's personality. The data were gathered from the men and women by asking them to recall past events and experiences. The accounts of childhood years are, therefore, subject to an unspecifiable margin of inaccuracy which attends all retrospective reports.

4

Families of Orientation

From birth to the present each husband and wife has been enmeshed in a network of family relations. Each was born into a family of orientation and, early in adult life, each established through marriage a family of procreation. During the childhood years the network of family relations is inescapable. It is a common belief among social scientists and psychiatrists that childhood experiences in the family of orientation have a marked effect on the personality development of the child. With this belief as a premise, we asked each individual a series of questions about the educational and occupational characteristics of his parents, the economic and interpersonal problems experienced during childhood, the composition of his family of orientation, and whether or not it was ruptured as a result of the death of or abandonment by a parent.

The 160 fathers and mothers of the 40 men and 40 women in the study were all born on the island of Puerto Rico. The offspring of these parents, the 80 men and women whom we studied, were also born in Puerto Rico; 17 per cent in the San Juan metropolitan area; 75 per cent in rural areas of the Island, outside the limits of the metropolitan area of San Juan; and 8 per cent in small towns on the Island.

Each person born in the metropolitan area began life in a slum. The neighborhoods outside the San Juan area in which the parental families lived were town slums, impoverished rural villages on the edge of sugar cane plantations, or mountain hamlets composed of a few families barely scratching a living from badly eroded hillsides. We found no association between the mental status of either the males or the females and the place of their birth.

Fifty-five per cent of the fathers were agricultural laborers who worked in the cane fields at least part of the year. During the dead time (the long season while the cane grows) a man did any work available to him. He crushed rock for a public road or cut wood to burn into charcoal to peddle in the nearby towns; if he lived near the seashore, he may have fished for his family's food and sold the extras to his neighbors; a man with a small patch of tobacco may have cured the leaves he did not sell to the local tobacco factory and made them into twists for local consumption. A man with a few carpenter tools may have combined working in the cane, vegetable gardening, and local construction work. To support his family, one father added bench- and chair-making to a series of odd jobs. Those who worked on the land toiled long hours under the tropical sun, their lives molded by the yearly cycle of planting, fertilizing, weeding, and harvesting the crops.

Nineteen per cent of the fathers were service workers: janitors, a truck driver, stevedores, street sweepers, grass cutters along the roadways, and a bottle washer in a brewery. Fifteen per cent were unskilled pick-and-shovel laborers, doing whatever hard, physical work was assigned to them; in a single day a man may have shoveled mud and rocks, handed lumber to carpenters, helped mix concrete, pushed it in a wheelbarrow, poured it into building forms, carried water to dampen the hardening cement, and cleaned up debris. These men were told by a foreman what to do, when to do it, and, usually, how to do it. Eleven per cent of the fathers were owners of very small businesses in which they peddled small items—thread, needles, cloth, local fruits and vegetables, fish, and soft drinks; three men distilled rum illegally, and one ran a bus line connecting several mountain towns.

Instability marked the businessmen's activities during the years the children were passing from early childhood to adolescence and on into young adulthood; none, in fact, remained in one business for very long. They alternated from worker to profit-seeker, to failure, to worker, to peddler. Failure in business was attributed to many things. Some men failed during the depression of the 1930's; some were ruined by sudden illnesses; the police ended the activities of others, particularly the bootleggers.

When Mrs. Gallardo's father first came to San Juan as a young man, he swept the docks and later became a stevedore. After he accumulated a few dollars, he peddled men's trousers from door to door. This was followed by the purchase of a pushcart from which he sold juices, beer, and rum in the streets. His third business, a small grocery store, failed because his nephew, a part-owner and co-operator of the store, wasted the store's money on rum and women. Mrs. Gallardo's father then returned to working on the docks, but he soon established a salvage business in which he washed used medicine bottles he found in rubbish heaps and sold them to drug stores. This business prospered to the point at which instead of using a fruit basket he once again acquired a pushcart so he could haul more bottles. Now he buys dirty bottles from other men who gather them from rubbish heaps. Recently, he was given a political appointment by the dominant Popular Party. As a *comisario de barrio*, his job is to see that problems in his neighborhood are alleviated; he is a man of prestige and power in the neighborhood.

Seventy-one per cent of the mothers were not employed outside the home during childhood. The 29 per cent who worked were employed in unskilled jobs, usually in domestic services such as cooking, washing and ironing clothes, scrubbing floors, and caring for children. The others worked in tobacco factories, pineapple canneries, or the coffee, tobacco, and cane fields. Some women not employed outside their homes did sewing to earn extra money, and a few sold home-cooked foods in the neighborhood. The gainful employment of the mothers outside the home was usually a result of the rupturing of the family by the death of or desertion by the father; 74 per cent of the working mothers had to enter the labor market because family ties had been ruptured. Three women went into business in their own homes following the departure of the father from the home. One started a boarding house, and the other two distilled rum at home illegally and sold it.

No association was found between the present mental status of either the men or the women and the principal occupations of the fathers. Neither the gainful employment of mothers outside the home nor their sole occupation as housewives is related to present mental status of either the males or the females.

Fifty-nine per cent of the fathers never attended school or did not complete 1 year of school; 20 per cent completed from 1 to 3 years of school; 14 per cent completed from 4 through 6 years of school, and the remaining 7 per cent had more than 6 years of schooling. Only one father attended high school. The formal education of the mothers is essentially the same as that of the fathers: 60 per cent either did not attend school or completed less than 1 year of school; 15 per cent completed from 1 through 3 years of school; 13 per cent completed 4, 5, or 6 years, and 12 per cent completed the seventh through the ninth grades. One man states that his mother completed high school. No mother of the women attended school beyond the ninth grade.

One man says his mother was an educated person who had taught school before her marriage, but, between 1900 and 1920, the school year was short, attendance irregular, and teachers inadequately trained. The shortage of teachers and the limited educational facilities in the villages and countryside, coupled with the fact that her father was "in politics," brought this woman an appointment as teacher in the local elementary school even though she, herself, had completed only elementary school. Two generations ago her village considered her to be well educated.

If at least 4 years of school is taken as a standard of reasonable literacy, four out of five of the mothers and fathers were illiterate or nearly so. No association was found between years of school completed by either the fathers or the mothers and the mental status of the persons in the study group.

Poorly educated and relatively unskilled fathers and mothers belonged to a segment of the society susceptible to economic problems. Consequently, each person was asked if his family had had economic problems during his childhood. The respondent answered this question according to his own definition of "problems," deciding for himself whether or not he had experienced them. Although the details of the stories told us vary, the central core of the subject matter does not. Mr. Aponte relates:

> My father had to cut grass on a whole acre to earn $1.25. There were seven people in the family. We had to live on what my father earned. We suffered from hunger. We had little clothing and no shoes. My father had to take us out of school in the fourth grade. My father did not work regularly. I still suffer from poverty.

The basic idea in this statement is repeated, with variations, by 85 per cent of the men. Low wages, unemployment and underemployment, misuse of money usually by the father, sickness and death, separation of the parents, and mental illness of a parent are the usual reasons given for economic deprivation in childhood. The lack of food and clothing is a repetitive complaint, but the failure to provide shoes for the children is considered the most galling sign of poverty.

Even young children were aware of the struggle to stay alive. From the time he was 6 years of age Mr. Santano was aware of his family's poverty. He relates:

> We were hungry. Each of us had only one pair of pants and one shirt —no shoes. The boys had to search for their own welfare. We shined shoes, sold newspapers and fruits. My mother made fritters and we

took them out to the streets to sell. My mother had to take in washing and ironing to help us.

The repeated recitations of deprivation in childhood are summarized by Mr. Urrutia: "Hunger was in me all the time. My feet did not know shoes."

Sickness and death accentuated the economic problems of the families. Mr. Fuentes recalls that when he was 8 years old his father, who worked cutting grass alongside the highways, died of pneumonia. Two weeks after his father's death, the mother and her small children were evicted from the house. Three months later, a brother of Mr. Fuentes died, and shortly after this a second brother died. Mr. Fuentes was the only male left in the family. He says:

> My mother had to work as a domestic servant. To do this she took the children to live with relatives. She got Sundays off to visit us. She could spend only a little time with each child.

Too many mouths to feed and too little food is the story of Mr. Núñez:

> There were eight children plus my father and my mother. We all lived on what my father made, and he did not make much. We lived poorly. My father was an agricultural worker; frequently he was unemployed for several weeks and we would have to get by on only one meal a day until he started working again. We ate breadfruit, bananas, codfish, bread, and coffee. We were always barefoot. Our clothes were repaired until they could not be repaired any more. This lasted 11 years.

The 15 per cent who do not report a series of economic problems come from families in which the father operated a small farm or a little business. Mr. Hidalgo, who is in this minority, recalls:

> On the farm where I was brought up we always had enough to eat. We had vegetables, meat, eggs. We had some milk, and whatever we had left we could sell. With the money, we bought clothes. We did not have any light and we did not have any water. We used to carry water from the river.

The economic situation in the families in which the women were reared was essentially the same as for the men. The proportion of women who believe there were economic problems is the same as for the men: 85 per cent report problems while 15 per cent do not. Women who do not remember economic deprivation during girlhood years sketch a picture of an existence with the bare necessities but with no tangible measure of affluence. Mrs. Cardona realizes her family was never "well off," but she does not list economic problems in her family when she was a girl:

> We did not have much clothing. When I went to the store or on errands I was always barefoot, but the other girls were barefoot also.

The six out of seven women who report economic deprivations phrase the problem in almost the same terms as the men. The need was for food first and clothing second. In Mrs. Herrero's family, illness created problems. Too many mouths for too little food is a poignant memory for Mrs. Oliver. Mrs. Ubarri who was born in a local slum and still lives there tells us:

> When I was born my parents were very poor. Three years after I was born my stepfather became paralyzed through bewitchment. When I was six years old my mother died. Life after this was one knock after another.

There is no statistically significant relationship between the presence or absence of perceived economic problems in the family of orientation and the mental status of the men or the women.

Each person was asked if there were interpersonal problems in his family during childhood. If the answer was "yes," the fieldworker asked about the nature of the problem. When a respondent said there were no problems in his family, the interviewer probed further. Usually, when a respondent stated that there were no interpersonal problems in childhood, he repeated the reply in the face of probes.

Four men and women out of five recall one or more interpersonal problems in their families of orientation during childhood years. Infidelity and heavy drinking were the most common issues of conflict in the family: 68 per cent of the men and 65 per cent of the women report infidelity on the part of a father, whereas the father's excessive use of alcohol is reported by 38 per cent of the men and 38 per cent of the women. Both men and women speak freely about their fathers' love affairs, as evidenced by Mr. Aparicio:

> My father had a concubine on the side. He also brought some kids that he had by this concubine to live at our place. There were three of us who were born of my mother, but there were two others who were living with us who were the product of my father's concubine.

Relationships between a father and his mistress frequently led to difficulty between the father and the mother. Mr. Espinosa tells of his father's affairs outside of the home:

My father used to fall in love very often. He had two or three extra women. Sometimes I accompanied my father to visit the other women. I ate in their homes. There were fights and arguments between my father and mother because my father had these other women. My father had other women from the time he married my mother until the day he died.

The infidelity of a father often resulted in economic deprivation at home. Mr. Lebrón says:

My father sometimes didn't bring anything home and we didn't have anything to eat because he spent his money on women. When my parents argued, it was over my father falling in love.

Mrs. Ubarri tells of her stepfather's infidelities and their aftermath:

My stepfather fell in love with a neighbor woman. This neighbor woman went over to my stepfather's store to purchase things. After a while, another neighbor told my mother that the woman was not actually paying for the things she purchased, because she was paying off by going to bed with my stepfather. One day my mother found the woman at the store with a lot of groceries in a paper bag. She noticed that the woman left without paying, and she jumped on her. She slugged her and ripped her clothes off. She pulled her hair and she spilled the groceries all over the street. She acted like an animal. She screamed at her and said, "That woman has no respect for marriage." My stepfather did not intervene as he was afraid of my mother. Then the woman sought vengeance by bewitching my stepfather and making him an invalid. He could not walk with his paralyzed legs, so he lost his grocery store.

Only three instances of infidelity on the part of a mother are reported. Mr. Cardona says:

My first stepmother was not faithful to my father. She was always walking around the neighborhood. The second stepmother was the same way. She didn't take care of Raúl [a brother]. She was always well groomed and always fighting with us. She didn't concern herself with the welfare of the home. She was a coquette with men and an immoral woman. The fights with us led her to abandon our home.

Mrs. Oliveras' mother had a series of affairs with men because, according to Mrs. Oliveras, "She was a woman of the world."

One man and woman out of three report that their fathers' excessive drinking was a problem during their childhood. Mr. Iglesias makes it clear that his father's drinking was the precipitating factor in fights between his parents.

> My father used to get drunk and my mother did not like this. She told him she didn't like it, and then they would have a big argument and fight.

The combination of "a woman on the left" and an empty rum bottle is stated simply by Mr. Padilla: "My father was a woman-chaser and a drunkard. His conduct killed my mother." Mr. Hidalgo's father chased women, drank rum to excess, and beat his wife.

A father's excessive drinking often embroiled a family in economic deprivation, debt, and, sometimes, troubles with the neighbors. Mr. Julía reports that his father was a chronic alcoholic:

> My father was always drinking rum when he was bringing us up. Everything he made at work was spent on rum. He had hardly anything left over for us. Sometimes he would spend several months drinking. He would lose his job and go into debt. Sometimes he would go away for several months. He also had fights with the neighbors. Once he was convicted of stealing and given five years in the penitentiary. He spent two years there and then he was put on probation.

Mrs. Oliver sketches a picture of heavy drinking in two generations. Her father stole hogs and goats from her mother and sold them to buy rum or have an affair with a woman. Whenever the mother noticed that an animal was missing she fought with her husband because she knew what had happened. Now Mrs. Oliver's two brothers drink as much as the father and are known as troublemakers in the neighborhood. Fights about drinking between the father and the mother, the father and the sons, and the mother and the sons have been going on for as long as Mrs. Oliver can remember.

Gambling is reported to have been a problem by only one man and one woman. Mr. Santano says, "My father was a gambler; he spent all his money on card games, dice, cock fights, and liquor." Whereas Mr. Santano links rum and gambling as the cause of family fights, Mrs. Tirado links gambling with rum and women in reporting that her father was a gambler and woman-chaser; on one occasion, he won several hundred dollars at the race track and spent it all on rum and women.

The intimate detailed stories of interpersonal problems were gathered to test the hypothesis that schizophrenia is related to disturbed interpersonal relations in the family during childhood. We assumed that schizophrenics had experienced significantly more family problems than nonschizophrenics. To test this assumption, we held sex constant and compared each type of interpersonal problem reported by those persons afflicted with schizophrenia with problems reported by those who do not have this illness.

Males and females who are not schizophrenic report as many interpersonal problems in their families of orientation as the males and females who are schizophrenic. There is no association between mental status in the present and the amount of interpersonal problems in the family during childhood. Specifically, when we compare what males and females who are schizophrenic tell us about infidelity with the recollections of males and females who are nonpsychotic, no association is revealed between infidelity in the family of orientation and present mental status. Likewise, there is no association between excessive drinking in the family of orientation and present mental status, irrespective of sex. The number of persons who report gambling in the parental family is too small to make comparisons between the sick and the well.

Interpersonal and economic problems are so intertwined that it is difficult to sort out the independent effect of each. In five out of six families there were economic problems in childhood; in approximately four out of five families there were also interpersonal problems. Families with economic problems usually report interpersonal problems, and in the homes where there were no economic problems ordinarily there were no interpersonal problems. A partially employed or underemployed man who was a drinker and had affairs outside the home had less money to spend on his family than a man who did not drink or did not have affairs. In eleven out of twelve families there were either economic or interpersonal problems. Either the twelfth family was free of problems or our respondent did not remember any problems in it; in all likelihood, there was far more tranquility in these homes. Mr. Soltero, who does not remember problems in his home, summarizes his childhood memories in the following words:

> My father was a hard-working man and a respectful man. He was responsible to his family. In all respects he was thoughtful.

The 80 families of orientation in which the spouses were born and reared are divided into intact families, in which the natural parents and children had social relations throughout the respondent's childhood, and broken or ruptured families, in which the respondent had one or two parental figures who were not his natural parents because of the severing of relations some time between the respondent's birth and his fifteenth birthday. Exactly 50 per cent of the respondents experienced the break-up of their families during childhood (43 per cent of the men, 57 per cent of the women). The families were ruptured by illness and death of or desertion by one or both parents. Twenty-seven of the families were shattered by the death of a parent (13 by the death of a father, 14 of the mother).

The rupturing of a nuclear family, either by death or desertion, was a dramatic event, usually recalled vividly, although in a few cases it occurred before the child was old enough to remember. Mrs. Feliciano was 10 years old when her mother died. She recalls:

> I took care of her when she was sick. I gave her medicine and nursed her. At the moment of her death she gave me one of her hands, and the other hand she gave to my father. I could not believe she was dead. My father kept telling me she was dead, and we cried. It was a hard experience for me.

In the 13 families ruptured by desertion, 10 were dissolved by the withdrawal of the father from the home; in three, the mother abandoned the father. Five of the 13 desertions occurred while the mother was pregnant with the respondent. In three others, the child was too young to remember the actual break-up of the family. In the five remaining families, the desertion occurred when the child was old enough to remember the circumstances. Mr. Gallardo tells of his feelings at the break-up of his parental family:

> Sometimes when I think of my father abandoning my mother to live with another woman, I feel hatred against him. Then I think I ought not to feel this hatred.

The usual cause of desertion was another sex partner. Infidelity was cited in 10 of the 13 families that were disrupted by desertion. There is strong presumptive evidence to support this inference in one additional family in which the wife abandoned the husband while she was pregnant.

Excessive drinking was the attributed cause of the break-up of two families, although this does not imply that excessive drinking did not create trouble in additional homes. There is no evidence of infidelity in these two families; in one the father abandoned the mother after a vicious fight; in the other it was the mother who left the home. We have a first-hand account from the woman involved, Mrs. Urrutia's mother. She recalls that alcohol and fighting ended her first marriage when she was 15 years old and the present Mrs. Urrutia was 1 year old. Her husband did not support his wife and child, he drank to excess, and demanded respect and obedience from his wife. One day he came home drunk and made sexual demands. When she resisted, he tried to beat her. In the mother's words:

> I would not put up with this. I grabbed a stick and hit him right on the prick. Then I slugged him over the head until he was knocked out. I picked up my daughter and left him. He continued to live in the place where we used to live. I took a lot of things from that man.

When a family was ruptured, the children were cared for by some person in the kin group; none was placed in an institution. The most frequent arrangement was for the remaining parent to keep the children in the home and call for help from the closest relatives. The phrase "the closest relatives" includes both geographic propinquity and social acceptance of the kinship obligation. If a mother died and the father was left with the children, he turned for help to whatever relatives were close by: his own mother or sisters or the deceased woman's relatives. If the father died, the wife did the same. Each member of the family is obligated to give whatever aid is possible during times of trouble. During the period immediately following the rupturing of a home, the nearest relatives either took the children into their homes or came to the home to help with the household duties. In 17 out of the 21 homes where there was a surviving parent, a stepparent was acquired at some later time. The arrival of a stepparent is not related either to the sex of the child or the sex of the surviving parent. The surviving parents who did not remarry were helped by the kin group.

The parental family was the most frequent source of support when a family was broken. In 15 out of the 40 ruptured families the orphaned child was reared by grandparents, aunts, and uncles; in eight cases it was the brother or sister of a parent, and in seven it was a grandparent. Sometimes the surviving spouse took the child to a parent's home or to a brother or sister while he worked to help support the child. In some cases it is difficult to determine exactly who reared a child from a ruptured family and for how long. Mrs. Rosado says that when she was 2 years old her father abandoned her mother. The mother gave her 9-month old son to one of her sisters to care for, and Mrs. Rosado and her mother moved to the home of her maternal grandmother. This grandmother and a maternal aunt raised her while the mother worked as a domestic servant to pay for her care. Although Mrs. Rosado's father lived with another wife a short distance away, he did not contribute to his children's support. Mrs. Rosado continued to live with her maternal grandmother and aunt after her mother took a second husband. The mother had 1 child with this husband who abandoned her after 4 years. She then married a third man with whom she had 4 children, but after 5 years she was abandoned again. The mother now lives alone with the 5 children from the second and third unions. During her childhood, Mrs. Rosado had a father in the home for 2 years. From that time on she lived within walking distance of her father's home, but she did not visit him. From 2 years of age until she was 10, her mother was in and out of her grandmother's home; then the mother established a new consensual union. Thus, Mrs. Rosado was reared by her mother, maternal grandmother, and maternal aunt. We cannot say whether the grandmother or the aunt did more of the rearing, but the fact is that Mrs. Rosado was reared by members of her mother's family of orientation.

In three of the four remaining ruptured families an older sister assumed the obligation of rearing a younger child when the family ties were ruptured. In the fourth family, an older brother cared for a younger brother when both parents died a few months apart. In these four families the younger sibling was of school age when the family of orientation was broken. In all but one family when a brother or a sister took a child to rear, either one or both parents had died. The exception was Mrs. Molína who had to be taken from her home at the age of 12 when her mother became mentally ill. The father took the girl to the home of a maternal aunt. From that time until she married, Mrs. Molína was passed from relative to relative.

The acceptance of children for rearing by a grandparent or grandparents resulted almost exclusively from the illness and death of a parent, usually the mother, when the child was less than a year old. In only one instance of a child being reared by a grandparent was desertion the reason given for the dissolution of the family of orientation.

There were twice as many children in the intact families as in the ruptured families. The essential data on family size, type of family, and mental status are summarized in Table 9. The schizophrenics, male and female, come from families of approximately the same size as the well men and women. This generalization is applicable to those who come from intact as well as from ruptured families. The intact families were large; the ruptured families were smaller.

When we turn from the number of children in a family of orientation to the number of persons living in a household in which an in-

TABLE 9 Mean Number of Children in Intact and Ruptured Families by Sex and Mental Status

	INTACT FAMILIES	RUPTURED FAMILIES
A. Males		
All families	9	4
Nonschizophrenics	9	4
Schizophrenics	9	4
B. Females		
All families	10	5
Nonschizophrenics	11	5
Schizophrenics	9	5

dividual was reared during most of his childhood years, we find no essential differences in size between the intact or the ruptured families because the children of ruptured families are raised by some other branch of the extended family group. The data on size of household by sex, family type, and mental status are summarized in the following tabulation:

	MEAN SIZE OF HOUSEHOLD	
	INTACT	RUPTURED
Male schizophrenics	11	10
Male nonschizophrenics	11	10
Female schizophrenics	10	13
Female nonschizophrenics	12	9

According to a variety of sociologic and psychiatric theories, experiences in the family during childhood are related to personality development. Thus, we assumed that an intact nuclear family is more likely to produce a mentally healthy adult than a family in which the parent-child relationship was ruptured. We now test a specific form of this general hypothesis: Is schizophrenia in the present related to the rupturing of the family during the childhood years?

The data summarized in Table 10 show no association between present mental status and childhood rearing in a home where the family ties were intact or ruptured. This finding applies to both the males and the females. We conclude that schizophrenia is not associated significantly with the gross fact of being reared during the childhood years in a family of orientation either intact or ruptured.

The composition of the household during the childhood years was examined to see if the presence of persons in the home other than the parents and their children is associated with mental status. To investigate this point, we divided the 80 families of orientation into two categories: (1) those composed of parents and children only, and (2) those that include no parent, one parent, or two parents plus other persons (the other persons include adopted children, children being reared because of a ruptured home in another nuclear family, grandparents, uncles, aunts, cousins, and so on through almost all members of the kin group by consanguineal or affinal ties).

In the families composed of parents and children only, two generations are represented; families composed of persons additional to the parents and children may consist of three or four generations. One family included five generations—a great grandmother, a grandfather, the mother of the respondent, the mother's sister and her husband, their children, two brothers of the husband, and two children of a daughter of the mother's sister. Another family contained an aged man and the children he had fathered from five different wives; in addition, two widowed sisters of the man and their children lived in the home. This man was 52 years older than his fifth wife, who at the age of 13 gave birth to his thirty-fifth child. This is an extended family, indeed!

TABLE 10 Intact and Ruptured Families of Orientation by Sex and Present Diagnostic Group

	SCHIZO-PHRENICS, %	NONSCHIZO-PHRENICS, %
A. Males		
Intact families	55	59
Ruptured families	45	41
N =	11	29
$p > .05$		
B. Females		
Intact families	31	52
Ruptured families	69	48
N =	13	27
$p > .05$		

TABLE 11 Family Composition during Childhood by Sex and Present Mental Status

	SCHIZO-PHRENICS, %	NONSCHIZO-PHRENICS, %
A. Males		
Parents and children only	55	28
Parents, children, others	45	72
N =	11	29
$p > .05$		
B. Females		
Parents and children only	55	52
Parents, children, others	45	48
N =	13	27
$p > .05$		

The family composition by sex and mental status is summarized in Table 11. The data presented reveal that the composition of the family of orientation in childhood is not linked to mental status in the present. This finding is applicable to both sexes. The slight difference in the percentage distributions in the different cells of the table are attributable to chance factors.

SUMMARY

The parents as well as their offspring, who compose the study group of this research, were all born in Puerto Rico. Practically all the husbands and wives were born and reared outside of the San Juan metropolitan area in small villages and hillside farms. Over one-half of their parents received less than one year of formal education. Many were employed in agriculture, but some were service workers, pick-and-shovel construction workers, and small-business operators. The vast majority of the husbands and wives recall having experienced serious economic hardships—a lack of food and poor housing and clothing—during childhood. An approximately equal number remember interpersonal problems in their families which resulted primarily from the infidelity and drunken behavior of their fathers. Economic and interpersonal problems were interrelated.

Exactly one-half of the husbands and wives come from "broken homes," defined as the absence of one or both parents because of death or desertion before the fifteenth birthday. The death or desertion of a parent presented a problem of care of the children which was solved by the assistance of relatives. The bonds of kinship were activated during the crisis, and obligations were transferred to relatives. Although there was no difference in the number of persons living in intact or broken homes, the intact families had twice as many children as those which were ruptured.

Economic and interpersonal problems are recalled by as many sick as well persons. Moreover, no relationship was found to exist between the economic level, education, composition, and stability of the families of orientation and the present mental status of the persons. Thus the sick and well persons come from a homogeneous background of fact and experience during childhood.

5
Parent-Child Relations

The authority or power the parent wields over the child is of central importance to the structuring of parent-child relations. Societies vary in the degree to which parental authority is exercised and the rapidity with which it is relinquished. Among lower-class Puerto Rican families, parental authority is exercised firmly and relinquished slowly. Often an adolescent child is able to attain some autonomy only through open rebellion against one or both parents. It is assumed by members of the extended family and neighbors that parents will enforce respect for and conformance with commonly accepted values of good behavior in their children.

Social distance between parents and children is maintained through an emphasis on *respeto* (respect), a concept employed time and again by interviewees to describe their childhood relationship with their parents. A respectful child obeys a parent immediately and without question. Failure to carry out work assignments, "back talk," "bad words," in fact any violations of the orders of either the father or the mother are viewed as evidence of disrespect. Respect is enforced by advice and example and, above all, by punishment.

Parents try to keep the children under control so the reputation of the family will not be tarnished by their children's misdeeds. Punishment is an ever present reinforcing agent relied on by parents to mold their children into acceptable members of the society. Children are taught in infancy that they will be punished for a failure to do what is expected in a given situation. How is this punishment now viewed by the men and women who were subject to it as children? Is the memory of punishments related to mental status?

Ideally, rigid discipline was maintained by a stern glance at the child, but few parents were able to command unquestioned obedience by such means. Parental punishment routinely consisted of reprimands, scoldings, standing in a corner, advice combined with threats, restriction to bed, a slap or spanking, and so forth. Beyond this, there was the punishment administered by a frenzied and explosive parent which was uncontrolled and furious and, consequently, went far beyond the bounds of routine punishment. On these occasions, the parent flew into a rage, comparable to the temper tantrum of a child, either with no regard for the safety of the child or, in fact, in an effort to injure, maim, or kill the child. We label this type of punishment *severe* to distinguish it from routine or *moderate* punishment.

Every man and woman was punished as a child by real or substitute parents for breaches in respect, parental expectations, and orders and for violations of social rules. Systematic questioning elicited stories of the misdeeds that led to the punishment, the form of punishment, and the parental figure who administered it. Mrs. Julía says:

> My father had no compassion for any of us. When we were young girls he would not let us go any place. He did not let us speak to anyone. If we even as much as climbed a fence, he hit us.

Defying the order of a father or father substitute meant swift and often violent punishment. Mrs. Domínguez remembers:

> When my brother was about six years old, he did one of those ridiculous things that boys do. When my father came home and found out what my brother had done, he grabbed a machete and tried to kill my brother. My brother ran into the woods, and my father looked for him for two days and nights. My father is a beast.

Mr. Padilla, who was reared by an uncle, recalls the uncle killing a neighbor's dog because the dog had killed his pig. He ordered Mr. Padilla to throw the dead dog into the river; when the boy refused the uncle beat him on the back, ribs, buttocks, and legs with the branch of a guava tree until he was bruised, torn, and bleeding. On another occasion, the uncle beat him until he lay on the ground bleeding from the contusions on his body and sobbing uncontrollably from the pain. He still carries the scars from this beating.

Although frequent punishment and rough treatment were the accepted ways of teaching children parental respect, mothers were more prone than fathers to enforce their authority with faultfinding followed by corporal punishment. Mrs. Escudero relates:

> My mother reprimanded me every five minutes. No matter how well I did things, she always found fault in it. She spanked us a lot. She wanted her children to behave as if we were grown up.

Mr. Santano tells us that his mother became "blind mad" when the children did not follow her orders or when the neighbors complained to her about the children. She used to call them "pigs," "damned ones," and other humiliating names. When she was angry she grabbed a child and pummeled him on the head, face, back, or legs with her fist, an open hand, or a stick until she was exhausted. When a child had done something particularly disrespectful she made him kneel on the grate (a piece of metal, perforated by a nail in a number of places, which is laid on the ground or floor of the house, so that when a child is made to kneel on it the jagged pieces of metal raised by the nail holes press into his knees). Mr. Santano recalls kneeling on the grate with a bucket of sand in each hand: "I had to remain in that position for a long time until she pardoned me."

The mother or the father who had a "loose arm" (one who slapped or hit frequently) is remembered vividly, as are kneeling on the grate and other painful forms of punishment: beatings with a man's belt, stick, or harness strap, often resulting in bruises that took a week or more to heal, and spanking with the sole of a shoe. Mr. Lugo remembers how he was whipped by his mother when "her bun stood on end":

> When my mother had those episodes she hit me hard with a whip. She hit me so hard I'd end up on the floor on all fours with welts all over me. It was as if my skin had been shredded. When she hit me with her fists she left black spots. She was really strong in punishment.

The memory of such beatings is accompanied by strong feelings toward the parents who gave them. Mr. Urrutia is open in his hostility toward his father:

> My father was a son of a bitch. He was shameless. He was like a Judas. He liked to punish his children as if we were animals. He was so hard on us that once my brother had to cut him to defend himself. After my brother did this, he had to leave home. That man used to beat my mother and my brothers and sisters as well as me.

Frequent punishment by the father or mother is linked with the rigid demands parents made of their children. Being reared "locked up" or in a parental "fist" is a common complaint. The boy's or girl's efforts to break out of the "fist" often led to violent retribution. Mrs. Molína recalls that when she was 12 years old her mother saw her speak to a boy in the yard. The mother called her into the house and accused her of disobedience. Words flew; the mother began to scream, slapped the girl, pulled her hair, and hit her with her fist; she grabbed a butcher's knife and tried to kill the girl, but, before she was able to do more than slash her arm, the girl's screams of pain and fright brought help from the neighbors.

Mrs. Domínguez relates:

> My father was very dominant and strict. He had us inside his fists. He did not even let us breathe. He did not punish us every day, but he treated us like animals. He had a very strong temper. One day when I was nine years old, my father came home from work and found me at the home of a neighbor. He had warned me not to visit this neighbor. He got so mad that he took some dry leaves from a banana tree and wrapped them around my legs and set fire to them. The neighbors rescued me and cured my burns.

The statements and recollections of the husbands and wives provide illustrations of both severe and moderate punishment. Now we attempt to determine if the kind of punishment received during childhood is related to present mental status. Sixty-eight per cent of the men and 65 per cent of the women recall being severely punished at some time during their childhood. The data for each sex, comparing well with sick persons, are summarized in Table 12.

Although the kind of punishment males received during childhood is not related to their current mental status, the sick males report more severe punishment in childhood than the well males. Among the females, severe punishment in the family of orientation is linked to the later development of schizophrenia. We cannot tell if the sick

TABLE 12 Type of Punishment during Childhood by Sex and Mental Status

	SICK, %	WELL, %
A. Males		
Punished moderately	18	38
Punished severely	82	62
N =	11	29
$p > .05$		
B. Females		
Punished moderately	8	48
Punished severely	92	52
N =	13	27
$p < .05$		

men and women were *actually* punished more harshly by their parents during their childhood years or if they only report that they were. Retrospective accounts, subject to unknown margins of error, do not allow a choice to be made or a clear inference to be drawn. All that can be said is that significantly more sick than well women claim that they were harshly treated in childhood. Among the men the trend is in the same direction. Future research may provide a firm solution to the problem of the possible etiological connection between harsh punishment in childhood and the development of schizophrenia in later years.

The vivid accounts of punishment in childhood should be viewed in relation to the findings derived from a series of seven questions designed to elicit the respondents' attitudes to their fathers and mothers or surrogate parental figures. These questions were asked to determine how the individuals now think they felt during their childhood about their parents. Each question is presented below as it was asked, followed by the findings pertinent to it.

1. How would you describe your mother?

The respondent was asked to characterize his mother when he was a child according to eight attributes on a list which was read to him. The respondent was free to assign all or none of the attributes to his mother. The attributes and the percentage of men and women who ascribe each one to their mothers are summarized below:

ATTRIBUTE	MALES, %	FEMALES, %
Respectful, serious	98	90
Affectionate, kind	93	83
Tolerant, understanding	78	53
Gay, lively	40	43
Moody, temperamental	38	30
Sorrowful, sad, shy	38	43
Dominant, strict	13	33
Responsible, resourceful	10	13

The men and women describe their mothers in similar ways on six of the eight attributes, the exceptions being tolerance and dominance. More men than women think their mothers were tolerant; more women than men think their mothers were dominant or strict. The men and women are in agreement and almost unanimous that their mothers were respectful. Likewise, they believe their mothers were affectionate and kind. Generally, the men have more favorable views of their mothers than do the women.

Nine men and ten women had substitute mothers during childhood. Owing to the similarity of views, we have combined the sexes in the analyses presented here. The percentage distribution on each attribute for the foster mother is:

ATTRIBUTE	PERCENTAGE
Affectionate, kind	68
Gay, lively	53
Dominant, strict	53
Tolerant, understanding	37
Moody, temperamental	21
Sorrowful, sad, shy	11
Responsible, resourceful	11
Respectful, serious	11

The foster mothers rate lower than the natural mothers on affection, tolerance, temperament, sorrow or shyness, and, above all, on respect. Foster mothers are sorely remiss in respect. They are viewed as being gayer than real mothers and more dominant.

When we compare the answers of the sick individuals with those of the well for each sex, attribute by attribute, we find that, in practically all cases, schizophrenia does not affect the person's description of his real mother. Only one attribute shows a significant difference between the sick and the well in each sex: the male schizophrenics view their mothers as sorrowful or sad; the female schizophrenics think their mothers *not* lively or gay. We interpret this to mean that more schizophrenics in both sexes than nonpsychotic men and women look upon their mothers as subdued.

The nine men and ten women, whether sick or well, who had foster mothers view them in similar ways. In seven of the eight attributes there are no significant differences in the ways the schizophrenics and the nonschizophrenics describe their foster mothers. The one category which shows a significant difference is affection or kindness; schizophrenics, men and women, think their foster mothers lacked affection.

2. *How would you describe your father?*

Five attributes were listed for the fathers and substitute fathers; each reflects a facet of the roles assigned to fathers in the culture.

ATTRIBUTE	MALES, %	FEMALES, %
Responsible provider	80	60
Strict, firm	73	60
Affectionate, kind	57	57
Dominant, abusive, unjust	45	45
Tolerant, understanding	38	25

Fathers are viewed similarly by the men and the women with two exceptions: more women than men think their fathers were intolerant, and more men than women think their fathers were responsible providers. The ten men and nine women who had substitute fathers viewed them in the following ways:

ATTRIBUTE	PERCENTAGE
Responsible provider	84
Strict, firm	63
Affectionate, kind	53
Tolerant, understanding	53
Dominant, abusive, unjust	37

As many substitute as real fathers are viewed as affectionate and strict; more are viewed as tolerant, fewer as abusive, and slightly more as responsible providers. In general, foster fathers are viewed as favorably as real fathers.

Schizophrenic men and women describe their fathers in the same terms as well men and women. The data show that attribute by attribute the two mental status groups in each set describe their fathers in essentially similar ways. The same finding applies to the men and women who had foster fathers. Irrespective of mental illness, real and foster parents are described in essentially similar ways.

3. Did your mother prefer one child over another?

The replies to this question are analyzed in three ways. First, we compare individuals in each sex and diagnostic group who believe their mothers preferred *them* to their brothers and sisters. Second, we compare individuals in each sex and diagnostic group who believe their mothers showed a preference for *some other sibling* with those who did not believe such a preference existed. Third, we compare individuals in each sex and diagnostic group who believe their mothers *did not show a preference* for any child with those who believe their mothers did show a preference.

These analyses reveal that a mother's bias for or against or lack of bias toward a child is not linked to mental status in either sex.

Each person who claims the mother had a preference for a particular child was asked why the mother preferred the designated individual. The most common reason given is that the preferred child was "sickly." The second most common reason differed among the men and the women, the men believing the oldest son was preferred by their mothers, and the women believing it was the youngest son who gained the mothers' attention. The only answer numerous enough to test for significance was that the preferred child was sickly. Differences were not found between the sick and the well in either sex regarding the sickly child. Sickly children are pitied; mothers feel sorry for them and show them preference. This preference is understood and usually shared by other members of the family including the respondents.

Regardless of whether or not the interviewee was the preferred child, each person who reported that his mother showed a preference for one particular child was asked how he felt about this preference. The replies to this question are coded into seven categories: the respondent (1) felt sad or worried, (2) considered himself inferior to his brothers and sisters, (3) was jealous, (4) was annoyed or discontented, (5) was angry at his siblings, (6) was understanding or not affected by this preference, and (7) was pleased or content with it. Only 19 women and 14 men report favoritism on the part of their mothers toward a particular child. For analytical purposes, the seven categories are combined into two distinct feelings: the first five categories are taken to mean a dissatisfied reaction and the last two categories as a satisfied reaction. These data are summarized in Table 13. The reported

TABLE 13 Reaction to Mother's Preference of One Sibling by Sex and Mental Status

	DISSATISFIED	SATISFIED
A. Males		
Well	7	5
Sick	0	2
$N =$	7	7
$p > .05$		
B. Females		
Well	6	4
Sick	2	7
$N =$	8	11
$p > .05$		

reactions to a mother's preferences for a particular child are not related to present mental status.

The nine men and ten women who had substitute mothers were asked if the substitute mother preferred one child. When the answer was "yes," we then asked how the respondent reacted to the preference shown to the particular child. The responses were analyzed to see if the schizophrenics, male and female, gave replies different from the nonschizophrenic males and females. No significant differences were found. Thus, an individual's reaction to a foster mother's preference for a particular sibling is not connected with present mental status.

4. How did your mother treat you during childhood?

The replies were recorded by the interviewer as the respondent told his story. During the analysis of data, a series of categories was constructed, and each person's statement about the way his mother treated him was placed in the appropriate category. Enough replies to enable us to compare the two diagnostic and sex groups were provided by six categories of treatment by the mother: (1) with affection, understanding, (2) tried to please, (3) took good care, (4) gave good advice, (5) scolded, punished fairly, and (6) taught good manners. A significant difference at the .05 level exists between the schizophrenics and the nonschizophrenics on one item—the schizophrenic males think their mothers lacked affection and understanding. In the other five categories there are no significant differences between the answers of the two sexes.

The profile of the ways the men and women describe the treatment they received from their mothers, stated in percentages for each category, is as follows:

TREATMENT BY MOTHER	MALES, %	FEMALES, %
With affection, understanding	70	58
Took good care	58	33
Gave good advice	53	28
Scolded, punished fairly	30	20
Tried to please	10	33
Taught good manners	3	13

There is somewhat more of a tendency for the males, in comparison with the females, to view their mothers' treatment as favorable.

94 The Childhood Years

The replies of the nine men and ten women who had substitute mothers were analyzed separately to learn if the sick and well persons, either men or women, differ in the treatment they think they received at the hands of their foster mothers. No significant differences were found between the two groups on any item.[1]

5. *Which parent, if either, did you prefer?*

Mothers are preferred to fathers by sick and well males and females. More well than sick males prefer their mothers, but this difference is not significant. The percentage figures for each group are given in Table 14. The "no preferred parent" category includes family members other than the natural father or mother as well as those respondents who did not prefer one parent over the other. The number of persons who preferred some parental figure, other than the natural father and mother, is too small to analyze by sex, mental status, and type of preferred parent.

TABLE 14 Preferred Parent by Sex and Mental Status

	SICK, %	WELL, %
A. Males		
Mother	46	72
Father	18	3
No parent	36	25
N =	11	29
$p > .05$		
B. Females		
Mother	62	56
Father	15	15
No parent	23	29
N =	13	29
$p > .05$		

[1] Because of an editorial oversight in the revision of the schedules used in the field, the questions on the respondents' treatment by their real and foster fathers were left off the final copy. This omission was discovered after the field work had been completed and all the data moved to New Haven. We decided to proceed with the analysis without the additional information the omitted questions would have provided about parent-child relations.

The reasons given for preferring one parent over the other or not making a choice between the parents are remarkably similar among the males and the females who are either sick or well. Neither illness nor sex has any appreciable effect on the data. This observation is clear from a glance at Table 15.

TABLE 15 Reasons Given for Preference of a Parent by Sex and Mental Status

	SICK, %	WELL, %
A. Males		
Preferred parent more affectionate, tolerant, responsible	52	58
Compassion for preferred parent	21	18
Both parents affectionate, tolerant, responsible	27	24
N =	11	29
$p > .05$		
B. Females		
Preferred parent more affectionate, tolerant, responsible	54	59
Compassion for preferred parent	31	28
Both parents affectionate, tolerant, responsible	15	13
N =	13	27
$p > .05$		

6. In addition to parents, was there some member of the family whom you preferred? If so, whom did you prefer?

The responses to these queries show no differences between the sick and the well persons in either sex. However, they do reveal a strong difference between the sexes. Among the females, three out of four named a preference for some other family member in addition to the parents, but among the males the corresponding figure is one out of four. Sisters led the preference list, 28 per cent; brothers were next, 20 per cent; and cousins, 3 per cent. The large percentage of women who prefer some other family member is probably indicative of the greater dependency of the women on the family.

96 The Childhood Years

7. What member of your family do you resemble most in character, behavior, and feelings?

Men think they resemble their fathers; women think they resemble their mothers. The second largest percentage of resemblances involves an older sibling of the same sex. Men identify with older brothers; women identify with older sisters. Two men (one sick, one well) think they resemble more than one family member. One believes he resembles his father and mother; the second thinks he is like his father and an older sister. Eight females (five well, three sick) believe they resemble two family members. Six of these dual identifications are with the father and the mother; two are with the mother and an aunt. The data on resemblance in character, behavior, and feelings are presented in Table 16. These data reveal no essential differences between schizophrenics and nonschizophrenics in either sex.

TABLE 16 Belief in Resemblance to a Particular Family Member in Character, Behavior, and Feelings by Sex and Mental Status

	SICK, %	WELL, %
A. Males' resemblance to		
Father	45	38
Older brother	27	30
Mother	18	17
Uncle	9	10
No family member	—	5
N =	11	29
B. Females' resemblance to		
Mother	54	56
Older sister	23	22
Father	23	15
Aunt	—	7
No family member	—	—
N =	13	27

SUMMARY

As children, all persons were punished by their real or substitute parents. Punishment ranged from light ridicule to humiliating denigration, from a slap to a violent beating. At some time during childhood, two-thirds of the men and women were subjected to at least one severe beating by a parent who had gone "blind" with uncontrollable rage. These beatings are remembered vividly and recounted with feeling. Significantly more sick than well women experienced such beatings; and although the direction of such a difference also applies to the sick and well men, statistical significance cannot be attached to this difference. Whether or not a person was punished severely does not appear to influence the way he answers the questions on his relations with his parents.

Men and women describe their mothers in similar ways as determined by the use of eight personality attributes. Contrary to what one might expect, the sick and well persons do not differ consistently in either sex in the descriptions of their mothers; the same lack of difference between the sexes and between the diagnostic groups is found in the persons' descriptions of their fathers' personalities during childhood. About the same number of sick and well persons in both sexes report that their mothers preferred a particular child in the family, most often because he was sickly and in need of special care; the sick of either sex do not register more frequent dissatisfaction over such a preference than do the well persons of either sex.

Men and women more often prefer their mothers to their fathers, but, again, this fact does not differentiate the sick from the well persons of either sex, nor do the reasons adduced for such a preference show a difference between diagnostic groups. Men believe they resemble their fathers and women their mothers, but in neither sex do the diagnostic groups show a significant difference in reporting a resemblance to family members.

In brief, there is no consistent and repetitive pattern of differences between diagnostic groups of either sex in reconstructing their interpersonal relations with their parents during childhood. Finally, we believe it is justifiable to question any conclusions regarding possible etiological significance for schizophrenia of the variables, conditions, and experiences embodied in the answers to the issues examined in this chapter.

6
Socialization

Socialization involves the transmission of a society's culture from the parental to the oncoming generation. The family of orientation, in the context of its class and national culture, is the primary setting in which the socialization process takes place in the childhood years. The family culture is transmitted consciously, as well as unconsciously, to the children. Children are given and taught their names by the parents. Simultaneously, parents teach them a language (Spanish in our study group), a set of values, expectations about how to behave, and so on through a complex myriad of acts that make them an integral part of the family, the neighborhood, the community of residence, and, in due course, of the larger society. The parents transmit their ways of thinking, acting, and speaking to their children. The children are taught to eat and to urinate and defecate in acceptable ways, at suitable times, and in approved places. The children learn much from parents and intimate associates. Socialization and personality formation are, therefore, inextricable parts of a single complicated process.

Not one mother in the parental generation entered a hospital for childbirth; all 80 men and women were delivered in the home by a midwife. If complications developed the midwife sent for a doctor, but this occurred only at one birth. In this instance, the mother was hemorrhaging and the midwife was having difficulty keeping the baby breathing. Although a female relative helped the midwife while the father went for the doctor in a nearby town, the mother died. Five per cent of the babies were reported to have been breech deliveries, 5 per cent to have been born 1 to 2 months prematurely. Difficulty in delivery was reported by 13 per cent of the group.

Toilet training occurred inside and outside the house. It began at 6 months in some families, although the modal age was 13 months. It was completed usually by the time the child was 5 years of age.

One comment was:

> In the country mothers did not always have to be teaching their children. When one felt like urinating, one squatted in the grass. When one felt like defecating, one simply went into the bushes. To wipe oneself, one got a stick. When one grew older he or she went to the latrine. Little ones were kept out of the latrine so they would not fall through the hole. We saw others go to the latrine to urinate or defecate. That is the way we learned. There was no trouble.

This report describes the experiences of some four out of five persons. The remainder, 18 per cent in both sexes, report difficulties in learning to use the latrines.

Some of the problems of learning to control one's bowels and bladder during the day and through the night are clearly shown in the answers to our questions on bed-wetting; 75 per cent of the men and the women were persistent bed-wetters when they were children. There is a sharp difference, however, between males and females who were bed-wetters after 6 years of age: 62 per cent of the women who report that they were bed-wetters as children claim they had stopped this practice before they were 7 years of age; 59 per cent of the males report they continued the practice after they were 7 years old.

Bed-wetting was punished in several ways by mothers, older brothers, and sisters; rarely did a father or father figure take an active part. Ninety-three per cent were scolded, slapped, or whipped for wetting in bed. This figure indicates that more were punished in childhood for this act than now think they were bed-wetters in the early years. Kneeling on the grate was another form of punishment for this offense, but public humiliation was the most effective punishment imposed on a persistent enuritic. One woman was made to drape the soiled and stinking bedclothes over her head and walk to school. Another now believes public humiliation is a sure cure: "Both my daughters were pissers until I made them walk around town with the wet sheets on their heads."

No relationship was found to exist for either sex between present mental status and trouble in toilet training.

Eating habits were examined to determine if there are differences between the schizophrenics and the well persons. One-third of the men and 43 per cent of the women state that they were selective, slow, or odd eaters in childhood. Twenty-three per cent of the males and 38 per cent of the females report the combination of selective eating and "delicate" stomachs. The difference between boys and girls also appears in responses to a question on vomiting in childhood: 18 per cent of the men, in contrast to 35 per cent of the women, claim they experienced repeated vomiting spells in childhood. When the stomach symptoms are viewed as a syndrome there is little difference between the sexes, 55 per cent for the females and 50 per cent for the males. These symptoms taken separately or in combination are not related to present mental status in either sex.

The age at which boys and girls began to walk and talk is not linked to mental status. Some began to walk when they were 9 months old— the majority between 1 and 2 years of age. Of the four women and one man who did not start to walk until at least age 3, the man and two of the women are mentally healthy; the two women who are schizophrenics think they did not start to walk until after they were 3 years old. A few men and women began to talk at 1 year of age, but the most common age at which to start talking was 18 months. One schizophrenic male claims that he did not begin to talk until he was 9 years old; this is balanced by a mentally healthy woman who says she did not speak until she was 5 years of age. These are very atypical reports, given here without any effort to evaluate their truth or falsity.

When we compare by sex and mental status those who report temper tantrums with those who do not, the differences between each group are not significant. Frequent temper tantrums in childhood are reported by 33 per cent of the males and 35 per cent of the females. Mentally healthy men and women report temper tantrums in childhood as frequently as those who are schizophrenic.

A systematic effort was made to elicit from each person how he thinks he was viewed by his family and play group. Fourteen questions were asked in this phase of the research, each designed to evoke a facet of the ways a person perceives others to have viewed him. From the responses of "yes," "no," or "don't know," we constructed a self-perception profile for each individual. These individual profiles were combined, in turn, into group profiles by sex and mental status. The positive responses on each item, stated in percentage form, were as tabulated on page 101.

Some self-perceptions are linked to the sex roles of boys: bad humor, hardheadedness, disobedience, lying, and cruelty to animals. Definitely associated more with girls than boys are the self-perceptions of obedience and affection. More than one-half of the men now perceive themselves as having been timid, sensitive, bad-humored, and hardheaded as well as disobedient, happy, active, affectionate, and liars when they

PERCEIVED TO HAVE BEEN	MALES, %	FEMALES, %
Timid	70	55
Sensitive	57	58
Bad-humored	53	33
Hardheaded	63	35
Spoiled	13	18
Disobedient	65	15
Obedient	35	80
Sad	35	48
Preoccupied	30	28
Happy	58	55
Active	78	63
Affectionate	73	85
A liar	68	33
Cruel with animals	25	10

were boys. More than one-half of the women perceive themselves to have been timid, sensitive, obedient, happy, active, and affectionate in their girlhood years. Relatively few in both sexes now see themselves as having been spoiled, cruel to animals, and preoccupied with their own thoughts.

The self-perceptions of the schizophrenics are similar to the self-perceptions of the nonschizophrenics in both sexes. It should be pointed out again that this is a retrospective view of self-perceptions in childhood. How these persons would have responded to the fourteen items when they were children is a matter of speculation, as is the way other persons, in fact, viewed them. All that can be said is that the schizophrenic males and females report now that as children they perceived themselves in the same terms as the mentally healthy persons.

Each respondent was asked a series of questions regarding his social relations with his age mates. Two persons out of three report they had many friends in childhood. Some three persons out of four believe they got along "well" or "very well" with their freinds. Those who had few friends claim they got along as well with their few friends as those who think they had many friends managed with theirs. Males and females, sick and well, report about the same number of friends, and approximately the same proportion think they were good friends.

We queried each person on the kinds of play he engaged in during the years when he was from 5 to 10 and from 10 to 15 years of age to learn whether the men and women who are now schizophrenic think they had, as children, the same play activities as or different ones from those who are now mentally well. The play activities in which they participated are typical of those in the culture and class level. Group activities predominated: hop-skip-and-jump for the girls, hide-and-seek for the boys; swimming in groups in the river was a favorite of the boys. Each person believes he had plenty of time to play, which is incongruous with the stories a number of men and women tell of how hard they worked as children. When asked specifically about play time, they state with few exceptions that they had plenty of time to play in the years before they were 15. Perhaps these individuals did not expect to play all the time.

The play activities of each person were grouped into one of three categories: (1) individual activity only, (2) individual activity sometimes, group play at other times, and (3) group activity only. The distribution by sex and diagnostic group is summarized in Table 17. This table shows that girls tend to be involved more in group games and in solitary activities than boys. The important point is that no significant difference appears between the types of play the sick and the well participated in for either sex.

We compared the number of different play activities each person reports to determine if well persons were more active in childhood than sick persons. We found that well men report a mean of 3.1 play activities in which they participated during childhood, whereas sick men report a mean of 2.6 activities. The well females report they en-

TABLE 17 Participation in Types of Play by Sex and Diagnostic Group

	SICK, %	WELL, %
A. Males		
Individual activities only	—	—
Individual and group activities	55	67
Group activities only	45	33
N =	11	29
$p > .05$		
B. Females		
Individual activities only	8	7
Individual and group activities	31	30
Group activities only	61	63
N =	13	27
$p > .05$		

gaged in 2.1 activities and the sick females 1.4. The differences for both men and women are not significant. It is beyond the scope of our data to infer if the slight difference in reported activities between the schizophrenic males and females and the nonschizophrenics means that schizophrenic individuals were less active in childhood. If the reports on the frequency and type of play activities are accurate, little or no evidence can be adduced to support the idea that schizophrenic persons were noticeably withdrawn or alienated from peer groups during childhood.

Eighty-five per cent of the men and 83 per cent of the women state that their parents approved of the kinds of games and play activities they engaged in as children. The few parents who disapproved are divided proportionately between the sick and the well persons. The only change in parental attitudes toward children's play activities occurs among the girls between the span from 5 to 10 years of age and 10 to 15 years of age. In the 10 to 15 years of age span the percentage of parents who disapproved of their daughters' play activities increased from 17 to 30. The disapproving parents are divided proportionately between the sick and the well females.

Slightly less than two boys out of five were prohibited from playing with some children in the neighborhood where the family lived. The figure for the sick males is 36 per cent, for the well males 38 per cent. Among the females, 33 per cent of the well group were limited by their parents to associations with selected children in their neighborhoods, while 62 per cent is the comparable figure for the sick females. Although the sick females report almost twice as many restrictions on their associations as well females, the difference is not significant.

Men and women, sick and well, are in agreement on the reasons for their parents' prohibiting them from associating with some children who lived in the neighborhood. The children who were proscribed as playmates are described as undisciplined, as using obscene words, and as violating the limits of decency. A few males say they were prohibited from playing with boys known to have visited prostitutes or who had been seen having sexual intercourse with animals. Three females were forbidden to speak to certain girls who were reputed to consort often with neighborhood boys. Gambling and the use of alcohol are not among the reasons given for the proscription of other children.

Each person was asked if, as a child, he was afraid of seven specific things. The answers to this series of questions are summarized in the tabulation below which shows the percentage of persons who experienced the specific fears:

FEARED	MALES, %	FEMALES, %
Thunder and lightning	73	75
Large animals	55	60
High places	43	53
Darkness	68	68
Dead persons	70	73
Being alone	55	63
Strangers	45	43
Other things	68	55

It is clear from these figures that the fears listed were common during childhood, and no fear is connected specifically with the biosocial role of being a boy or girl; the same fears were shared by boys and girls. Theoretically, a person could have claimed he was not afraid of any of the listed fears, or he could have said he was fearful of every item on the schedule. One woman and two men report they were not afraid of any of the situations presented; no one admitted fear of all the situations presented. The mean number of fears reported by males is 4.8; the mean number reported by females is 4.9. This is further evidence that there was little difference among the ways these men and women remember the fears they had in childhood.

We compared the schizophrenics and the nonschizophrenics in two different ways. First, we compared them serially on each fear to determine if more schizophrenics report being fearful of a specified thing in childhood than the nonschizophrenics. An item by item comparison reveals no significant differences between the schizophrenics and the nonschizophrenics in either sex for any fear in the list. In the second analysis we compared by means of the T test the matrix of fears reported by each mental status group for each sex. The difference between the schizophrenics and the nonschizophrenics was not significant. The male and female schizophrenics, however, report slightly more fears than the nonschizophrenics.

Nightmares represent another dimension of fear. An individual may be troubled during his sleep by fears he does not consciously experience during his waking hours. Although he may not understand the meaning of his tumultuous and frightening dreams, he is often able to remember at least some of the more spectacular details. Our queries on nightmares reveal that 58 per cent of the men and 50 per cent of the women have memories of bad dreams in childhood. Those who report the nightmares recall the content of their nocturnal fantasies. Similarity in the dreams from person to person is apparent, the underlying theme being fear of attack and destruction of the self or its dignity. For example, Mr. Cardona began to have recurrent nightmares at the age of 7, after his mother's death and the entrance of his first stepmother into the home. This woman, who was much younger than the father, had a roving eye. Mr. Cardona recalls:

> This stepmother used to make me mad. She did not take care of the house and she did not take care of my brother. I began to have these dreams. I dreamed there were heavy rains, but it would not be water —it would be rocks that were falling.

Similarly, Mrs. Gallardo's mother died when she was 4 years old. Some time afterward, the mother called to her in her dreams. She dreamed she went to her mother and kissed and caressed her; then she woke up crying. She also had nightmares about falling and woke up very much frightened; sometimes she fell out of bed. She had nightmares that she was flying but fearful of falling, or that she was fleeing from bad people who were chasing her. Upon awaking, she was very tired and very much afraid. (She still suffers from nightmares about her mother.) The context of nightmares reported by other individuals was similar. They dreamed of faceless persons chasing them, of animals, of evil spirits, of death.

Individuals who report that they had nightmares during childhood were asked if the nightmares occurred rarely or frequently. Twenty per cent of the males and 30 per cent of the females experienced nightmares frequently. The memory of frequent nightmares is linked to mental status. Schizophrenic males and females report significantly more nightmares than the nonschizophrenics in both sexes. The responses to the questions on nightmares are summarized in Table 18.

The history of physical illnesses each person experienced during his life was elicited by systematic questioning. The schedule asked for the respondent's identification of the illness by name, age when it occurred, duration of illness, length of treatment, and if the treatment was at home or in the hospital. Any surgery reported was recorded with the age when it occurred, the number of days of hospitalization if any, and the length of time until recovery.

All physical illnesses that each person experienced from birth to

TABLE 18 Reports on Childhood Nightmares by Sex and Diagnostic Group

	NIGHTMARES FREQUENTLY, %	NIGHTMARES NEVER OR RARELY, %
A. Males		
Schizophrenics	63	19
Nonschizophrenics	37	81
N =	8	32
$p < .05$		
B. Females		
Schizophrenics	83	11
Nonschizophrenics	17	89
N =	12	28
$p < .01$		

his fifteenth birthday were categorized into one of three groups:[1] infectious illnesses, noninfectious illnesses, and traumatic illnesses. Infectious illnesses include the commonly experienced childhood diseases: measles, mumps, whooping cough, respiratory infections, worms; and less commonly encountered infections such as filariasis. The noninfectious illnesses include such disorders as fatigue (asthma), diabetes, and rheumatism. Traumatic illnesses include broken bones, knife cuts, and injuries from accidents such as head wounds resulting from a falling coconut or the kick of a horse.

The number of each type of illness each person experienced was recorded. We then summed the number of illnesses experienced in childhood, organizing the data by mental status in each sex. The number of each type of physical illness was then divided by the total number of years each sex and diagnostic group of persons had been exposed to the hazards of illness. In this analysis the number of illnesses experienced is the numerator, the years of possible exposure the denominator; the quotient is expressed as the rate of illness experienced per 100 years of risk. By stating relations between illnesses experienced and the number of years of exposure to illness in each group as a rate, we are able to control for the variable amount of time involved in each sex and mental status group. Moreover, by stating the ratio of illnesses experienced to the years of exposure or risk as a rate within

---

[1] This classification scheme was suggested by our colleague, Raymond S. Duff, M.D. He assisted us also in placing specific illnesses in each category.

TABLE 19 Types of Physical Illness Experienced in Childhood by Sex and Diagnostic Group *

	SICK	WELL
A. Males		
Infectious	7.8	9.4
Noninfectious	1.6	1.7
Traumatic	3.3	2.9
Total	12.7	14.0
B. Females		
Infectious	11.6	10.3
Noninfectious	2.8	1.6
Traumatic	3.3	4.2
Total	17.7	16.1

* Expressed as a rate per 100 years of exposure.

each mental status group, we can make direct comparisons between types of illnesses from one mental status group to another.

The rates of illnesses experienced during childhood, given in Table 19, are similar for each group of illnesses for the mentally well and mentally sick. Well males report slightly more infectious illnesses than the sick males, but sick females have a higher rate of infectious illnesses than well females. The same kind of minor variation occurs in the other groups of illnesses. The total rate pattern is likewise variable: the well males have a higher rate than the sick males; however, the sick females are higher than the well females by the same amount. In sum, mentally healthy persons claim to have suffered as frequently from physical illnesses in childhood as schizophrenic persons.

Treatment at home by folk remedies and practices was the rule; by a doctor or a public health nurse the exception. A child was taken to a doctor or a hospital only when the family realized it could not cope with the illness or accident. One woman relates how she suffered from a rash on her body when she was 10 years old; this was followed by nodules and fissures on her face, then boils filled with pus on her forehead and cheeks. After several months of home treatment she was taken to a public health clinic in a town some miles from her rural home. The physician assigned to the clinic diagnosed her affliction as syphilis.

Only in extreme cases did the family resort to hospitalization. One man tells of a severe enteric infection when he was 7 years old. He remembers his stomach was bloated and sore and "turned black." He passed blood for a week before he was taken to a doctor who hospitalized him for about a week, the second longest hospitalization reported. The longest one, for a month, was occasioned by an automobile accident. The victim was a 9-year old boy whose leg and ankle were crushed when he was run over by a car. He was taken to the hospital in an unconscious state, but as soon as he was well enough to be cared for by his family he was taken home. Six males and four females spent some time in hospitals before they were 15 years of age. These individuals are divided proportionately between the sick and well groups.

Surgical procedures by a physician were even rarer than hospitalizations. Four women and three men experienced surgery when they were children. Only one was hospitalized, a girl who underwent an appendectomy when she was 9 years old; the others were operated on for minor ailments: a tonsillectomy, two circumcisions, a tumor in an infected hand, an infected scalp and skull, and an infected foot. The performance of surgery is not related to schizophrenia in either males or females.

Accidents during childhood were experienced by twelve men and nine women, ranging from minor cuts and bruises to having been run over by a car. Only three persons were treated by a physician after an accident: one was the boy mentioned above who was hospitalized after an automobile accident; one was for a dog bite; the third was for foreign matter in the eyes. Home remedies for accidents, in a few cases, involved minor surgery. One man says that he was hit on the head with a coconut at the age of 14 and knocked unconscious for 2 hours. He was carried home and cared for until his recovery. Some weeks later a growth was seen on his head. His father decided it should be removed and he cut the growth out with a red-hot razor blade. A woman relates a similar tale: An abscess formed after she cut her hand on a rusty wire; an aunt performed home surgery with a heated razor blade.

Accidents that gave rise to dislocated fingers, ankles, and shoulders were treated at home. The dislocated member was pulled back into place by an adult, and the child was told he was "cured." One woman dislocated her right shoulder twice as a child; in both instances her father set it back in place. One man was thrown from a horse when he was 11 years old and broke his collarbone which was set at home by his father. Accidents serious enough to be remembered are distributed proportionately between the sick and the well men and women.

The only formal institution outside the family with which these men and women came into contact in childhood for varying lengths of time is the public school. A generation ago, tax-supported elementary schools were located close enough to a child's home so he could walk to school easily, go home for lunch, and return for the afternoon's session. As is the case today, many schools met for only half a day. The level of education attainable in a local school varied widely: in some schools only the first three grades were taught; in others there were four grades. Whether or not a child went beyond the grade limit provided by his neighborhood school is related to the location of schools. If a child was to continue in his studies after completing the curriculum at the local school, he had to face a long walk or a bus ride to a school offering either six or eight grades, usually located in a town or city.

All the men and 95 per cent of the women attended elementary schools; two women never attended any kind of school. The boys and girls averaged seven-and-one-half years of age when they started school. The girls, on the average, completed the fifth grade before they left school; no differences exist between the sick and the well women and the last grade completed. The average age at which the girls left school, 12.8 years, shows no difference from one diagnostic group to the other. The mean number of years of school has a similar pattern, 5.5 (average) for both sick and well females. These figures indicate a remarkable similarity between the well and sick women insofar as it applies to the temporal aspects of their school experience.

The sick males completed seven grades of school and the well males five grades.[2] This difference is significant, but its interpretation is a matter of speculation. The average age at which the boys left school varies with mental status: the sick males were older than the well males (a mean of 14.7 years of age compared to 13.3) when they quit school, but the age difference is not significant. Likewise, although the sick males spent 7.4 years in school and the well males 6.0 years, the difference is not significant.

The school years are viewed as a pleasant experience by 82 per cent of the men and 70 per cent of the women. There are no differences in the ways the sick and the well men look back on their years in school,

---

[2] $T = 2.367$; 38 degrees of freedom; $p < .05$.

but among the women the way the school experience is viewed is related significantly to mental status; 92 per cent of the sick women liked school very much, but only 59 per cent of the well women view their school years with this much favor.

The sick males had significantly more "difficulties" or "problems" while in school than the well males. This difference is summarized in the following tabulation:

	SICK, %	WELL, %
Males		
Difficulties in school	82	24
No difficulties in school	18	76
N =	11	29
$p < .01$		

There is no meaningful relationship between reporting problems in school and present mental status among the women: 27 per cent of the well women and 38 per cent of the sick women report one or more difficulties in their school years. Frequent absences and low grades were seldom viewed as problems. Most of the difficulties reported involve interpersonal relations with either the teacher or other students. Fighting with other students was the most common difficulty among all the females and the well males, whereas the sick males' difficulties clustered around arguments with the teachers. Reciprocally, a significant proportion of the schizophrenic males were afraid of their teachers whom they viewed with apprehension. The teachers were usually women, and the boys who later developed schizophrenia experienced difficulties centering around their authority relations with these women.

Males and females, sick and well, give almost identical reasons for leaving school. Therefore, the data on leaving school are discussed without distinguishing between the sexes or the sick and well persons. The reasons given for withdrawal from school are summarized in six categories as follows:

REASONS FOR LEAVING SCHOOL	PERCENTAGE
Economic problems in the home	53
Father's desire	13
No advanced school nearby	10
Did not like school	10
Marriage	8
Illness and death in the family	6

Some of the details given were:

> My father started to chase women and he would not buy me the things that I needed. My mother would not send me to school poorly dressed, so she took me out.
>
> I had to stay at home and take care of my brothers and sisters while my mother went out to work as a domestic servant.
>
> My mother could not buy me pencils and paper. I had few clothes and no shoes.
>
> I used to eat with the money I was given to go on the bus. Oftentimes I did not go because there was no money at all.
>
> My father was always fighting me. At school they asked for things my father said he could not give me. He would not buy me clothes or shoes. I had to go to school with nothing.
>
> I quit school because I had no money for food. To attend school that way was too humiliating.
>
> When I finished the fourth grade I did not have shoes to put on for graduation. I left school so I could start working and buy the things I wanted to have.
>
> The economic situation was very bad at home. When my mother could no longer make money from washing and ironing, things got worse. I was 13 years old and I did not dare go to school with such worn-out clothes. I had been wearing those clothes for a long time.
>
> When my father died everything changed. We were very poor. We had to move. Then I had to start school again. I got into the first grade again. They asked for books. I did not have any money. So I had to leave school at the age of seven.

More than one-half the group attribute their leaving school to economic reasons. The most humiliating problem was the lack of shoes. Simple clothing, well washed and ironed, can be tolerated; hunger does not shout its misery for all to hear, but when a child lacks shoes and cannot buy pencils, a pad, and the required books, everyone concerned witnesses his degradation.

The category "father's desire" as a reason for leaving school also reflects the family's economic plight. The father's desire for the boy or girl to leave school often resulted from the family's need for additional help on the little farm or for a young hand and a loud voice on the pushcart. Some fathers made their sons quit school so they could carry the fathers' lunch to the distant cane field and eventually earn 50 cents a day as a water boy for the workers in the cane. Some fathers, however, wanted their daughters to leave school out of concern for the girls' morality. As a girl nears adolescence the parents develop anxiety about her associations and activities away from home. To go to a school removed from the neighborhood makes the girl vulnerable to approaches from males. Girls were needed at home to take care of the younger brothers and sisters. Moreover, a girl who could read and write was considered to have enough education for a "humble person."

Some children did not live within walking distance of an advanced school, and either there was no bus or their families did not have bus fare. Dislike of school and poor grades took their toll, as did loss of interest in school, falling in love, and marriage. As many boys as girls claim they left school because they were in love.

The linkage between a recognized need for the necessities of life—food and clothing—and a desire to leave school is related to the next step in the life histories of these young people. Two boys out of three went from the classroom to an unskilled, physically demanding job with low wages. The other one-third were employed by their families. The boys who worked at home were mainly from rural families who tilled a few acres of land. As a family hand, these boys either worked at agricultural tasks with their fathers or took over such tasks at least several months of the year while the father, or father substitute, worked for a cash wage for a sugar plantation or the government.

The pattern of gainful employment upon leaving school is summarized by diagnostic group in Table 20. The significant difference be-

TABLE 20 First Employment upon Leaving School by Sex and Diagnostic Group

	SICK, %	WELL, %
A. Males		
Gainful employment	64	66
Employed at home	36	34
N =	11	29
$p > .05$		
B. Females		
Gainful employment	62	22
Employed at home	38	78
N =	13	27
$p < .05$		

tween the well and the sick females calls for some discussion. The well girls tended to remain at home and help their families with the household and farm chores; they cared for children, washed, ironed, carried water, fed the livestock, and worked occasionally in the coffee, tobacco, and vegetable fields. This was a transitional period in their development. The girls who became schizophrenics in later years stepped almost directly from the classroom into someone else's kitchen or into a local factory.

The data on the first full-time paid job of the different individuals range over a quarter of a century: some boys began to work in 1929 and some girls in 1930; those who are younger began to work outside their homes as late as 1951 for the boys and 1955 for the girls. Drastic changes occurred in the Puerto Rican economy during the years the young people entered the labor force, and these changes are such that comparisons between the beginning of the time span 1929–1930 and the end of 1951–1955 would be hazardous. Therefore, the starting years of the work careers were divided into two periods: the first extends from 1929 to 1941, the era of the Great Depression; the second covers the years from 1942 through 1955, the era of World War II and its aftermath.

The most commonly held first job in both periods for males was that of an agricultural laborer, hoeing the cane, irrigating and fertilizing cane, and cutting stalks for the grinders when the cane was ripe. After several years "in the cane," the typical young man drifted to San Juan where, in the words of one, "I changed the hoe for the hammer [in a factory]." Boys who did not start their work careers in the cane fields found a wider assortment of jobs that required some strength but no skill. Four boys began as "assistant ambulatory merchants," boys who push the cart for a peddler selling wares in the street and hawk the wares in a raucous voice. Other boys were employed loading and unloading trucks, on road crews, as janitors, messengers, or on odd jobs.

The mean age for a boy's first full-time job during the depression years was 13.2 years; he earned 67 cents a day (mean). The age at which boys were employed on their first job increased slightly to 13.9 years (mean) from 1942 through 1951; the starting wage in this period was $1.40 per day (mean). Boys who developed schizophrenia in later years began work at approximately the same age as boys who have not developed a psychotic illness. Likewise, there is no difference in the average earnings on the first job between those who are now mentally ill and those who are mentally well.

The first jobs for the women follow a different pattern from that of the men. The average age at which a girl took her first job before World War II was 12.0 years; the girls started their work careers as domestic servants or as agricultural laborers in specialty crops such as coffee, tobacco, pineapples, or general farming, rather than in the cane. After World War II, the average age to begin work was 15.8 years; these girls were employed most frequently in factories where they became sewing machine operators or workers in small plants that had moved to the Island. Nondomestic service employment drew a number of girls; such jobs included beautician's aid, sales assistant, waitress, steam presser, and nurse's aid. Some girls still found employment as domestic servants and agricultural workers; however, these jobs were in the minority in the post-World War II years.

Girls who began to work after 1941 earned more than five times as much as girls who began to work before then. In the more recent period the mean wage earned was $2.18 per day in comparison with 41 cents per day in the earlier period. After the war the girls earned an average of 78 cents per day more than the boys, which is probably attributable to the changes that have taken place in the occupational structure of Puerto Rico since World War II.

Girls who later became afflicted with schizophrenia began their first jobs at about the same age as those who have remained mentally well. This generalization is applicable to those who began to work before the war as well as since the beginning of World War II. The only difference is that the girls began to work at an earlier age in the 1930's than in the 1940's and 1950's. The wages of the girls who later became mentally ill were not significantly different in either period from those who have remained mentally well.

A higher proportion of the males than females were employed before they were 15 years of age, 75 per cent in comparison with 53 per cent. The data on the first jobs show that being employed before 15 years of age is not connected with a diagnosis of schizophrenia in later years. We may conclude that the age at which boys and girls began to work is not related to whether they were to be diagnosed in their adult years as suffering from schizophrenia or as mentally healthy.

SUMMARY

No association was found to exist between present mental status and problems in childhood of toilet training, eating habits, or temper tantrums. Based on a list of fourteen attributes, sick and well individuals have essentially similar ideas of how others viewed them in childhood. Sick and well persons are alike also in the number of friends they report having during childhood and in the quality of relations they had with their friends. The findings do not support the inference that in childhood the schizophrenics were estranged or removed from social relations with peers.

An analysis of childhood fears indicates that as many sick as well persons experienced them during childhood. Frequent nightmares during childhood, however, afflicted more schizophrenic than nonschizophrenic men and women.

The type of physical illness, the amount of it in proportion to years of risk, and the frequency both of accidents and hospitalization from birth to the fifteenth birthday are not unduly concentrated in the schizophrenic group. Variations in each of these dimensions of health are not related to psychiatric diagnoses.

Sick men completed more years of school than their well counterparts, but no such difference is to be found among the women. Even though sick men went to school longer than the well, they experienced more difficulties in school, particularly problems with teachers, a difference not observed among the females. On the other hand, more sick than well women liked school very much, a difference not found among the men. Men and women, sick and well, left school primarily because of pressing economic problems at home requiring their help in the house or gainful employment outside of it. The sick women more than the well were gainfully employed immediately upon leaving school. The employment history of the men does not reveal a relationship to present mental status.

PART III BECOMING AN ADULT

The second period in the life history covers the years from an individual's fifteenth birthday until marriage. The boys and girls had almost all left school before they were 15 years of age. They wanted to earn their own money and to spend it in their own way. They sought freedom from parental domination in their choice of friends and leisure activities. The males desired to prove they were *machos* (real men). The females wanted to be *señoritas* (young ladies romantically sought by marriageable men). Both the boys and girls aspired to adult roles; they hoped to play them and to be regarded as grown up. Three crucial steps in the young person's search for adult identification are a job, a mate, and a home of his own.

The years of becoming an adult stretched from the fifteenth to the twenty-second year among the males and from the fifteenth to the nineteenth year among the females. What happened to these young people during those years? Were the men and women who now suffer from schizophrenia different in this time period from the men and women who are now mentally healthy? Are we able to recognize definite behavioral signs of the onset of schizophrenia during this phase of the life cycle?

We seek answers to these questions by a detailed examination in Chapter 7 of job histories, geographic movement, and experiences with physical illness. In Chapter 8 we examine courtship and marriage. In these chapters we present the data on geographic movement from birth to the present and the story of courtships and remarriages for persons who have had more than one marriage.

7
Jobs, Geographic Mobility, and Illness

During childhood boys and girls are integrated into the inner world of their families of orientation. As they begin adolescence, subtle changes occur in the way they are viewed by their parents; reciprocally, they acquire new attitudes about themselves and their relations with adults and peers. They desire more freedom from parental control than they were allowed as children. They develop new interest in persons of the opposite sex, and their leisure activities change.

In childhood, girls participate in individual and group games at or near home. As adolescence arrives they look for entertainment away from home, visiting girl friends, walking in small groups on the main street of the town, eyeing boys, and occasionally going to a dance or movie accompanied by girl friends and female relatives. The girls become interested in attracting boys, but only for amusement or harmless flirtation since they must guard their chastity to be desired as *señoritas*. To achieve their immediate objectives they want attractive clothing and greater independence from parental domination.

The primary entertainment of adolescent boys consists of joining street-corner peer groups which gather on sidewalks, in the main *plaza* surrounding the town church, and at bars and *cafetines* where the older men play cards and dominoes. Occasionally, they go to a dance or movie. Boys who live away from the town walk or hitchhike several miles to participate in these activities. They have learned from the conversation of older men and from their own friends that it is pleasing to have a woman sexually. Girls are very much the center of their attention. At this age the boys begin to test themselves by approaching girls, addressing *piropos* (compliments) to them, engaging them in apparently casual conversations, and inviting them for *paseos* (walks). These new interests accentuate the need to earn money.

A generation ago, before boys and girls entered the labor market, they were expected to do unpaid work at home. Country boys walked the hillsides picking up stray pieces of wood for cooking fires at home. Town and city boys gathered driftwood from the lagoons, boxes from stores, and crates from factories. Boys and girls carried water from a nearby creek, well, or public faucet. Girls took care of their younger brothers and sisters, washed and ironed clothes, helped scrub the floors, washed the dishes, sewed, embroidered, and sometimes cooked the family meals. Boys carried the noon meal to their fathers who were working in the cane or other field crop, did the chores connected with the care of livestock, worked in the family garden, and repaired fences. Town boys carried lunches to their fathers at the factory or helped with the family pushcarts. In addition, they sought jobs that would pay them in cash: in the country carrying water to workers in the fields, in the city shining shoes and carrying messages. The need to earn money for personal necessities was continuous in the life of the lower-status boy. As he reached adolescence, the need became imperative. To live, to have money for clothes and entertainment, a boy had to work at a job that paid him a cash income; this meant searching for a job outside his family.

All the males entered the labor force before they reached their fifteenth birthday. They were employed predominantly in unskilled, casual jobs. The country youths, working on farms or plantations, were assigned to menial, hard, outdoor jobs such as cutting weeds, planting, hoeing, and cutting cane, building fences, hauling manure, cleaning brush from hillsides, and cutting wood for charcoal. City and town youths found jobs as janitors, helpers on pushcarts or trucks, laborers on construction projects, delivery boys, bus boys, and messengers. There was no relationship between the type of job first held or earnings on the first job and the present mental status. Both sick and well males earned mean monthly wages of $57.80.

The females show a sharp difference in the rate of entry into the labor force before 15 years of age: 92 per cent of the sick females were working outside of their homes on their fifteenth birthday, whereas only 41 per cent of the well females were gainfully employed outside of their homes at 15 years of age. The types of jobs the two groups of girls held were not different. The employed girls did housework, farm work, and sewing. Some two out of three girls started to work as domestic servants, cleaning floors, washing dishes, helping to cook, and caring for children. A few girls worked in the tobacco fields and curing sheds; some picked coffee beans during the harvest. Girls employed in the needle trades either sewed at home from materials and patterns brought to the house by a contractor or went to a factory where they operated sewing machines. Two girls found employment in beauty parlors. The mean monthly earnings at 15 years of age for the employed girls who later became sick were $33.41; for those who remained mentally healthy the mean monthly wage was $37.20. This difference is not significant.

The job experiences of the sick and the well persons between 15 years of age and marriage were similar. An examination of the figures summarized in Table 21 substantiates this generalization. These data show that the work careers of the schizophrenic males were no different from those of the well males. The work patterns of the well females were very close to those of the schizophrenic females. In each sex group, the job histories of the sick and well persons are almost identical during the transition from childhood to young married adulthood.

The monthly earnings figures by sex and mental status in Table 21 are mean figures for the phase of the life history which extends from the fifteenth birthday to marriage. To test the possibility that there might be observable differences in the life histories considered, we calculated the percentage of each sex and mental status group *employed at the time of marriage* and the mean earnings of each group. These

TABLE 21 Job Experiences between 15 Years of Age and Marriage by Mental Status and Sex

	SICK	WELL
A. Males		
Mean number of years worked	6.9	6.9
Mean number of jobs held	3.2	3.4
Mean number of months on a job	26.0	24.0
Mean monthly earnings	$81.88	$88.96
Percentage of jobs left voluntarily	77.0	73.0
Percentage of unskilled jobs	64.0	62.0
B. Females		
Mean number of years worked	1.9	1.8
Mean number of jobs held	2.6	2.5
Mean number of months on a job	8.0	7.5
Mean monthly earnings	$48.95	$52.51
Percentage of jobs left voluntarily	86.0	93.0
Percentage of unskilled jobs	75.0	71.0

figures are presented in Table 22. All the men were working when they got married. The sick men earned almost as much as the well men. A higher percentage of sick than well females earned less, but the differences between the percentage working and the mean monthly amount earned are not significant for the sick versus the well females.

The typical male, sick or well, worked approximately 2 years on a job. When he left one job to seek another, he did so voluntarily three times out of four. The reasons given for leaving a job indicate widespread dissatisfaction. Mr. Cardona, for example, always worked in motion-picture theaters. Before marriage, he had advanced from usher to assistant operator of the projection machine. When he asked for a raise, the theater owner refused. He quit and obtained another job as an assistant motion-picture projector operator.

Mr. Dávila's first job which paid very little money was caring for livestock on a farm. He decided to leave the job and come to San Juan where he obtained work as a laborer on a construction job. He says:

> It was very dangerous, especially when I had to go to the top of a building. One time I pinched my finger and it was very painful. I decided to quit this job.

He later obtained a job as a machine operator on the night shift of a factory. He found he could not sleep during the day so he quit this job.

Mr. Espinosa, a bus boy, left "the best job" he ever had in a tourist

TABLE 22   Individuals Gainfully Employed at Time of Marriage and Mean Monthly Earnings by Mental Status and Sex

	SICK	WELL
A. Males		
Percentage employed at time of marriage	100	100
Mean monthly earnings at time of marriage	$110.15	$111.57
B. Females		
Percentage employed at time of marriage	85	74
Mean monthly earnings at time of marriage	$64.39	$68.85

hotel because "... there was a change in headwaiters. We didn't get along. I quit before he fired me." Mr. Gallardo had a "good job" as a delivery boy for a bakery: "I got up at 3:00 AM to carry the bread to the stores and houses." He quit because his boss was "too mean." Mr. Ramos was a pushcart operator's assistant. He relates, "I grew too old for that job. I found work as a waiter in a hotel." Mr. Urrutia specialized in unskilled construction labor. Several times he walked off jobs because he could not get along with his fellow workmen. He says, "I didn't get along with them, and they didn't get along with me. I just walked away."

Trouble with the boss was the recurrent complaint of men who were fired from jobs. Trouble on the job was reported by several men. When "trouble" occurred, the young man quit or was fired. Mr. Iglesias was a servant in the home of a wealthy family. He reports that his mistress was mean and unjust; she made him work hard, paid him very little, and showed her anger quickly and violently. He claims she fired him one day in anger.

Mr. Quintero, who was employed as a bus driver by his father, hit and killed a man while he was driving the bus. The next day, a passenger was hurt as he stepped off the bus. The father blamed him for both accidents, so Mr. Quintero left to seek his fortune in San Juan. Mr. Ubarri was employed as a truck driver's helper. The driver came to work one day drunk and insulted him. A fist fight ensued. Mr. Ubarri knocked the driver down with a rock. He quit the job before he was fired. Mr. Soltero was working as an orderly in a private hospital in San Juan when his father died. He asked the physician who owned the hospital for an advance on his salary so he could bury his father. The physician refused and Mr. Soltero was so angered that he left this job.

The women had fewer jobs than the men, and they did not stay on a job as long as the men. In general, they viewed their jobs with dissatisfaction. Those employed as domestic servants complained about the long hours, hard work, low pay, and poor food. Girls in the needle trades were unhappy about the long hours, irregularity of the work, and the low pay. Mrs. Janer, whose jobs were all domestic, illustrates all of the reasons for leaving a job. The first one was "too much work." She was expected to cook, clean the house, and care for the children of two families. "Many times at 12 o'clock at night, I was still in the kitchen. I quit." The next domestic job proved to be no different:

They went out and left me alone. I was very lonesome. I had to get up at 5 AM to prepare breakfast. I left after 7 months. My next job lasted 10 months. The husband of the woman of the house fell in love with me. I slept alone, but he came in to visit me many times. He woke me up with his fondling. The brother of the lady of the house was also in love with me. He used to visit me at night. One day they were away from home and I took the children bathing. The children told their parents, and I was fired.

A number of women report sexual approaches by the man of the house combined with sexual jealousy by the lady of the house. When Mrs. Quiromo was 15, she noticed that the lady for whom she did housework was very jealous. One day Mrs. Quiromo went into the bathroom to clean it and found the husband there. He made a fast approach. The lady of the house rushed into the bathroom, grabbed the girl by the arm, and pushed her outside. Thereafter, whenever the husband was at home the wife kept her eye on the maid. When Mrs. Quiromo told her mother about her experience, the mother made her quit.

Domestic servants were not the only ones subjected to sexual approaches. It is not unusual for a male boss to make a pass at a female employee. A woman is expected to know how to respond to familiar advances. Several women report that in the factories where they worked the male bosses were having sexual affairs with female workers. Some women left jobs to avoid being seduced by their bosses.

At the time of her marriage, every woman who was gainfully employed left her job. The most common reason given by the women is: "My husband did not allow me to work;" the second is, "I left to go with my husband"; finally, "Shortly after I went with my husband, I became pregnant."

A detailed examination of the job histories of the men and women between the fifteenth birthdays and their present marriages indicates that schizophrenia is not a discernible factor in employment or nonemployment, the kind of work done, the length of time individuals stayed on a job, their wages, and the circumstances surrounding an individual's separation from a job. Sick and well persons in each sex group relate almost identical stories of their job experiences. These stories focus on the menial nature of the work, the long hours, the insensitivity of the boss, the low wages, fights on the job, and a search for a better job. There are no significant differences between the males or the females who did or did not become psychotically ill in later years.

The securing of gainful employment introduces a new factor into the assumption of an adult role: the freedom to move from place to place *buscando vida* (in search of life). Possible interrelations between migration and mental illness have been of interest to psychiatrists and sociologists for many years. Is geographic movement linked to the development of schizophrenia? To answer this question, we queried each person on the moves he made in the course of his life. The data we gathered enable us to reconstruct the migratory history of each person from birth to the present. In the presentation of these data we depart from our stated discussion of the period of the assumption of the adult role. We focus on geographic mobility not just in the years from 15 to the present marriage, but throughout the entire period of the life history. Our data on geographic mobility are divided into the three time sequences: from birth to the fifteenth birthday, from 15 to marriage, and during the present marriage. We are concerned with the possibility of a significant relationship between geographic movement during each of these periods and mental stability in the present.

One person in every six was born and reared in San Juan; five out of six migrated to San Juan from the community in which they were born. Migration to San Juan from other parts of the Island is unequally distributed in the three sequences of the life history. The data are summarized in Table 23. Movement to the city occurred in each life history sequence. Individuals who came to the city during the childhood years were brought to San Juan by their parental families or were sent there to live with some member of the kin group. In both sexes the largest proportion of migration occurred before the fifteenth birthday. Among the males, migration in childhood accounts for 42 per cent of the net movement to San Juan from the outlying areas of the Island. The comparable figure for the women is 50 per cent. The next largest net migration for the males, 39 per cent, occurred during the adolescent and early adult years; the females experienced less movement in these years, 23 per cent. This differential migration for males in comparison with females may be attributed to the greater freedom of males to move from place to place.

Migration to the city previous to the current marriage may be viewed as an independent move, that is a move by the male independent of the female. After marriage this is not the case. Migration since the present marriage is similar in both sexes, which results from the couple moving as a unit.

Migration from the outlying parts of the Island to San Juan is

TABLE 23 Residence in San Juan by Period of Life History, Present Mental Status, and Sex

	SICK, %	WELL, %
A. Males		
Became residents of San Juan		
At birth	9	10
Before 15 years of age	27	41
Between 15 years of age and present marriage	45	31
Since present marriage	18	17
N =	11	29
$p > .05$		
B. Females		
Became residents of San Juan		
At birth	38	19
Before 15 years of age	15	47
Between 15 years of age and present marriage	24	15
Since present marriage	23	19
N =	13	27
$p > .05$		

not associated with mental status in either sex. Moreover, when we examine the data from the perspective of the time in the life history at which the migration occurred, no significant relationships appear. Mental status is not connected with the fact that practically all individuals moved into San Juan sometime between birth and the present.

Even though no association exists between mental status and migration for the time sequences we are using, it is possible that there is a relationship between the exact ages at which individuals moved to San Juan and their present mental health. To test this idea we determined the age of each person when the move to San Juan occurred. The ages of the persons at the time they moved to San Juan were compared by diagnostic groups and sex. The test shows that the age at which persons moved to the city is not related to the presence or absence of schizophrenia in either the males or the females.

A third type of test of the migration hypothesis involved an examination of the data from the viewpoint of the length of time each person lived in San Juan. The mean length of residence in the city by sex and diagnostic group is as follows:

MEAN YEARS OF RESIDENCE	SICK	WELL
Males	18.9	19.0
Females	17.9	17.1

The impressive fact about these means is that they are so similar in each diagnostic group and in each sex. In terms of the length of residence in the city, the four groups are remarkably similar.

If movement to the city entails cultural shock, the sick males and females and the well males and females on the average have endured it for approximately the same length of time. The idea of cultural shock was pursued one step further to see if trips off the Island were related to mental status. A large difference between the sexes might be expected because the males are obligated to the United States for military service. All the males were of draft age during either World War II or the Korean conflict; some had experienced military service, but the proportion was small. More males than females, 25 per cent of the men and 17 per cent of the women, have been to the United States or some place other than Puerto Rico; however, no relationship was found in either sex between trips off the Island and present mental status.

Every residential move each person made between 15 years of age and his present marriage was tabulated separately. These data were analyzed from two points of view: (1) the number of different residences a person occupied in this phase of his life and (2) the amount of time he lived in each residence. In these analyses we are concerned with determining the possible relationship of the amount of residential mobility to mental status in the present. The data on the number of moves by sex and mental status are as follows:

MEAN NUMBER OF MOVES	SICK	WELL
Males	2.4	2.2
Females	1.7	1.6

The means of the diagnostic groups within each sex are not significantly different. We conclude that the number of moves in the years before marriage is not related to mental status in the present.

The length of time a person lived in a given residence presents a similar picture. The sick and the well males lived almost the same length of time in each residence, 4.4 years. The women lived almost the same length of time in each residence, 4.2 years. The amount of time the sick women lived in a given residence is not significantly different from that of the well women. The interesting point is that the mentally ill men and women followed a residential pattern that is essentially the same as the one experienced by those who are mentally healthy. The mental status groups are equally residentially stable in the years under review.

Movement from residence to residence since marriage follows a pattern very similar to that exhibited before marriage. The sick and the well are almost equally stable. No significant differences appear when the number of moves mentally healthy individuals have made are compared with those the mentally ill have made since marriage. Moreover, the length of time each person, whether male or female, sick or well, lived in a particular residence shows little variation from one group to the other. The few differences that do appear are not significant. Finally, when comparisons are made by families rather than individuals, no significant differences appear; the sick families and the well families are equally stable in their dwelling places.

To list the possible effects of the onset of schizophrenic symptoms on the residential experience of a family, we tabulated the data by the number of months each family lived in its present and previous residence. The results of these analyses are presented in the following tabulation:

MEAN NUMBER OF MONTHS IN	SICK	WELL
Present residence	42	44
Previous residence	27	29

The sick and the well families have lived approximately the same length of time in their present homes, three and one-half years. They lived a shorter time in the previous home, some two and a half years. In both periods the well families lived in their homes a mean of 2 months longer than the sick families, but the difference is not significant in either time period. We conclude that the onset of schizophrenia in either the husband or the wife is not accompanied by a change in residence. The mentally healthy families move almost as frequently as the mentally ill.

In the preceding analyses we focused attention on the number of moves a person made in each of the three phases of the life history from birth to the present and on the length of time he lived in each residence in each phase of his life. It is possible that this division obscures the overall mobility pattern of an individual's lifetime. To test this possibility, we examined the data on the number of times each person had moved in the course of his life. We found no significant differences between the sick and the well for either sex. The men had moved an average of 7.3 times, and the females had moved an average of 7.1 times.

The length of time the two diagnostic groups had lived in each residence was not significantly different for either the males or the females. The males averaged 4.6 years in each residence. The females averaged 4.4 years in each residence during their lives. The figures presented here indicate that the residential mobility pattern for the males is very close to that for the females. We conclude that sex and mental status are not correlated with residential mobility.

A third point of interest to us concerning the years between 15 and the present marriage is the physical illnesses experienced. Each person experienced at least one physical illness during this period, and some persons had several illnesses. Are physical illnesses in adolescence related to mental status in the adult years? We investigated this question by grouping the physical illnesses each individual reports he experienced into one of the three categories of illnesses discussed in Chapter 6, page 106. The data on illness experiences during the youthful years are summarized in Table 24. The total illness experi-

TABLE 24 Types of Physical Illness Experienced between 15 Years of Age and Present Marriage by Sex and Mental Status *

	SICK	WELL
A. Males		
Infectious	7.8	9.1
Noninfectious	—	1.0
Traumatic	5.2†	2.2
Total rate	13.0	12.3
B. Females		
Infectious	11.3	10.7
Noninfectious	1.6	4.9
Traumatic	6.4†	2.9
Total rate	19.3	18.5

* Expressed as a rate per 100 years of exposure.
† $p < .05$.

ences of the sick males are no different from that of the well males. The same generalization is applicable to the females. Females, however, report more illnesses than the males.

In both the mentally sick and mentally well groups the females report slightly more infectious illnesses than the males. The kinds of infectious illnesses they experienced are sharply different from those the men claim they had. The males are infected most frequently with venereal diseases: 45 per cent of the men state they suffered from a venereal disease before they were married; 60 per cent of the first infections occurred before the individual was 18 years of age; 31 per cent of those who suffered from venereal disease were infected more than once. Venereal infections are more frequent in the years before marriage, but 30 per cent of the males report they contracted a venereal infection for the first time subsequent to their marriages. Multiple venereal infections were as frequent after marriage as before marriage. Infections of venereal diseases are not linked to mental status in the men either before or after marriage. Venereal infections are rare among females. Less than 10 per cent of the women admit infection with venereal disease before marriage. Venereal infection among the women is not associated with mental status.

The very large differences between the percentage of men who claim venereal infection and that of the women are attributable, in good measure, to the double standard of sexual behavior. A young man who looks for sexual conquests usually finds them among prostitutes and unattached women. These women ordinarily have a wide variety of heterosexual contacts, and we may infer that a considerable number are diseased venereally. A young woman's sexual contacts are limited, however, by the ideal of the virgin *señorita*, to the boy friend she marries. When she has sexual contact with him she considers herself to be married and sexually his property. If she remains true to the ideal of a faithful wife, her sexual life is restricted to intercourse with her husband. This limits the possibility of a woman becoming infected with venereal disease before marriage; after marriage, she is vulnerable to infection from her husband.

The disproportionate amount of venereal disease among men is overbalanced by the tendency of the women to report other kinds of infections. These include worms, malaria, impetigo, schistosomiasis, and enteric disorders of one kind or another. More women than men report infectious diseases usually associated with childhood such as chicken pox, measles, whooping cough, and mumps. The reporting of infectious diseases is not linked to mental status.

Noninfectious diseases are rare among the males. The rate is higher for the females, but it is lower than for either infectious or traumatic illnesses. The higher rate among the well females is worth noting.

Traumatic illnesses are composed of two major types of events, accidents and surgery. Accidents are limited largely to the males, but five females report accidents during this period of the life history; four out of the five were among the sick group. Likewise, among the males significantly more mentally ill ones had accidents than well ones. Accidents involving motor vehicles and machines used on the job account for most of the traumatic experiences. Surgical repairs are usually associated closely with the accidents, but in a few cases men and women underwent surgery for nonaccident-connected difficulties. These include an appendectomy and an excision of a stomach ulcer. The interesting point is that there is significantly more traumatic illness among both the schizophrenic males and females from 15 years of age to the present marriage than among the well men and women at the same age.

SUMMARY

Significantly more schizophrenic than well women were employed away from home at the age of 15. This difference does not apply to the men, as all of them entered the labor force by the time they were 15 years of age. A detailed analysis of the number of years employed, jobs held, months on each job, monthly earnings, percentage of jobs left voluntarily, reasons for leaving jobs, and employment in unskilled work of the men and women between age 15 and marriage indicates that the sick and well persons had essentially similar employment histories. At marriage, the percentage of persons gainfully employed and the monthly earnings of those who were employed in each sex group did not distinguish the well from the sick.

The same lack of consistent differences is to be found in the history of geographic mobility of schizophrenic and nonschizophrenic persons. Although five out of six persons migrated to San Juan, the sick and well persons do not differ with respect to birthplace in or out of San Juan or in migration to San Juan before 15 years of age, between 15 years and marriage, and since marriage. Nor do the sick differ from the well in the age at which they migrated to San Juan, the length of time they lived in the city, and whether or not they have lived outside of Puerto Rico. The number of residential moves and the length of time lived in each residence do not separate the sick from the well of either sex, irrespective of the span of time in the life history which is considered.

From 15 years of age to the present marriage, more schizophrenic than well persons, in both sexes, had accidents, but during this period the sick and well of each sex experienced in equal numbers infectious and noninfectious illnesses. The few and infrequent differences in employment, geographic mobility, and physical illnesses during adolescence do not permit general inferences to be made about the social processes which may have culminated in the development of schizophrenia.

8

Courtship and Marriage

Inculcation of socially approved attitudes toward sex and sexual behavior is a very important aspect of child rearing. Boys and girls are taught two different sexual codes. Mothers, older sisters, and other female relatives take an active part in the transmission to boys of cultural values, beliefs, and practices associated with maleness. The code of the *macho* is transmitted to little boys by fathers, older brothers, and male members of their peer group. The socialization of girls to sex is sharply different from that of boys. Chastity is the central theme of the values that revolve around female sexuality. Mothers and fathers may differ in the ways they view the transmission of sexual values and customs to their sons, but they are in agreement on how daughters should be taught to behave in such matters. Parents teach girls consistently and systematically the attitudes they ought to hold toward males as well as the precise ways they ought to conduct themselves in their associations with them. Sex is charged with heavy emotional meaning from the earliest childhood years until old age.

The preservation of chastity is the ultimate objective of the careful training a girl receives in her family of orientation. Although girls are instructed forcefully about the dangers of sex, particularly the attractions of young males, they are not taught the nature of the harm that can be done to them by violating sexual mores. The following statements by women are typical:

> My father told me that a man would always try to get everything he could out of a woman. He told me that merely to be alone with a man was dangerous. In the presence of men I should sit correctly by not spreading or crossing my legs; also I shouldn't wear low-cut dresses.

> My mother told me that men are not to be trusted; they are bad; they try to feel you up and talk you into doing bad things.

Whenever there were boys in our yard, my parents would not let me out of the house.

My parents told me not to stand too close to men as this would provoke them.

My mother reprimanded me because my father had seen me talking to a boy. He said that I should feel ashamed.

My mother told me all men are tempted by the devil, and if I allowed a man to place his hand on my head, my hair would fall out.

The negative attitudes taught to girls regarding males are authoritative. As a consequence, girls acquire a set of defensive beliefs that order their relationships with males before they learn the underlying reasons for these rules of behavior. For a parent to explain the "whys" is alien to the *respeto* pattern in the family relationship; respect makes sex an inappropriate topic of conversation between parent and child. To discuss sex would inculcate *malicia* (a term referring to forbidden desires and cunning drives—usually meaning some aspect of sex). In contrast to girls, boys are commonly believed to be born with *malicia* or to acquire it at an early age.

The intensity of parental controls over a girl's behavior stems from the parents' fear of having their daughter's reputation damaged. Parental controls may include forbidding the daughter to visit girls who mingle with boys. Her brothers and other relatives may have to accompany her as chaperones whenever she goes out. The girl's normal desire to see boys clashes with the restrictions imposed by the parents; she resents not being allowed to leave the house to speak to boys, and with the onset of adolescence she fights back; she actively seeks opportunities to see boys when she goes on errands for the family, visits friends or relatives, and travels to and from school.

The intermittent, rather casual training about sex given to boys differs sharply from the carefully deliberate training received by girls. The parents of a boy do not emphasize the proper ways to think about and act toward girls. Boys acquire from their parents stylized ways of treating girls, but this is largely a product of incidental, not deliberate, training. Boys, in general, have fewer restrictions imposed on their personal behavior than girls. The differences in permissiveness are rationalized, in part, by the assumption that boys have "stronger characters" and are less pliable than girls, but of central importance is the fact that boys do not have to guard their virginity and behave according to the strictures of modesty that are applied to girls. Occasionally, parents advise boys to treat girls with respect, cordiality, and politeness ". . . as if they were your sister or your mother." This advice is given casually; only mild sanctions are invoked if the boys disregard it. Such advice is not supported by their contacts with either adults or peers.

From an early age, boys overhear their fathers talking to other men about the pleasures of sexual relations with *mujeres de la vida alegre* (women of the happy life); they are aware that their fathers have extramarital affairs. Adolescent boys talk to one another about naked women and couples who have been seen having sexual relations. The size and shape of a woman's vagina are topics of conversation among boys and men, and younger boys learn from older males that women are objects of sexual gratification. As a consequence, they orient their thoughts and behavior in accordance with what other males expect of them as young, on-the-make *machos*.

A *macho* is an aggressive, domineering male who glories in his masculinity. He asserts his authority by physical strength, fist fights, drinking, and sexual triumphs. Conversation about baseball, boxing, cock fighting, horse racing, gambling, drinking, and one's exploits, whether they are with women or besting other males, are parts of the accepted pattern. A male who fights, stands up for his personal dignity, and realizes potential conquests with women is said to be a "man with balls." A youth who fulfills accepted male standards of behavior is highly regarded; he is a *macho!*

A *macho* is alert to sexual opportunities which are defined, in the extreme case, as occurring any time a man and a woman are together in a situation where sexual intercourse can be carried out. A girl adrift from her family presents a clear sexual opportunity, but since she has been conditioned to protect herself against the approaches of men she may not comply immediately with the advances the *macho* invariably makes. To the *macho*, an unused but unmistakable sexual opportunity represents a failure to fulfill an important aspect of social role and self-concept that could return to haunt his daydreams.

During our interviews with men who were integrated strongly into the *macho* pattern, we observed that they described fist fights and sexual adventures in similar terms and with similar physical gestures. A man is considered and, indeed, expected to be sexually stronger than a woman; this is the central creed of the *macho*. To be bested by a woman in sex is a humiliating defeat comparable to losing a fist fight, as both activities involve a physical encounter.

Parents understand thoroughly the role and the creed of the *macho*. Just as they take pride in a son who is a *macho*, they likewise attempt by training and surveillance to guard their daughters from the approaches of *machos*. The double standard of conduct prevalent in the culture is symbolized by the proverb: "I let loose my rooster; you coop up your hen."

The sharp differences between the freedom allowed boys to wander and seek sexual adventures and the rigid controls imposed on adolescent girls create strong emotional problems for the girl, her parents, and young men who may be interested in her. Social contacts with a young man present serious hazards for a girl and her family. Courtship is a dangerous experience for everyone concerned. During adolescence, one-half of the girls were prohibited by their parents, under threat of punishment, from having *any* social contacts with boys or men who were not immediate relatives; the comparable figure for the boys is 5 per cent.

Two distinctive patterns of courtship occurred in the families of orientation: approved and clandestine. There is no compromise between the two forms. Each is related to the attitudes the parents of the girl adopt toward a young man. Parents are seldom indifferent toward their daughter's possible acceptance of a husband; they either outlaw a prospective groom or they accept his attentions to their daughter conditionally, uneasily, and, whenever possible, under their critical and suspicious eyes. A man who is not outlawed by one or both parents is granted *la entrada* (the privilege of visiting the girl at her home). By tacit agreement, visits to the home are steps in the direction of getting married; for the boy to treat them otherwise would outrage the parents and would be an insult to the family. In playing the role of a suitor it is important that the boy present himself as an *hombre serio* (a responsible man with a sense of honor and dignity). Courtship is too serious a matter and *la entrada* too serious a trust to be placed in the hands of a frivolous, irresponsible young man. In granting *la entrada*, the parents are not completely relieved of their apprehensions; a girl's reputation is in jeopardy until the marriage is consummated. They say, "*Hasta los hombres pendejos se defienden*" (even men who are harmless capitalize on their interests).

Neither the boy nor the girl views her home as a desirable place to court, but it is the only one available to them. The home is the center of the family's social life. The furniture in the living room, if there is one, consists of a couple of old chairs that have long needed paint, a small keg, an orange crate, and perhaps a two-seat, wrought-iron sofa with cushions that are in a state of disrepair. Relatives and friends come in and out and engage one another in rapid-fire conversation. Infants, in the diaper stage, crawl on the floor, tug at the furniture, and cry. The mother may be carrying an infant straddled on her hip and held with one arm while she uses the other arm to emphasize what she is saying. Younger boys scuffle outside the door. A husky feminine voice singing a *bolero* and the noise from radios tuned to different programs come through the unglazed window. The odor of boiling *bacalao* (codfish) drifts through the house. Conversations are spontaneous, expressive, and frequently punctuated by joking and laughter, but should the courting couple even whisper in secrecy the suspicions of the adults are aroused. In a family scene that is not puritanical, puritanical controls are exercised.

Courtships approved by *la entrada* are more apt to result in legal marriages than clandestine courtships in which the prospective groom is outlawed by the girl's parents. Marriages following parental approval of the groom are more likely to be planned; the girl usually accumulates some linen, towels, a table cover or two, and a few cooking utensils which she may store in a cardboard box under her bed in preparation for the establishment of her new home.

Parents often do not allow visiting privileges to a youth. By their refusal to allow the young man to see their daughter they are setting the stage for a clandestine romance. When one young man came to ask for *la entrada* at the home of the parents of a girl, the irate mother hit him on the head with a kerosene lamp and chased him out of the house. One father responded to such a request by threatening to hit the youth with a club if he ever showed up again. Another mother told a suitor that she didn't believe in "the *entrada* business" at all and that if he wanted to see her daughter he would have to marry her immediately even though the girl hardly knew the young man.

A girl whose parents prohibit her from talking to boys often enters a surreptitious courtship. She communicates with her boy friend by clandestine messages sent through a mutual friend; a circuitous route is taken on an errand to the store to catch a glimpse of him or to have a secret moment with him. A smile, a wave of the hand, a couple of rhythmic beeps on an automobile horn directed toward a girl standing on the sidewalk often mean more than is apparent.

In spite of efforts to hide such a relationship, it is probable that the girl's parents are aware of a boy's interest in their daughter. In each neighborhood there is a network of observation, talk, and gossip that keeps all residents of the area informed about who does or says what with whom, when, and where. Talk is focused especially on the behavior of adolescent girls. One father who was told that his daughter was being secretly courted looked for the boy, beat him up, and threatened his life if he ever saw his daughter again. The older brothers of this same girl responded in a similar way when she started seeing another boy. The more usual reaction, however, is for the parents to restrict their daughter's further contacts with boys. This forces the girl to make a decision of fundamental importance to her future.

When parents refuse visiting privileges to a young man, a young woman is confronted with a serious dilemma: Should she remain under parental control or should she defy her family and entrust herself to the hands of her boy friend? The women who faced this dilemma resolved it by leaving their families. Their departure was precipitated by an argument, usually a fight, with their parents. The decision to leave was taken in anger on the spur of the moment. The break was rarely foreseen by either parents or daughter.

Mrs. Urrutia describes the controls of a bad-tempered mother who brought her up *dentro del puño* (inside her fist). One day after her mother beat her savagely, the girl left home angrily vowing never to return. She went to a girl friend's house and sent for a young man who had twice said "pretty things" to her as she walked by him on the sidewalk. (This a common custom in Puerto Rico.) Mrs. Urrutia recalls:

> When he came I asked him to take me to live with him. At first he said he couldn't do this because he didn't know me well enough. I stayed with my girl friend for two or three days. She lived in a very small, crowded home that did not have sufficient room. I couldn't return home because my mother was so angered at me when I left, and she would have been worse if I attempted to return home. He returned on the third day and took me away. He took me to live with his father and mother, and we have been living together ever since. If it hadn't been for my mother's bad temper, I would never have left with this man who became my husband.

As an adolescent girl Mrs. Quintero was popular with a number of boys who sent her messages. One day her mother whipped her, and says Mrs. Quintero:

> I was angry. I took a bus to another town where I found my boy friend. I told him what had happened at home and he proposed that we run away together.

Mrs. Ubarri says:

> When my husband started to court me I was a little pile of shit, thirteen years old. My uncle did not like him for he thought I was too young and he was too old. In our neighborhood my husband was known as a drunkard, a woman-chaser, a lazy man, and a gambler. My relatives opposed the match and did not allow me to see him. One evening my uncle and aunt reprimanded me and stayed up half the night giving me advice, advice, and advice about why I should avoid this man. The next day my uncle and aunt went visiting and I sent for my boy friend who walked by often to peek at me while I scrubbed the floor of the house. He proposed that we elope. We left, but before this I stole some mangoes and oranges from my uncle and we ate them during our honeymoon.

One day Mrs. Julia was talking to her boy friend in the back yard when her father ordered her to come inside the house. Because she delayed in coming, her father slapped her. She says:

> I was infuriated by this, so the next day I put my clothes in a paper bag which I took to the factory where I worked. When I got out in the afternoon I met my boy friend and I left with him. I wanted vengeance against my father.

Mrs. Hidalgo's family withdrew from her because of alleged immoral behavior. One night her parents allowed her to go to a supervised party at a neighbor's house. There she met a boy who asked her to dance. She had so much fun she lost track of time; suddenly she realized it was past midnight. The boy with whom she had been dancing hurriedly accompanied her to her home next door, but the door to her house was locked. She was afraid to knock on it lest her father scold her in front of the boy. She went back to the dance and spent the night with the woman of the house in which the party was held. The following day when she went home, her mother would not accept any explanations:

> My mother reprimanded me severely, for the neighbors were gossiping about me. My mother would not accept me in the house. I returned to the neighbor's house, for my mother insisted that I had been discredited in front of the whole neighborhood. I had not slept with this boy at all.

Soon after this, Mrs. Hidalgo entered a consensual union with her boy friend.

The lower class does not provide a variety of acceptable roles for a young woman living away from her family of orientation. Once a girl departs from her family as the result of a fight or an alleged sexual misdeed, she confronts a limited number of alternatives. She cannot go to other relatives because they are concerned about her soiled reputation. She has a hard time finding a place to live. If she is not already working, employment is difficult to find because she lacks marketable skills in a scarce job market. She has the choice of becoming a servant, a prostitute, or of entrusting herself to her boy friend.

Two alternatives face a young couple when they decide the time has come for them to assume adult sex roles. They may be married legally or they may simply start living together. Morally and socially, there is little difference between these two types of union. The partners in either a legal or consensual union do not view themselves as "living in sin," nor do they suffer public disgrace. To form a consensual union, a girl believes she need only participate in sexual intercourse with a male friend with whom she lives. To form a legal union the couple must engage in an impersonal transaction with persons who are relatively peripheral to their lives; they must go to a civil official, fulfill a number of bureaucratic requirements, and undergo a civil or religious ceremony. The partners in such a union are referred to as being *casado casado* (the word *casado* means married); in referring to a consensual union the word is not repeated. A consensual union is not a "trial marriage" if by this is meant an implicit or explicit agreement by the partners to test their compatibility.

At the beginning of a legal or consensual union most couples live with relatives of the husband, usually his parents. The bride wants and expects her husband to provide her with privacy, preferably in a house of her own, but this happens very rarely because the cost of renting or buying a house is prohibitive. For almost every wife the desire to be mistress of her own household is a dream; the reality is sharing a small, overcrowded home with some part of the kin group. This is a disappointment to the new wife as her husband's parents suffer from the same pressing economic hardships she experienced at home; they are unprepared for a new daughter-in-law, but custom impels them to share their home with her.

After their first marital night, and probably a row with the boy's parents over his precipitous marriage, the young couple face their new life with little or no privacy; their bed, which was probably vacated by three or four siblings or cousins in the household who now have to sleep on the floor or in hammocks, is separated from the living quarters only by a curtain, sheet, or blanket hung about it. In the crowded household, the members of the family see and hear each other during all hours of the day and night. (Only adult males, because of employment or other activities outside the home, escape family observation.) Physical privacy is seldom achieved for months or years; psychological privacy is invaded by questioning relatives from the first hour the family learns of the new marriage. Mrs. Janer says that on the day following her legal marriage, her husband's aunt asked him, "How did it go?" thus expressing her husband's relatives' doubts about her virginity. Mrs. Janer reports:

> I got mad when she asked this. I ripped off the sheets from the bed and showed her the blood. By doing this I hoped to assure her of my virginity.

Another woman told us that one morning while she and her husband were having sexual intercourse in their bed, her mother-in-law pulled aside the curtain which shielded the bed from the rest of the room and said, "That looks pretty good." New wives resent the fact that their in-laws recognize little distinction between family business and the private affairs of the couple.

The wives repeatedly complain about in-laws who try to make servants out of them. Much criticism is directed at the new wife because she is reluctant to assume the obligations thrust upon her. She is expected by both her husband and her in-laws not only to be respectful to them, but also to scrub the floor, wash dishes, wash and iron clothes, and cook. The wife does not want to be subordinate to adults with whom she feels little or no sense of emotional identification; she tries to persuade her husband to establish a household for her, independent of his parents, but most often money is not immediately available for this purpose. "All I wanted," says one woman, "was a house of my own even if it were in a swamp." In a consensual union, the man may not feel a responsibility to provide his spouse with separate quarters and economic support. The bonds that link him to his mate are tenuous; he does not consider himself to be a husband. If the couple is legally united, however, the husband tries to comply with his wife's wishes to move to a separate household.

Eighty-five per cent of the men and 7 per cent of the women had sexual intercourse prior to marriage. The mean age of the men when they had sexual intercourse for the first time is 17 years; for the women it is 19. This coincides with the age of marriage for the women, but it is 5 years before marriage for the men. The premarital sexual experiences of the men are with prostitutes, "women of the happy life," and divorced and separated women who do not live with their families, have lost their virginity, and are not the sexual property of a particular man, therefore providing a socially safe, sexual outlet. A relatively small number of such women is sufficient to provide numerous men with premarital sexual experiences.

The first sexual intercourse of the women is either with men they have married legally or with whom they have eloped. When the union is not legal, women consider their marriages to have been effected by the sexual intercourse. The men, however, do not consider sexual intercourse to be symbolic of marriage. In other words, the women *get married* by having sexual intercourse; the men *become married* by gradually assuming the obligations of a husband.

We asked each person to describe his or her feelings during the first sexual intercourse. The replies were analyzed in terms of the content of the themes they emphasized. Four themes appeared repeatedly in the individual stories. The following tabulation summarizes the eighty replies to the question: How did you feel during your first sexual intercourse?

THEMES IN REPLIES	MEN, %	WOMEN, %
Nervous, frightened, restless, painful	18	83
Sad, remorseful, ashamed	5	40
Pleasant, happy, joyful	85	5
Manly (for men), womanly (for women)	40	0

Eighty-seven per cent of the themes in the replies to this question are included in this tabulation. The percentages do not total 100 since some replies had more than one theme.

Stated briefly, women view their first sexual experience in unfavorable terms, whereas men view theirs in favorable terms. The views held toward first sexual intercourse are based on more than the physical pain for the women and the physical pleasure of the men; most of the women had little or no knowledge about the rudimentary mechanics of intercourse and were reluctant students when their more worldly and experienced husbands tried to explain. Some of them had strong fears and reacted in terror when confronted with the prospect of their first sexual intercourse. They screamed, wept, and struggled to keep their husbands away.

Mrs. Medina had her first sexual relations with her husband at the age of 16, when she started to live with him consensually. Before this she had thought girls lost their virginity by holding hands with a man.

I didn't know what I was supposed to do on the wedding night. I felt uncomfortable and ashamed. I didn't know my husband very well, for we hadn't seen one another very much. I was afraid of sex, but my husband was understanding. Today I laugh about how little I knew on that night. I couldn't laugh about it then.

Mrs. Julía, who ran off with her husband at the age of 16 after a bitter fight with her father, reports that her husband tried to take her to a hotel but she refused to go as she believed only prostitutes went to hotels.

. . . so my husband took me to his mother's place and for three nights I only let him put a little bit in, for it hurt. On the fourth night he put it all in. I bled a little. I was ashamed. I also was afraid his mother would hear us doing all that business in bed. I was so ashamed I couldn't look him in the eye on the following day. I couldn't face anyone for several days.

In legal or consensual unions, the first sexual experience is unpleasant to the girl; she responds with shame, humiliation, and terror to the violation of carefully inculcated, internalized norms of modesty. What has been learned has to be unlearned, and what was morally unacceptable behavior has to be enacted in the process of trying to bridge a sharp discontinuity in social conditioning. Many women do not overcome this barrier successfully, and the tensions surrounding sexual activity become marital problems.

The men had varied reactions to their first sexual intercourse. Mr. Cardona had his first sexual relations at the age of 18 with a 30-year old divorced woman. He recalls:

We went wild with one another. We did it in a hotel four times. Then we went out and did it on the beach, in the bushes, or any place we could lay down. We did it about eleven times the first night and I hit eight times. Although my knees shook after that, I felt good.

Mr. Lebrón reports:

At the age of 14 I had an 18-year old whore. It was a pleasure. While I was having this woman I was achieving the dreams I had had while I was masturbating—here I was actually having a woman! I told my friends about it afterwards. I felt I had passed the test of real manhood. After this experience I had sexual relations with about ten women, most of them divorced or whores.

For a number of men, sexual intercourse is a test of their *macho* identity. Mr. Hidalgo, for example, is a real *macho* in demeanor and attitude; his posture and gestures are consciously the antithesis of the *pato* (literally, a duck, but in the vernacular, a homosexual). He tells us that when he was 15 years old, and a skillful baseball player, a woman married to a prominent man invited him to visit her sick mother. This was only a lure, for when they arrived at her house the woman took him into her bedroom, closed the door, took off her clothes, and invited him to bed. He says:

> I was scared, and I told her that my only experience had been fondling the genitals of girls my own age. That woman had me in bed for five hours and when we were through I felt weak and limp. That damn woman couldn't get enough. When we were through she called me a *pendejo* [pubic hair]. That day I got my diploma as a man. Having had her made me believe in God and heaven. Though I was happy, I was mad at myself for not having given her all she needed. If I could get her today, it would be a different story. We'd see who the pubic hair is!

Consensual unions are believed by both men and women to be more unstable than legal unions. They are formed, from the viewpoint of the wife, when a man and a woman have sexual intercourse and begin to live together. Consensual unions are dissolved, from the perspective of the husband, when the couple cease to live together. The dissolution of a consensual union usually consists of the husband simply leaving the household. Abandonment presents the woman with a series of problems: she generally has the burden of supporting herself and her children, if any; symbolically, she loses her "representative in society," her husband; sexually, she is "damaged goods" and, therefore, is vulnerable to advances from marauding males; her parents are less concerned with enforcing their interest in relation to a potential mate, and thus her "bargaining power" is restricted when she enters a new union. The woman who is abandoned, divorced, or separated suffers the penalties that accompany her status. Women more than men are concerned with the kind of union they enter and with justification as the figures in Table 25 show. These data reveal two points of interest: first, 55 per cent of the wives and 66 per cent of the husbands established consensual unions the first time they were married; second, among the females but not the males significantly more consensual first marriages dissolved than legal ones. The consensual unions that dissolved lasted 2.3 years, whereas the legal unions that

TABLE 25 Type of Union at Beginning of First Marriage and Instability of That Marriage

	LEGAL UNION, %	CONSENSUAL UNION, %
A. Males		
Dissolved	8	32
Did not dissolve	92	68
N =	13 *	25
$p > .05$		
B. Females		
Dissolved	0	32
Did not dissolve	100	68
N =	18	22
$p < .01$		

* One case was excluded because the wife died and another because the respondent gave ambiguous information.

dissolved lasted 3.8 years. Our classification of unions which dissolved includes divorce, separation, and abandonment, but not the death of a spouse. The first marriages that have remained intact are classified in the table as "Did not dissolve"—these marriages are a portion of the group of 40 on-going marriages that we studied directly.

As attrition weeds out the fragile consensual unions, the stable consensual unions that remain hardly differ from the legal unions in their unity and harmony.[1]

Seven women who had been consensual partners in a first marriage had experienced its dissolution. All these women remarried at a later time, and all of them contracted a consensual union the second time. Twelve men had encountered a broken first marriage. When these men remarried, one-half of them entered into consensual unions; the other six contracted legal marriages.

Remarriages occur among persons who have not dissolved their legal ties to former spouses. One woman and three men are legally wed to persons with whom they no longer live. The first marriage

---

[1] A variety of approaches was used to study the solidarity and interpersonal harmony of legal unions in comparison to consensual unions. The following points were analyzed: (1) the commitment that the spouses have toward each other; (2) the fieldworkers' appraisal of the cohesion of the families; and (3) the qualitative case studies of the families.

of the woman was forced by her family upon a reluctant groom who allegedly raped her; after a month he left her. This woman now feels she cannot control the infidelity of her consensual husband, the father of her eight children, because she is not "really married" to him. Two of the three women who are living consensually with men legally tied to other women are trying to convince their husbands to divorce their earlier mates and marry them legally.

Public recognition is given to the greater strength of the conjugal bonds in legal unions. Sixty-eight per cent of the first marriages of women that *begin consensually become legal* at some later date; the comparable finding for the men is 45 per cent. One-third of all first marriages changed from a consensual to a legal status. A girl may have eloped in the midst of a bitter conflict with her relatives, but immediately after she enters into a consensual marriage these same relatives, irate because of the elopement, form a united front to pressure the groom into marrying her legally. To be effective, family constraint must be brought to bear immediately; if some time elapses, the girl's family loses interest and power to legitimize the union.

Consensual wives are concerned over the possible instability of their marriages. One wife introduced this topic into the interviews many times. This wife's anxieties are exacerbated by the fact that her husband is having affairs with other women. She is unhappy about his philandering and fears he is going to leave her. She does not accuse her husband openly, as this could provoke him to leave her. "I have absolutely no rights," she comments. "I have suffered much in this matter." Some women mask their grievances and suffer in silence to avoid open confrontation with their husbands.

Inner doubts often accompany the husband's resistance to legal marriage. One husband, whose wife is trying to persuade him to marry her legally says:

> I think it would be good to get married [legally] because of the children. At the same time, I feel that if my marriage is not convenient to me or not to my liking I can abandon her. If I were married to her legally, I could not do this.

The change from a de facto union to a de jure marriage often depends on how such an ambivalence is resolved. A couple may decide to legalize their union after the arrival of children. Concern for each other's welfare and that of the children is important in making this decision, as children can be baptized and employment benefits, such as medical care, can be secured only upon the presentation of a marriage certificate. One husband made the decision because, as he says, "My wife has been such a good woman. I owe her a lot."

Courtship behavior is not related to mental status. Proportionately as many men and women who are now mentally ill had clandestine romances as those who are now mentally healthy. Proportionately the same number of men and women who are now well experienced an explosive disengagement from their families through a precipitous marriage as those who are now sick.

Mentally healthy men had their first heterosexual experiences at the same age as men who are now schizophrenic; that is, when they were 17 years old. Likewise, mentally healthy women and those who are schizophrenic had their first sexual intercourse at the same age, 19 years.

The kind of marriage—consensual or legal—is not associated with present mental status. However, the *kind of remarriage* a man who later develops schizophrenia contracts *is* related to his present mental status. The preschizophrenic man is as romantic, impetuous, and as much on-the-make as the mentally healthy man before he acquires his first wife. When his first marriage fails, he becomes cautious. Typically, a man who later becomes schizophrenic is reluctant to enter into a series of secret meetings with a potential marriage mate. He makes a formal approach to a girl's family, asks for visiting privileges, and is often granted them, as he usually makes a good impression on the girl's parents. The preschizophrenic, previously married man is likely to seek out a woman his own age or older by a few years. Actually, 45 per cent of the schizophrenic men, in comparison to 14 per cent of the nonschizophrenic men, who have remarried are now married to women their own age or older.[2]

Mr. Herrero courted the girl who became his legal wife under the supervision of her mother. According to the psychiatrist, Mr. Herrero presents almost all of the symptoms and signs of a person suffering from schizophrenia, including blunted emotions, suspiciousness, and hallucinations. He expected and wanted to marry a girl who "would take care of me and give me love and affection." He saw in his prospective wife a vigorous, resourceful person on whom he could depend. Although his behavior might have had significant meaning to a person experienced in the reactions of the mentally ill, it created a good impression on his prospective mother-in-law who had an unusual degree of enthusiasm for the young man. If he remained silent for a pro-

---

[2] This difference is significant and in the expected direction.

longed period during his visits, this was seen as the sobriety desirable in a husband; the suspicious questions he asked the girl were interpreted by the mother as the understandable possessiveness of a young man in love. His manner was seen as evidence of a serious, responsible character by the mother, and she encouraged her daughter to marry him.

The experienced preschizophrenic man's quest for support obligates him to the girl he is courting and to her parents. His desire for support becomes interwoven with the *entrada* relationship. As a result, schizophrenic men establish legal unions significantly more often than men who are not now afflicted with schizophrenia.[3] The number of remarriages into which the persons have entered is not related to mental status in either sex. The 40 men have had a total of 58 marriages; one man in three has been married twice and every eighth man three times. The women have had 47 marriages; seven women have had two marriages; none has had more than two. Proportionately as many mentally healthy men as sick men have taken second or third wives, but their unions are consensual rather than legal.

SUMMARY

Every effort is made to control the courtship of adolescent girls. Chaperoned courtship is the ideal, but clandestine romances are frequent. The *entrada* pattern of courtship takes place under the jurisdiction and control of the girl's parents and leads to a legal union more often than clandestine courtship which takes place outside the purview of the girl's parents. Clandestine romances are almost always accompanied by violent conflict between the girl and her parents, from which the girl escapes by eloping with her boy friend. In doing this, she takes an irrevocable step toward the assumption of the role of married woman. For the females consensual unions are more unstable than legal unions; a larger number of consensual unions dissolve than do legal unions. Gradually, differences between the two types of unions disappear as attrition disproportionately dissolves consensual unions.

Both men and women perceive consensual unions to be less stable than legal unions, but women, more often than men, are interested in

---

[3] Seventy-three per cent of the schizophrenic men are united legally to their current wives; only 28 per cent of the men who are not schizophrenic are legally married. This difference is not attributable to chance; the probability is less than .05.

binding their consensual unions legally. The dissolution of a union presents graver threats to women than to men, which is reflected in the fact that more women than men enter into consensual unions in their second marriages. These women have no choice, unless they marry a man who is later subject to mental illness. In these marriages the wife has "the rope and the goat." Legalization of consensual unions is accompanied often by the inner reservations of men who want to enjoy the benefits of marriage combined with the freedom entailed in the role of the *macho*.

PART IV BECOMING A SCHIZOPHRENIC

Part IV is focused on various dimensions of illness in the study group. At the time the field work was begun, each person was given a mental status examination by a fully trained psychiatrist, and a psychiatric diagnosis was made of the individual's personality structure. In twenty families, the husband, the wife, or both are diagnosed as suffering from schizophrenia. In the other twenty families, neither the husband nor the wife is afflicted with a psychotic illness. All the schizophrenic persons became ill before we began to study them, but none of them had been a psychiatric patient in a clinic or a hospital. When and under what circumstances did they become mentally ill? How do the life conditions of the sick families differ from those of the well families?

These questions are answered in Chapters 9 and 10. In Chapter 11 we focus our attention on the ways mental illnesses are viewed in this stratum of Puerto Rican society. We also examine the ways in which sick persons conceive of their illness and how their spouses look upon it. Chapter 12 demonstrates that psychotic illnesses are handled, in large part, by nonmedical institutions, more particularly by spiritualistic mediums.

9
Illness and Death

The physical illnesses each person experienced in childhood and adolescence were discussed earlier. This chapter presents findings relevant to three questions: (1) Is mental illness attributable to members of the family of orientation linked to the psychiatric diagnoses of the spouses in the present family of procreation? (2) Are physical illnesses connected with mental status? (3) Are the deaths of children related to the psychiatric diagnoses of the parents? The material from the interviews enables us to give an answer to each of these questions.

From childhood, each person has been aware of mental illness. He has seen irrational, wild, and violent behavior by persons who babble and wander aimlessly. When it is a relative who behaves in such a manner, the experience is more meaningful and painful than are the tales about persons who have "lost their minds." We examined each life history to see if mental illness attributed to one or more members of the family of orientation is related to a person's present psychiatric diagnosis. Although reports of a parent, a brother, or a sister who is assigned the mentally ill role by a second family member are not as good evidence as diagnostic evaluations made by a psychiatrist, persons who are reported to be mentally ill probably are, in fact, ill. However, not all persons who are mentally ill are viewed as sick; for this reason we take these reports as imputations of mental illness.

Evidence to support ascribed mental illness in a family of orientation ranges from hospitalization to allegations of "nervousness." To be hospitalized for mental illness in the recent past, a person had to be not only mentally sick but also a constant threat or extreme nuisance to the community. Ten husbands or wives report one or more commitments in their families to a mental hospital. Figures on commitment, however, are understatements of the extent of severe mental illness, as several persons report unsuccessful efforts to have a disturbed member of their family admitted to a mental hospital.

Mr. Janer reports that his mother had been subject to "attacks" since she was 18 years of age. In her early years, during an "attack," she became "foolish," "daydreamed," and "wandered"; in later years she became violent to the point that she used to "chase her children with scissors and knives." Several times she pursued her husband around the neighborhood with a machete. When the "attacks" passed, she could not explain why she acted this way. After Mr. Janer married and had children of his own, his mother periodically chased his children with a knife. Once she choked a 1-year old child until it was unconscious and tried to bury it in a shallow grave; although she was discovered before the burial was completed and the child was revived, the neighbors demanded that she be committed. The son and the father took her to the psychiatric hospital where the attending doctor allegedly stated that she could not be admitted because "these are not the type of cases in the hospital. The mental attacks are only momentary." The doctor advised the family to lock the mother in a room when she had her "attacks." It has been hazardous to follow this advice, and the family continues to be terrorized by the mother.

A number of persons who report mental illnesses in their families recall that no efforts were made to obtain psychiatric care or to have the mentally ill person admitted to a hospital. One man reports his sister "lost her mind" after the birth of a child. For 2 years the sister threw herself on the floor, screamed, talked incoherently, fainted on the street, and repeatedly escaped from a locked room. (This woman was cured, allegedly, by her husband who, following the advice of a spiritualistic medium, gave her cold baths before daylight.)

Several persons say a father or mother was "nervous." When we probed for examples of "nervous" behavior, serious emotional problems came to the fore. One woman told us her mother is subject to "nervous attacks"; when an attack occurs, the mother starts to scream; she clenches her fists and doubles her arms in a belligerent gesture. The screams may go on for hours, and she may hold her arms flexed for 2 or 3 days. When the "attack" subsides, she resumes her family duties. Evidences of depressions severe enough to disturb family routines also are described as "nervousness."

Behavior that is not too deviant from the norms of the subculture is viewed without concern by our respondents. How it would be judged in other socioeconomic groups in this society, or in other societies, is a matter of speculation. Moreover, there is probably a marked difference in the ways it would be judged by members of the family concerned, by their neighbors, and by officials such as the police or public health nurses and psychiatrists. The point to remember is that the kinds of behavior psychiatrists label as mental illness are an integral part of the lives of the people we are studying.

Although we cannot classify the kinds of mental illness ascribed to members of the families of orientation, we can determine which family member was reported to be mentally ill. The member who was or was not mentally ill, by generation, gives rise to four groups of families: (1) families free of mental illness, (2) those with mental illness in the parents only, (3) those with mental illness in the parents and siblings, and (4) those with mentally ill siblings only. The percentage distribution of these 4 groups of families between the well and the sick series is as follows:

ASCRIBED MENTAL ILLNESS IN FAMILY OF ORIENTATION	PERSONS IN SICK AND WELL FAMILIES OF PROCREATION	
	SICK, %	WELL, %
No mental illness	40	57
One or both parents	17	10
Parent and sibling	18	13
Sibling(s) only	25	20
Number of individuals	40	40
$x^2 = 4.341$ 3 df $p > .05$		

This tabulation shows no association between family members who are, or are not, reported as mentally ill in the family of orientation and the present diagnosed mental status of the 80 individuals who comprise the 40 spouse pairs in the families of procreation. When the three groups of families in which mental illnesses are ascribed are summed into a single group and compared with the families in which there is no reported mental illness, we have the following tabulation:

FAMILY OF ORIENTATION	PERSONS IN SICK AND WELL FAMILIES OF PROCREATION	
	SICK, %	WELL, %
Some ascribed mental illness	60	43
No ascribed mental illness	40	57
Number of individuals	40	40
$x^2 = 2.4514$ 1 df $p > .05$		

Ascribed mental illness in the family of orientation tends to be weighted toward the sick group but the association is not significant.

Is ascribed mental illness in the family of orientation related significantly to the mental status of individuals who are espoused into families of procreation? To answer this question, we describe each spouse pair in terms of the psychiatrist's diagnosis of the two partners' mental status and compare this with the presence or absence of ascribed mental illness in the parental family. The four groups of families that emerge from this type of classification are the ones we use in subsequent analyses: (1) neither the husband nor the wife is suffering from schizophrenia (control families); (2) the wife is a schizophrenic, the husband not (wife-schizophrenic families); (3) the husband is a schizophrenic, the wife not (husband-schizophrenic families); and (4) both the husband and the wife are suffering from schizophrenia (double schizophrenic families). The exact pairing of spouses is summarized in Table 26. Statistical analysis of each of these combinations of spouse pairs

TABLE 26 Ascribed Mental Illness in Family of Orientation by Diagnosed Mental Status of Husband and Wife

FAMILY OF ORIENTATION	HUSBAND'S, %	WIFE'S, %
A. Control Families		
No mental illness	60	55
Some mental illness	40	45
$N =$	20	20
$p > .05$		
B. Wife-Schizophrenic Families		
No mental illness	56	11
Some mental illness	44	89
$N =$	9	9
$p > .05$		
C. Husband-Schizophrenic Families		
No mental illness	14	71
Some mental illness	86	29
$N =$	7	7
$p > .05$		
D. Double Schizophrenic Families		
No mental illness	75	25
Some mental illness	25	75
$N =$	4	4
$p > .05$		

reveals that the relationships are not significant: the presence or absence of ascribed mental illness in the parental family is not related to the present mental status of the various spouse pairs.

Chapters 6 and 7 demonstrated that there is no association between physical illnesses in an individual's childhood and youth and his mental status at the present time. By examining the illness experiences of individuals during their present marriage, we can determine if the more recent physical illnesses are associated significantly with mental status.

In a preliminary analysis of physical illnesses we followed the threefold life history scheme discussed earlier: the childhood years, adolescence, and the years of the present marriage. We find that physical illness rates, per 100 years of exposure, increase markedly among the schizophrenic males and the schizophrenic females after marriage, but there is little change among the nonschizophrenics, male and female. It is clear that something happens after marriage that increases the rates of physical illnesses among the families in which one or both spouses are now suffering with schizophrenia. Does this increase in the physical illness rates among the schizophrenics occur gradually or is it related in some way to the onset of the mental illness?

Further examination of the data indicates that the time immediately preceding the onset of the mental illness in a given individual is the key to an explanation of this increase in physical illness. To avoid a series of dates dependent on the time at which a particular individual developed manifest symptoms, we decided to divide the years of marriage into two periods: from the beginning of the marriage to 5 years before our field work began, and the 5 years immediately prior to the field work. This division coincides with the time at which the onset of symptoms was noted in the behavior of most sick persons. The mean number of years that elapsed between the onset of psychiatric symptoms for the males and the time of our field work is 2.7 years; for the sick females it is 4.1 years.

The rates for infectious illnesses are essentially the same for mentally ill males and females as for mentally healthy males and females in each sequence of the life history until 5 years before our field work began. During this period infectious illness rates increase sharply for both sexes. The rates for infectious illnesses are given in Table 27.

The rates for noninfectious illnesses in each phase of the life history by sex and mental status are given in Table 28. The data show that the onset of schizophrenia appears to have a clear-cut effect on the noninfectious and infectious disease rates.

TABLE 27 Infectious Illnesses Experienced during Sequential Phases of Life History by Sex and Mental Status *

	SICK	WELL
A. Males		
Birth to 15 years of age	8	9
15 years to present marriage	8	9
Present marriage to 5 years before field work began	4	5
During 5 years prior to beginning of field work	26	5
B. Females		
Birth to 15 years of age	12	10
15 years to present marriage	11	11
Present marriage to 5 years before field work began	3	4
During 5 years prior to beginning of field work	24	6

* Stated as a rate per 100 years at risk.

TABLE 28 Noninfectious Illnesses during Sequential Phases of Life History by Sex and Mental Status *

	SICK	WELL
A. Males		
Birth to 15 years of age	2	2
15 years to present marriage	—	—
Present marriage to 5 years before field work began	4	4
During 5 years prior to beginning of field work	9	2
B. Females		
Birth to 15 years of age	3	2
15 years to present marriage	2	5
Present marriage to 5 years before field work began	8	11
During 5 years prior to beginning of field work	45	14

* Stated as a rate per 100 years at risk.

Traumatic illnesses exhibit a life history pattern similar to those of the infectious and noninfectious illnesses. Mental status and sex are not related to traumatic illnesses before 15 years of age. After age 15, the rate increases consistently for sick males. Among the well males the rate is relatively stable until 5 years before the field work began; during the 5 years prior to the field work it almost doubles. In the most recent period, the rate for the well males is one-half that for the schizophrenic males. Among the sick females, the rate doubles between 15 years of age and their present marriage; after marriage it drops by almost one-half. In the last period, however, the rate increases threefold. The well females show a sequence similar to that of the mentally healthy males. Their rate is relatively stable from childhood until 5 years before the field work began; then it increases moderately.

During the 5 years before the field work began the rate for traumatic illnesses among schizophrenic males is twice as high as that for the well males. The rate for schizophrenic women is almost two and one-half times higher than that for the mentally healthy women.

Traumatic illnesses are composed of accidents and surgery. Accidents are largely limited to the males and are linked directly with motor

TABLE 29 Traumatic Illnesses during Sequential Phases of Life History by Sex and Mental Status *

	SICK	WELL
A. Males		
Birth to 15 years of age	3	3
15 years to present marriage	5	2
Present marriage to 5 years before field work began	8	4
During 5 years prior to beginning of field work	13	7
B. Females		
Birth to 15 years of age	3	4
15 years to present marriage	6	3
Present marriage to 5 years before field work began	4	3
During 5 years prior to beginning of field work	12	5

* Stated as a rate per 100 years at risk.

vehicles and machines used on a job. Forty-five per cent of the males, since they were 15 years of age, experienced some kind of accident severe enough to remember. Significantly more mentally ill males had accidents than healthy males. The number of females reporting accidents is much smaller, only 12 per cent, but four of the five who had accidents are in the sick group.

Surgery is concentrated almost as heavily among the females as accidents are among the males. The surgery most commonly performed among the women is on their reproductive systems. Childbearing is not considered as an illness experience, although complications connected with it, such as albumin in the urine, stitches to repair uterine tears during childbirth, or a Caesarean section, are counted as illnesses. Albumin in the urine is classified as a noninfectious illness. The most frequently encountered traumatic illness experience of these women is surgical sterilization—38 per cent were sterilized, all during the present marriage. There is no difference between the sick and the well women in their ages at the time of sterilization (24.3 years mean for both groups) or as to the time the sterilizations occurred (for the well women a mean of 4.7 years before our field work began, and 4.6 years for the sick women). Significantly more sick than well women were sterilized, however—62 per cent in the sick group and 26 per cent in the well group.

When a possible relationship between the onset of symptoms and surgical sterilization was examined, none was found. In one-half the mentally ill women the sterilization operation preceded the onset of the symptoms; in the other half, it followed the mental breakdown. Among the women who were sterilized before the onset of symptoms, the time interval between their operation and their breakdown averaged 4.3 years. The women who were sterilized after their schizophrenic break averaged 2.8 years between these illness experiences.

The general physical illness patterns for each sex and mental status group through the several phases of their life histories are depicted graphically in Figure 1. This chart shows how the three types of physical illnesses are relatively stable in each sex and mental status group from childhood until 5 years before the field work began. The rate for schizophrenic males increases slightly after marriage, whereas that for the schizophrenic females drops! During the 5 years prior to our field work, the rates for both the schizophrenic males and females increases dramatically. The nonschizophrenic males have a rate pattern that is stable from childhood to the present. The nonschizo-

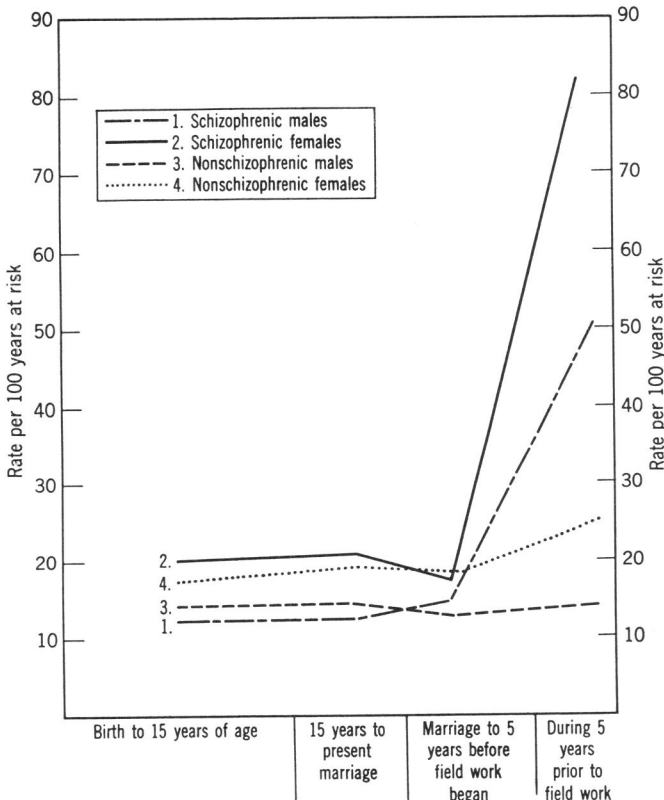

Figure 1. Physical illnesses experienced during sequential phases of life history by sex and mental status, stated as a rate of illness per 100 years at risk.

phrenic females' rate curve turns upward in the last period for each type of illness group—infectious, noninfectious, and traumatic.

There are two salient points in Figure 1. First, the rate curves for each sex and mental status group from birth to marriage parallel one another; after marriage there is a slight shift among the males and females who later developed schizophrenia, but it is small in magnitude and in opposite directions for the two sexes. Second, the upward sweep of the curves for the sick males and females during the 5 years prior to our field work demonstrates that schizophrenia has a marked effect on physical illnesses.

Hospitalization experiences during the present marriage are congruent with the data on experiences with all physical illnesses. From the date of marriage to 5 years before the field work began, there is relatively little difference between the rates of hospitalization for the sick and well females. In the early years of marriage the mentally ill men and women were hospitalized more frequently than the mentally healthy men and women, but the difference is relatively small in each sex. The males, both sick and well, have higher rates than the females.

During the 5 years prior to our field work the rate for the sick males increases three and one-half times in comparison with the rate in the earlier years. Among the well males the rate drops to one-third of what it was previously. Comparison between the male mental status groups is far more striking, as it shows that the hospitalization rate is fourteen times higher among the sick males than the well males.

The rates for the females are different in one respect from the rates for the males. The well females were hospitalized more frequently in recent years in comparison with earlier years. The well females' rate increased almost threefold in the most recent 5-year period. In other respects the rate pattern is the same in the two sexes. The sick females were hospitalized almost five times more frequently in the 5 years immediately prior to the field work than in the earlier years. A comparison between the sick women and the well women in recent years shows that the sick women were hospitalized three times more frequently than the well women.

Every hospitalization among the women in the 5 years prior to our

TABLE 30 Hospitalization Experiences since Present Marriage by Diagnostic Group and Sex *

	FROM PRESENT MARRIAGE TO 5 YEARS BEFORE FIELD WORK BEGAN	DURING 5 YEARS PRIOR TO BEGINNING OF FIELD WORK
A. Males		
Sick	8	28
Well	6	2
B. Females		
Sick	5	24
Well	3	8

* Stated as a rate per 100 years at risk.

field work involves the genitourinary system. Practically all hospitalizations were for surgical sterilization, Caesarean section, or repair of tears during childbirth. No male or female was hospitalized for mental illness. Probably a certain proportion of the physical illnesses indirectly reflects the mental illness. Our data do not enable us to prove or disprove this point; all we can say is that the increase in hospitalization among those afflicted with schizophrenia during the 5 years prior to our field work is not the result of mental illness per se.

In the preceding section, which deals with the illness experiences of individuals in sick and well families, the interactional effect of marriage and mental illness on physical illness within the family is the center of our interest. The analyses assume that the close interactions which take place day after day between husbands and wives may have some effect on the illness experiences. Mental illness in the married couple is taken as the independent variable and physical illness experience the dependent variable. To isolate the effects of the interactional matrix we divide the spouse pairs into four groups: control families, husband-schizophrenic families, wife-schizophrenic families, and double schizophrenic families. By separating the spouse pairs into these groups and looking at the data by sex, we may determine how mental status affects each combination of spouse pairs from marriage to 5 years before the field work began and during the 5 years immediately prior to the field work. The data in Table 31 summarize our findings.

The effect of the mental status is clear in each sex and each time sequence. Briefly, for the males it is as follows: (1) Men afflicted with schizophrenia married to women also suffering from schizophrenia have the highest physical illness rates in both time periods; in the 5 years prior to the field work, however, the rate is two and one-half times higher than it was previously. (2) The rate for sick husbands married to well wives is midway between that of the double schizophrenic and wife-schizophrenic families; the rate for sick husbands with well wives more than doubles in the most recent time period. (3) The rate for well husbands married to sick wives is almost the same as the control families' to 5 years before the field work began; during the 5 years prior to the field work their illness rate has increased about one-third. (4) Well men married to well women show no change from the earlier to the later period.

Mental status also has a marked effect on physical illnesses among the females. (1) The double schizophrenic families exhibit the highest physical illness rate from the beginning of the present marriage to

164 *Becoming a Schizophrenic*

TABLE 31 Physical Illnesses Experienced by Spouses since Present Marriage by Sex and Mental Status *

	FROM PRESENT MARRIAGE TO 5 YEARS BEFORE FIELD WORK BEGAN	DURING 5 YEARS PRIOR TO BEGINNING OF FIELD WORK
A. Males		
Control families	14	14
Husband-schizophrenic families	18	40
Wife-schizophrenic families	13	18
Double schizophrenic families	24	60
B. Females		
Control families	11	14
Husband-schizophrenic families	27	51
Wife-schizophrenic families	23	76
Double schizophrenic families	33	60

* Stated as a rate per 100 years at risk.

5 years before the field work began; then it doubles in the 5 years prior to the field work, from 33 to 60. (2) When the wife is schizophrenic and the husband is not, the physical illness rate is lower than in the double schizophrenic families, but it is twice as high as for families where both spouses are mentally healthy. The largest increase of any spouse group in the 5 years prior to the field work occurs among the families in which the wife is schizophrenic and the husband is not; here the increase is from 23 to 76. (3) Well women married to schizophrenic men have a physical illness record similar to the preceding group: in the early years of marriage they have almost as many illnesses as the sick wives of mentally healthy husbands; then in the 5 years before the field work began their illness experiences double. Well women burdened with the care of schizophrenic husbands have developed many more physical illnesses than well women married to well husbands. (4) The control families reveal an illness record for the females that is almost identical with that for the males; a second

similarity is that in both sexes there are no sharp differences between the years from marriage to 5 years before the field work began and within the 5 years immediately prior to the field work.

The rates presented in Table 31 demonstrate that schizophrenia has a discernible effect on the physical illness experiences of one or both members of a spouse pair. The one group in which this effect is not clear-cut involves schizophrenic wives and well husbands. The relatively minor effect on the well husbands' illness rates of schizophrenia among the wives may be attributed to the fact that the well husbands, as Part V demonstrates, do not internalize the problems of their sick wives. The well husbands leave their schizophrenic wives at home, usually under orders to stay there, and lead lives of their own outside the home. The wives' response to this may be reflected in the highest rate of physical illness for any group.

When we examine the illness experiences of all the members of the sick and well families, we find there are more physical illnesses per year of risk in the sick families than in the well families. The illness rates for each group are presented in Table 32. During the 5 years prior to the beginning of the field work, the physical illness rate is 278 per cent higher among the spouses in the sick families than among the spouses in the well families. The rate of 9 physical illnesses per 100 years at risk may be viewed as what we would expect to encounter among a lower-status group of mentally healthy young adults. The significantly higher rate among the spouses in the sick families is associated with schizophrenia. Although the differences in the illness are not as great among the children there is a difference in both age groups. The difference between children 6 years of age and younger in the two groups of families is significant. Clearly, the younger children in the sick families experience more illnesses than the children in

TABLE 32 Physical Illness Experiences during 5 Years Prior to Beginning of Field Work for Specified Family Members by Family Diagnostic Group *

	SICK	WELL
Children 6 years of age and under	111	80
Children over 6 years of age	53	44
Spouses	34	9

* Stated as a rate per 100 years at risk.

the well families. These illnesses occurred largely during the years when one or both parents were suffering from schizophrenia.

Fear of death is a constant threat. Whenever a member of a family becomes ill, latent fears become manifest. A fear of death when a child becomes ill is realistic: within the study group there are twelve deaths of children, all of which occurred during the present marriages of the spouses. Eleven of the twelve deaths occurred in the sick families; ten of the twelve children who died were born to schizophrenic mothers. In one family both father and mother are schizophrenic. In only one sick family which experienced the death of a child is the mother mentally healthy. The one family in the well series that lost a child received a mixed diagnosis: the father is mentally healthy; the mother shows nervous symptoms. The clustering of deaths in the sick families, more particularly in the families in which the mother is schizophrenic, reveals that the mental status of the mother is related to the death of a child.

The linkage of childhood deaths to the present mental status of the parent raises an important point: the child's death may have been a consequence of the parental illness, particularly that of the mother, or a parent's mental illness may be a sequel to the child's death. We have information on the date of the death of each child and behavioral data regarding the development of the parents' psychoses or nervousness which enable us to date accurately the perceived onset of the parents' mental illness. In every instance, a child's death preceded the onset of the parent's overt symptomatology.

Interrelationships between the death of a child and the onset of psychiatric symptoms are best illustrated in the words of those who faced bereavement. When we learned that a child had died, we asked the father and the mother independently: "What effect do you think this death had on the family?" This query elicited several types of responses. Sometimes one spouse gave a brief answer, whereas the other went into considerable detail on the circumstances of the child's death and the way each parent reacted to it. Mr. Berríos, one of the two schizophrenic men who saw one of their children die, simply states that a son had died of asthma when he was 2 years old: "The asthma drowned him. He was wanting for air." Mrs. Berríos fills in the details of the child's death:

> ... for three days this child could not eat. He was somehow out of this world. He got very weak. He could not respond to anything. He died of fatigue [asthma]. It was a terrible blow.

Illness and Death 167

While the child was suffering from asthma, the mother and father took him to the municipal hospital. Mrs. Berríos believes the child was killed by an injection he was given at the hospital:

> I don't know the name of the shot, but I recall he was feeling pretty good. Right after they gave him this shot, the child died. My husband continued to drink liquor as it was his custom, and he could not sleep at night after the death of the child. A few days after my child died my husband took me to visit a sister of mine who lives in Santurce. The following day he came to get me. He was drunk, and he wanted me to return to take care of the home. He continued to drink as he had before; the only change was that he kept seeing things that were not there. He went to bed in the evening, and suddenly he would jump out of bed and hurl himself on top of me so I would not see the vision on the ceiling that he had seen a moment before while lying in bed. He said there were many things he was seeing, but he couldn't identify them. I couldn't see anything.
>
> Our other son suffered a great deal because of the death of his brother. He also suffered when he saw how desperate and weak I was as a result of this death. My son began to feel a fear of his father. My husband was seeing things that were not there, and he was jumping out of bed at night. These spells lasted a number of weeks. They scared my child.

Mrs. Berríos makes a direct connection between the death of her little son, the beginning of her husband's hallucinations, and his fear of being alone.

For these people, death is hard to understand; sudden death is beyond comprehension. Its dramatic effects are illustrated in the Feliciano family. On the afternoon of a bright May day, the 10-year old son of the Felicianos hurried home from school. He changed from school clothes into his baseball suit, said good-bye to his mother, and hurried out the door and down the path to the baseball field. On his way to the playground he crossed a wide, heavily traveled highway and was hit by a truck. A crowd gathered, and someone went to tell the mother her son had been in an accident. Since the bearer of the news arrived only a few minutes after the boy had left, the mother could not believe it was her son. Mr. Feliciano was summoned and he and Mrs. Feliciano were taken to the municipal hospital. The authorities would not permit Mrs. Feliciano to enter the room; the father was taken into the morgue to view the boy's body. Mrs. Feliciano recalls:

My husband informed me. When I first heard him I could not believe it. Then I did. I had to believe it. From that moment on I felt as if I were in another world. It is the most horrible thing that has ever happened to me. That has been the greatest shock I ever experienced. Although it had this effect on me, I carried the coffin to the burial.

I had not experienced the death of a child before. I lost weight and became very skinny. I began to have dizzy spells. I tried to resign myself to it.

The father felt very close to this son; they had talked together of baseball and of the son's hoped-for future. Mrs. Feliciano remembers:

They had a great love for one another. My husband was very fond of him. He used to look at pictures of our son and say this was a boy who was going to be somebody; the one who was going to be really good. Four or five months after the death of our son, my husband began to act differently. His character changed. He began to speak bad words around the house and he cursed God. He lost his love for his other children. He says that the one child he had hopes for was gone. He is disillusioned with all the children. All this occurred after my child was killed.

Mr. Feliciano substantiates his love for the dead son:

When I saw my son's crushed body I was out of this world. But I am a person who has learned to exercise control, and I was able to dominate my feelings. This happening had such a strong effect on me that when I think of my son the tears come to my eyes.

Mr. Feliciano was very quiet when he said this. His voice was choked and very low. As tears came to his eyes he lowered his face to mask his strong emotions. When he regained his composure he went on:

With respect to my wife, I would not want her to hear us talk about this matter. Whenever she thinks about it, it damages her a lot. After the boy's death my wife acted like a *loca* for more than a month. I believe this experience was so shocking that it contributed to her illness.

Mr. and Mrs. Feliciano both date the onset of her illness from the death of this child.

The Iglesias family has had four children die. The sequence of deaths was as follows: When Mrs. Iglesias was 9 months pregnant with her first child she went to the hospital with labor pains. A doctor examined her, gave her a hypodermic injection, and sent her home.

Several days later labor pains began again. Mr. Iglesias' account of this experience supports that of his wife with more details:

> The child began to be born in the house. It was coming out of my wife's vagina. We rushed her to the municipal hospital. The child finally came out there. The child was dead. The doctor commented that had there been any delay my wife would have died. She was gravely ill. She developed gangrene.

Mrs. Iglesias adds, "The child was dead in my stomach for three days." Mr. Iglesias goes on:

> After the child's birth my wife was very sad. I used to find her crying or thoughtful, thinking about the death of this daughter. I do not believe I suffered as much as my wife. I have learned to control myself. I always beg of God that he let me accept things like this with resignation.

The second death followed an accident. Mrs. Iglesias was scrubbing the floor of her home when:

> ... one of the boards on the floor broke. I fell down through the floor with my pail of water. I was seven months pregnant. They took me to the hospital. The child was born alive, but he died two days later. The doctor told us that he died of fear. I did not suffer as much from the death of the first child because she was born dead, but I did not feel well either, for I cried very much. When a child is born alive and one has fed him from one's breast, it is something different. I suffered much. Since then I have felt very nervous, and I have been the way I am now.

Mr. Iglesias independently stated:

> After this injury I noticed that she behaved the same way as she had at the time of the other death. She was very nervous, thoughtful; she wept a lot. For about a year she used to scream as if she were a *loca*.

While the field work was in progress Mrs. Iglesias was pregnant with her eighth child. She was caring for her home and five living children. She was especially fond of a 7-year old boy. The mother and father decided this boy was particularly bright and should be given special advantages. They enrolled him in a private Catholic elementary school, but to reach the school the boy had to cross a heavily traveled, main street. The parents were afraid he would be injured or killed on his way to school, so Mr. Iglesias wrote to a sister in New York City explaining the problem. The sister agreed to send them

8 dollars a month for the boy to take the bus to and from school. Mrs. Iglesias made arrangements with a bus driver to stop for the boy at the entrance to the slum where the family lives. The driver dutifully took the boy to school daily and returned him in the afternoon.

One day the boy came home with a high fever which modern medicine, prayer, and spiritualistic *pases* (gestures) could not reduce. Two days later he died. Mrs. Iglesias, in an advanced stage of pregnancy, was distraught. The new child, delivered in due course, appeared to be healthy until fatigue (asthma) and a fever overcame him. His death at 7 weeks of age was too much for the disturbed mother to bear. She experienced a serious psychotic break and was "out of this world" for several weeks. Yet, she managed to keep her family together, and they coped with her illness. When we visited the home after we had completed the field work, Mrs. Iglesias was sad but resigned to the burdens she had to bear.

The temporal sequence of the death of a child followed by severe psychological disturbances in the family is not a chance factor. The significant relationship between the death of a child and the mental status of one or both parents is summarized in Table 33.

TABLE 33 Experience of Child's Death in Sick and Well Families

	NO DEATHS, %	DEATHS, %
Family sick	42	86
Family well	58	14
N =	33	7
$p < .05$		

These stories of the effects of a child's death on the spouses indicate that mothers react more sharply to a child's death than fathers. This fact is summarized in Table 34.

TABLE 34 Experience of Child's Death by Mental Status of Mother

	NO DEATHS, %	DEATHS, %
Mother schizophrenic	25	71
Mother nonschizophrenic	75	29
N =	33	7
$p < .05$		

SUMMARY

The data presented on the preceding pages give clear answers to the three questions posed at the beginning of this chapter. Mental illness is a fact of life among these families. In 80 per cent of the present families some person in either the husband's or the wife's family of orientation was said to be mentally ill. Mental illness was ascribed to one or more members of the families of orientation by 39 of the 80 individuals in the study—a remarkable finding! Detailed analyses of which member of the parental family was said to be mentally ill did not show any significant associations with the choice of marital partner in the four types of mental status groups of families. Schizophrenia in the present families of procreation is not linked to ascribed mental illness in the parental families.

The rates for each type of physical illness change very little in the years after marriage for all mental status groups until 5 years before the field work began. During the 5 years immediately prior to the field work, the rates for each type of physical illness increase markedly among schizophrenic individuals. The rates increase very little among the nonschizophrenic men, but they increase slightly among the control women. When we examine the interactional effect of schizophrenia on spouses by holding sex constant, we find no change in the rate of physical illnesses since marriage for males in the control families. The females in the control families show a moderate increase during the 5 years immediately prior to the beginning of the field work. The males in the husband-schizophrenic families show a physical illness rate, during this period, more than double what it was earlier. The females in these same families have a rate in recent years almost double that of the earlier years of marriage. Husbands in the wife-schizophrenic families have had more illnesses in the most recent period than in preceding years. The wives, however, have the largest increase of any group in the 5 years prior to field work. Their rate more than triples, an increase from 23 to 76 per 100 years at risk. Physical illness rates for the husbands and the wives in the double schizophrenic families are twice as high in the most recent years as they were earlier. The interactional effect of schizophrenia on physical illnesses is clear in all the sick families except among the males in the wife-schizophrenic families.

The death of children is linked significantly to the mental status of the mother. Twelve children died in seven families. Ten of the twelve deaths were in families in which the mother is suffering from schizophrenia. Six of the seven families who have faced the death of a child are in the sick group. All the deaths preceded the onset of mental symptoms in the parents. This generalization includes the one mother in the control group who developed manifest neurotic symptoms subsequent to the death of her child.

The data presented in this chapter enable us to draw some conclusions regarding interdependencies between schizophrenia and physical illnesses. The sharp rise in the rates of physical illnesses among the sick men and women during the 5 years immediately prior to our field work indicates that schizophrenia is accompanied by a series of physiological symptoms. Our data do not enable us to draw any inferences as to whether the linkage between schizophrenia and physical symptoms is a causal phenomenon, a concomitant one, or a sequential one. We can observe only the clustering of physical and mental symptoms in the most recent segment of the life sequence. Deaths of children are another issue. Here the connection between the death of a child and the onset of schizophrenic symptomatology is sequential. In every instance, the death of a child preceded the eruption of mental symptoms. This sequential effect leads us to infer that the shock of a child's death triggers internal strains in the personality of mothers subjected to the anxiety and emotional pain of burying a child. The effect is not so evident among the males. The differential effect of the death of children on fathers and mothers might well be the subject of a future research project in sociology and psychiatry.

10
The Problematic Year

This research postulates a relationship between the stressful experiences through which an individual has lived and the onset of schizophrenic symptoms. The personal-social situations an individual faced shortly before he became overtly psychotic could be crucial to the development of manifest symptomatology. To examine this idea empirically, we designed an interview schedule to enable us to gather information systematically on the problematic experiences of each individual during a one-year interval. This schedule was administered to each person after the other interviews had been completed. For each nonpsychotic person the problematic year focuses on the 12 months preceding the date on which the fieldworker began to administer the Problematic Year Schedule to the respondent. For each of the twenty-four schizophrenics the problematic year is the 12 months immediately preceding the onset of an individual's clinical symptoms. Before the data on the schedule were gathered from the schizophrenics, the field staff made a careful review of all the information we had accumulated on each sick person and his spouse. From the evidence on the several schedules we were able to determine when the first psychotic episode occurred.

The Problematic Year Schedule was administered to each person by the fieldworker who had been collecting information from him or her from the beginning of the study. Schizophrenic individuals were asked the same questions as the nonschizophrenics, the only difference being the time around which we focused our queries. No respondent was told why we asked intensive questions about a particular period of his life. The repetitive nature of the questions and the close rapport the fieldworker maintained with the respondent probably minimized biases in the information collected from the sick and well persons.

The definition of a problem was left to the respondent. If he believed that the question asked designated a problem he experienced during the specified year, we accepted as a problem what he considered to be a problem. A given individual's definition of a problem depends on his experiences, what he views as problematic to him, and his recall of meaningful happenings in the year under review.

Our questions were focused on six areas of the person's life: illness, employment, relations with spouse, relations with members of the extended family, relations with neighbors, and frustrations of aspirations. We queried each person also on any other types of problems we might have missed in our formal inventory. The respondent was asked to describe each problem he experienced, the date when it began and ended, his level of preoccupation with the problem, and what he perceived as the level of preoccupation of his spouse with the same problem. The level of preoccupation was ranked as: very much, much, average, very little, not at all.

Because of the methodological difficulties of dealing with a personally experienced problem which is later recalled as a dimension for classification, we have chosen to present these data as case histories rather than as statistical comparisons. By means of case analyses, the unfolding, sequential problems which affected the families can be reconstructed and portrayed. One family in each diagnostic group—control families, husband-schizophrenic families, wife-schizophrenic families, and double schizophrenic families—has been selected as typical of the families in that group. The problems this family encountered during the problematic year are related in detail. The psychiatrist's assessment of the mental status of each spouse at the time of the psychiatric examination is presented before the discussion of the family's problems so that the reader is provided with the psychiatric dimension of the personalities involved in the problematic situations recounted in the paragraphs that follow it. Immediately after the presentation of the problems each family enumerates, we summarize the main points of tension the spouses emphasize in their accounts of circumstances they faced during the problematic year.

A CONTROL FAMILY: THE FUENTES FAMILY

The Fuentes family was selected as representative of the twenty families in the control group. Mr. and Mrs. Fuentes were diagnosed as mentally healthy individuals. The psychiatrists' statements on each spouse is as follows.

Mr. Fuentes. There is ability to evaluate his present situation and his adaptive limitations. He dreams rarely, and during the interview he did not recollect any dreams. Most of his thought content is about his work, his family, his welfare, his health, and what he reads or hears through the newspapers and the radio.

There is no evidence of distorted thinking. Situations and events affect him most. He says that other people's bad deeds are what stimulate him adversely. He shows no evidence of inappropriate emotional responses; his mood changes are rare and only short-lived and mild.

He feels friendly toward other people, gets along well with others, and likes to get together with people. There is no evidence of unrealistic attitudes toward other people. He has no negative feelings toward superiors. He has a healthy attitude toward his peers, his superiors, law, and authority. He has changed jobs in order to better himself and has had no trouble at all while at work. He is a good provider, a good husband, and a good father. He is very respectable and responsible.

He has no distortion of his body image; he sees himself as he is. His attitude toward himself and others is realistic, as also are his plans. He makes good use of his spare time in constructive endeavors. There is no evidence of ego rupture. He states he has sexual intercourse with his wife about once a week.

There is no confusion of the love-hate conflict. There are no evidences of ambivalence; we see only positive feelings governing this personality. Because of the demands of his job he has little time for play and recreation, but he does not ignore his wishes for recreation; when he channels some energy in this area he can fully enjoy recreation without any guilt feelings.

The analysis of his replies shows an organized, well-integrated personality. He sees himself as happy and with a place in life he can successfully meet. The only area in which he is inhibited is in the sexual sphere, but there is no pathology. He is a good listener and also a fairly good performer.

We see no definite pathological trends, signs, or symptoms in this man.

Mrs. Fuentes. She is functioning adequately within normal limits. Her dreams are usually related to her children and their health. She hopes to be able to have a piece of land big enough for her to raise her children and for her husband to do some planting.

She is able to react to other people and tolerate them without any difficulty. There are no outstanding reactions to persons, events, or situations. She performs smoothly throughout the situations that face her. There are no evident outstanding mood changes. Her main concern is the care and protection of her children and her husband. She is able to tolerate frustrations adequately.

She participates in community activities. She attends religious services but shies away from political activities. She is able to get along with people of the same sex and of the opposite sex. She accepts people in authority without any difficulty. She expresses a capacity to love which surpasses any hate she may have for her husband or her children.

Although she has expressed desires to move to a bigger house, she is attached to the home they have because they own it. She accepts work and responsibilities cheerfully. She is able to participate with others in the neighborhood and in group activities whenever the care of the children permits it. She is able to express her emotions without any apparent difficulty. She is a good listener and is able to assimilate without apparent difficulty whatever she is told. She appears well adjusted.

There are no symptoms of outstanding psychopathology in this woman.

The Problematic Year. Mr. Fuentes earns $162 a month as a janitor in a municipal building. Social security, dues to the employees' association, benefits for the employees' association, and payment on a loan borrowed from the credit union are deducted from his gross earnings. With his take-home pay of $108 a month, he supports his wife and 5 children, but, in addition, he is expected to help his wife's relatives. Mr. Fuentes is more optimistic over his economic situation than his wife. He states:

> I am happy with what I have. I dress. I eat. People should live within their means. I do not borrow a penny. [This is contradicted by his statement that a sum is subtracted from his check each month to pay off a loan.] To borrow . . . is a bad habit. He who borrows keeps borrowing and goes more into debt until the day comes when he doesn't even own his own shirt.

Mr. Fuentes does not think his wife worries over the financial situation.

> My wife is *conforme* with whatever I bring home. We take care of the household expenses. My wife does not desire to have luxurious dresses. She does not pretend to raise our children as if they were rich.

She's never shown any lack of accepting our economic condition. She knows me as a poor person. She knows that I offer her all that I can.

Mrs. Fuentes believes her husband's earnings are hardly enough to enable them to eat, not really enough for clothing or for things in the house, but she is not disgruntled. She says:

We buy the same things at the store every time. Now that the children are going to school I have not been able to buy them uniforms. I worry very much about this. We need more money for clothing for the children; also we need more money to feed the children. Things are expensive. My husband worries about this. He notices that he does not make enough to buy the things that are needed, but he can't make any more.

Mrs. Fuentes hopes eventually to take a job and increase the family's income so their essential needs can be met.

Mr. and Mrs. Fuentes are adjusted to one another. He says he has had only one girl friend in his life, the one he married. Mrs. Fuentes states that she had only one boy friend (her present husband) whom she picked out when she was 13 years of age, and this is the way she thinks it should be. Whenever the boy came to the house, Mrs. Fuentes' grandmother sat between them on the sofa. The grandmother told her not to have any affairs with men and to insist on a legal marriage in the Catholic Church. Mrs. Fuentes tells us, "This is the way it was." She prepared for her wedding for years by keeping a cardboard carton as a hope chest under her bed. From the meager earnings she made as a servant and as a worker on the small farm her grandmother owned, she saved a little money. Whenever she had a few cents she bought a pot or pan so that she would have her own cooking utensils when she was ready for marriage.

Mr. Fuentes also prepared for his marriage; he, too, worked on a small farm located in the rural neighborhood where he grew up. As he was able to accumulate a few dollars, he bought lumber, nails, cement blocks, and cement for the house he planned to build on some land he had inherited from an uncle. Eventually, he assembled all the supplies and built a small house. When it was ready, the marriage ceremony was performed in the local Catholic church, and after the wedding he took his bride to their new home.

Mrs. Fuentes was not prepared for the marital night. Since nobody had told her what to expect, she thought it would be just like when they were sweethearts. After they were in the house and darkness came, they prepared for bed. At this point the husband began to make sexual approaches to her; she says that she loved him and he loved her but she was horrified and scared. Later at night, she allowed her husband to have sexual access to her. She reports that even though ". . . he was gentle," intercourse was very painful and she bled; she was also very embarrassed and very surprised. Both of them were sore the next day, and they did not have further intercourse for 3 days. She was so humiliated and frightened that she did not go out of the house for 9 days. After the first 4 or 5 days, they both enjoyed having sexual contact.

Mr. Fuentes had his first heterosexual experience during the wedding night. At the age of 13 he started masturbating; he used to watch the animals have coitus and then he masturbated with pleasure. He reports that he never chased women because a neighbor's story instilled a fear of venereal disease. This neighbor, a young man, told Mr. Fuentes that he had gotten a very painful disease from contacts with prostitutes; he had pus and bleeding from his penis. The neighbor told him to stay away from women unless he wanted to suffer the same way.

Mrs. Fuentes enjoys intercourse, and she reports, what is rare among the women in the study, that upon occasion she stimulates her husband to the sex act. She believes this is proper because this is a woman's way to show a man that she appreciates him. Mr. Fuentes believes a man should initiate the sex act, but he does not object nor does he think anything derogatory about his wife when she does so; he seems to enjoy it more when she does. Both are in agreement on the importance of sex in their marriage, although Mrs. Fuentes believes it is more important to her husband than it is to her. She says, "A woman can get along without sex, but a man cannot." She was told by a woman ". . . a man will go crazy if he does not have sexual intercourse with a woman."

There are no allegations of unfaithfulness on the part of either spouse. Both believe that once married a person should be faithful to his mate throughout life. As a result, there has been no marital conflict about amorous affairs outside the home. The husband and wife have great respect and affection for one another, for their children, and for their relatives.

During the year preceding the field work, the Fuentes family was confronted with problems of illness in the immediate family and the extended kin group. The oldest daughter developed influenza. She had a high fever, vomiting, and dizzy spells, and she was very weak. Mrs. Fuentes worried about it: "I even thought she might die." Mr.

Fuentes also was afraid the girl might die although the doctor assured him the illness was not serious; he always worries when the children are ill.

A son then developed dizzy spells, headaches, and vomiting spells. The parents took the boy to the municipal hospital. The attending doctor, who diagnosed the difficulty as "worms," gave him medicine but the boy did not improve. The parents thought it might be malaria. They then took the boy to a private doctor who charged them for his services; they also had to pay for the medicine he prescribed. The boy soon began to improve, but at the same time the parents were happy that the doctor had cured him they were worried about the cost of the illness.

Later on the oldest girl caught whooping cough. The parents took her to the municipal hospital where she was given medicine that did not help her. Mrs. Fuentes lay awake all night thinking about the child's illness; she could not sleep because the child had coughing spells and choked up. Both parents held her, rubbed her, and soothed her. "Finally," says Mrs. Fuentes, "I just stuck her under the faucet and turned the water on her, and her cough disappeared."

Shortly after the girl developed whooping cough, one of the boys came down with a fever and shortness of breath. The parents took him to the municipal hospital where a doctor diagnosed his illness as whooping cough and prescribed medicine that the hospital did not have. The parents were very concerned about the boy's illness so they bought the prescribed medicine even though it was an added expense. The expense was of minor concern, however, because the boy soon improved.

In addition, a maternal aunt of Mrs. Fuentes, who had raised her from the age of 2 years, caught influenza. Every day Mrs. Fuentes went to her aunt's home which was nearby and cared for her throughout the illness. Mr. Fuentes looked after the children while his wife took care of her aunt. He recalls, "She cried very much thinking her aunt was going to die."

A serious health problem dominated the thoughts of Mr. and Mrs. Fuentes throughout the year. Mr. Fuentes' mother developed schizophrenia many years ago. In 1942 she was committed to the insane asylum because relatives who were caring for her could no longer cope with her behavior, and she has been in the insane asylum since that time. Although Mr. Fuentes visits her periodically, his wife has never met her mother-in-law. Both are very careful not to let their children know that their grandmother is in the insane asylum. Whenever her illness is discussed, they see to it that the children are not around. Six months before we began the field work, the attending doctor at the asylum decided that the older Mrs. Fuentes could be discharged. Since Mr. and Mrs. Fuentes have no room for her and no other relative is willing to keep her, the old mother remains at the insane asylum. Mr. and Mrs. Fuentes talk of adding a room to the house so the old lady can live with them, but nothing has been done about it. Mrs. Fuentes would be willing to have her mother-in-law move in if they could afford to build a room in which she could be locked securely. Mr. Fuentes agrees with his wife.

Recently, Mrs. Fuentes' younger brother and his wife came to live with them. Now Mr. and Mrs. Fuentes sleep in one room with their 5 children, and the two relatives sleep in the combination living room-dining room-kitchen. The brother was unemployed and had no home when he was united consensually with his young wife. According to the norms of the kinship system, Mrs. Fuentes and her husband are obligated to accept her brother and his wife. Even though they have fulfilled their responsibilities, Mrs. Fuentes is not happy about having her relatives in her home. She thinks that her brother neither worries about unemployment nor knows how to get a job; not once has he brought money into the house. She looks upon his wife as a "lazy young woman, an ignorant country girl." She has to do the work for both the brother and his wife because the sister-in-law has done nothing but wash a few of her clothes since she has been in the house. Deliberately, to insult the sister-in-law, she told the interviewer in a loud voice, "When I was married I was taken to my own home."

There are no problems with the neighbors; Mrs. Fuentes reports: "My husband comes straight home from work and he doesn't visit anyone, so we have no problems." Similarly, her husband says:

> My wife has a good understanding of the neighbors. She is devoted to me and the children, and she doesn't concern herself with the neighbors' affairs. My wife does not want to live in this neighborhood, but she understands that I do not make enough money for us to live in a better area. The neighbors behave well toward her. They do not interfere in our affairs, and we do not interfere in theirs.

The neighbors visit the Fuentes family once in a while, and they visit the neighbors, especially when there is illness or when they celebrate a holiday such as Christmas. When Mrs. Fuentes is ill or about to give birth, the neighbors always offer their services, but Mr. Fuentes does not like to accept their offers. He prefers to take time off from his job to look after his family and care for the house. Mrs. Fuentes is careful not to get too close to the neighbors. Although there are no neighbors with whom she would not associate, she does not believe it is a good neighborhood in which to raise children: "Here they hear bad words; children and adults steal. You have to lock up everything." As a result, Mr. and Mrs. Fuentes have a cordial, friendly, but relatively distant, relationship with other families in the neighborhood.

Mr. and Mrs. Fuentes do not think any specific problems during the year preceding the close of the field work blocked their aspirations. Mrs. Fuentes is not happy about the amount of money her husband earns, as it severely limits what she can buy for the children, especially food and clothing. She would like to live in a different neighborhood, and above all she would prefer to have her brother and his wife move out of her home. Mr. Fuentes is concerned about his mother's confinement in the insane asylum and the possibility that the children will learn about it. Both accept the problems they face with passivity and resignation. Illness of the children, the problem of the old mother, the low income, the unemployment of the brother, and the overcrowded home are viewed as the normal burdens a "poor family" carries. The two psychiatrists who examined the spouses in this family assessed them as adjusted to themselves, to one another, and to their lot in life. They possess elementary dignity within the confines of dire poverty.

A HUSBAND-SCHIZOPHRENIC FAMILY: THE TIRADOS

The Tirados are representative of the seven families in which the husband is afflicted with schizophrenia and the wife is not. The psychiatrists who examined them summarized the mental status of each as follows.

Mr. Tirado. The subject is confused at times. He says he feels as if he is "walking over space." He sees things getting bigger and bigger; he feels as if "the world is on top" of him; his head feels "heavier and bigger." He gives evidence of auditory hallucinations; voices told him, "Go kill that lieutenant." He also exhibits evidence of gustatory hallucinations ". . . tastes like vinegar in my mouth."

The subject lacks insight. He says that he is not the same man he used to be: he has changed, but he is not able to define in what way he has changed. He states that he is more limited now and his ability is lower; he does not understand why this is so.

He has daydreams about things that happened long ago. His night dreams are sexual in tone; one, about a woman on a wall calendar in his room, is a repetitive dream which obsessed him so he had to burn the calendar. He dreams about his body being full of holes and blood oozing out, about trying to kill somebody but the victim runs away, and he wakes up hitting the bed.

The subject shows evidence of autistic thinking. He has tremendous preoccupation with his body. He is plagued with somatic delusions about his body—that he is an invalid and very weak. He is obsessed with suicidal ideas, marital worries, his inability to work, and his invalidism. He has many conflicts. He has feelings of anger, and then he freezes; he cannot walk. Very frequently he feels he has to do something or go somewhere right away; he feels an excessive degree of energy which has an intensive quality; this compulsion and the fits of energy are followed by feelings of excessive weakness. He is plagued with insomnia.

The subject is ambivalent; he has hostile angry thoughts about his father but takes care of him daily; he hates his wife and must stay home with her each day; he loves his children but is unable to provide rightly for them. When angry, he is unable to control his hostile feelings and thoughts.

He cannot tolerate hostility outside of himself. He is dominated by hatred; his aggressive feelings are so strong that his adjustment is impoverished. He has extremely strong hostile feelings toward his wife, his father, people around him, his children, and so on. His hates are oceanic. He is unable to enter relationships with other people. He is afraid of people in the neighborhood, relying on a sister who accompanies him wherever he goes. He cannot tolerate the nearness of other people because he cannot control his aggressive feelings which make him freeze almost to the point of paralysis. He is hostile toward his wife and argues with her nearly every night in bed so there are no sexual relations for weeks.

At present, the subject is suffering a very marked disintegration of his ego. Therefore he is unable to have a favorable attitude toward familiar things. His life is so constricted that his adjustment is impaired markedly, and his functioning as a member of society is at its lowest. He is both a poor performer and a poor listener. He is unable to give, and what he receives he begrudges. He is not satisfied, yet he wants more. He exerts great energy attempting to control the expression of his emotions and bodily actions.

All this leads to a diagnosis of schizophrenia, undifferentiated type.

Mrs. Tirado. This woman is aware that her physical ailments are related to her dealings with her husband. She is very upset by his behavior, although she claims she does not argue about it. She says he frequently berates her, calling her names which she would not repeat.

She becomes very upset on witnessing or taking part in arguments of any kind. She can move from happiness to anger on short notice. There are incongruities between her moods and actions. She becomes angry at her husband but retreats and claims to be submissive to him. She has often thought of leaving her husband, but she does not do so because she thinks she would not find a good man; besides, she could not abandon her children.

She reacts to her husband's philandering with gastrointestinal symptoms, such as pains in the anus, urgency, anorexia, and discomfort. When she becomes angry she has desires to void and defecate and cannot do so in spite of her repeated attempts. She claims she does not need sexual satisfaction.

She is very conscientious toward her domestic responsibilities and accomplishes them without objection. She has little recreation outside the home and does not participate in group activities, although she says she gets along well with people in the community and has no difficulty in getting along with either male or female acquaintances. She avoids the women who have affairs with her husband.

She occasionally attends Catholic church. Mostly she stays at home and away from people except to visit her mother and a very close neighbor, claiming her husband objects to her visiting others.

This woman changes her moods rapidly. She claims to forgive neighbors who have had affairs with her husband. She definitely makes an effort to suppress her inner feelings. Although she cannot verbally express anger toward her husband, she does so through gastrointestinal and gastrourinary symptoms.

The conflict in this woman and its attempted suppression lead to the conclusion of psychophysiological neurotic difficulties.

The Problematic Year. Mr. Tirado's mental illness is the culmination of a sequence of stressful experiences he encountered during the year under review. The beginning of this sequence was marked by an accident while he was a soldier in the United States Army. Mr. Tirado was stationed in the United States when the accident occurred. While he was target shooting on the rifle range with his company, a bullet hit his left hand; bones were broken, muscles torn, and nerves cut. He was hospitalized for 6 months during which he underwent seven operations. When he had recuperated from the surgery he was returned to Puerto Rico. (It is not clear from the record whether he was discharged from the Army at this time or later.)

While he was in hospital in the United States he received news that an unmarried sister in Puerto Rico who was a deaf-mute had become pregnant. The sister was afraid to tell anyone who was responsible for her pregnancy. Mr. Tirado recalls:

> We had to find out who the father was. I was upset, restless, and ashamed. It was an effrontery to the family; there was gossip about it. This was a horrible thing to occur in a family. My father, my brothers, cousins, even two in-laws were suspected. My parents were very fond of this daughter.

When Mr. Tirado returned to Puerto Rico, his sister indicated to him that she was pregnant by a 14-year old cousin. When confronted, the boy admitted his guilt and was sent to the United States.

Soon after this, Mr. Tirado's hand became infected. He was hospitalized in a clinic under contract with the Veterans Administration. The doctors in the clinic decided on an eighth operation to amputate the middle finger of his left hand. The infection had spread so that a ninth operation was ordered, during which a metal rod was put in his hand and metal clips were placed in his fingers. Three more operations were necessary to graft muscles, nerves, and skin. After these operations were completed and feeling had returned to his hand, still another operation was needed to remove the metal clips.

At the time of these operations Mr. Tirado became restless and began to feel sick. He developed a limp in his left leg; he claims he could no longer dance as a result of the weak leg. His wife unexpectedly became pregnant and this added to his worries. From the time he was discharged from the Army until the onset of his mental illness he was unemployed and had no income. Mrs. Tirado's father, who had a wife and 5 dependent children to support, was trying, in addition, to help Mrs. Tirado and her family, but there was not enough money to feed the Tirados. They owed money to the grocery and rent on the house where they lived. Mr. Tirado recalls:

> All of these things made me restless, preoccupied, worried. I couldn't eat, couldn't sleep, lost weight; I went down to 88 pounds. I don't know what we would have done if our relatives had not helped. My wife couldn't eat thinking about all those debts. She was ashamed to owe rent on the house. She could hardly sleep. Just at that time she gave birth to our youngest child.

Shortly after the birth of this child, Mrs. Tirado developed complications and had to be hospitalized. She was in the hospital 9 days and had three operations performed: appendectomy; curettage, cauterization, and replacement of the uterus; and sterilization. While she was in the municipal hospital, her husband was in a clinic maintained by the Veterans Administration and the children were cared for by her mother and sister. While Mrs. Tirado was convalescing from her hospitalization, her father, an itinerant handy man, had no work for 10 weeks. There was not enough to eat and his family was encumbered with more debt.

During this phase of the family difficulties, Mr. Tirado became fearful that he had tuberculosis because he had lost so much weight. He apparently convinced the doctors at the clinic that this might be so, and they gave him permission to transfer from the clinic where his hand was being treated to one concerned primarily with the care of tuberculous veterans. On the day he was to go to the new hospital he went home for some clothing. While he was there his father had a heart attack. The father was rushed to the hospital where the family was told he was not expected to live.

Mr. Tirado was taken to the veterans clinic, but he became so worried about his father's condition that he asked the doctors to allow him to visit his father in the city hospital. Although the doctors warned him not to do this, he went against their advice. Seeing his father, lying so quiet and white in the bed, affected Mr. Tirado extremely; he thought his father was dead. When he returned to the clinic, a series of tests were made, all of which were negative. He was then discharged from the tuberculosis clinic.

Mr. Tirado had applied for a disability pension, but he did not receive word he was eligible for it for several months. The Tirados were completely dependent on their parents and other relatives and neighbors for over a year. Mr. Tirado recalls: "We had little income. The only money we got was collected from the family. They sent us what they could afford." When the family could not help, both Mr. and Mrs. Tirado borrowed small items from the neighbors, some food and, in extreme instances, a dollar now and then. Mr. Tirado began to avoid the neighbors in embarrassment, and they reciprocated by staying away from him. Worry over their impoverished condition made him restless and preoccupied and he could not sleep. In addition, his father was paralyzed after the "heart attack." He says, "I was on a roller skate."

During this period Mr. Tirado developed sexual dissatisfaction with

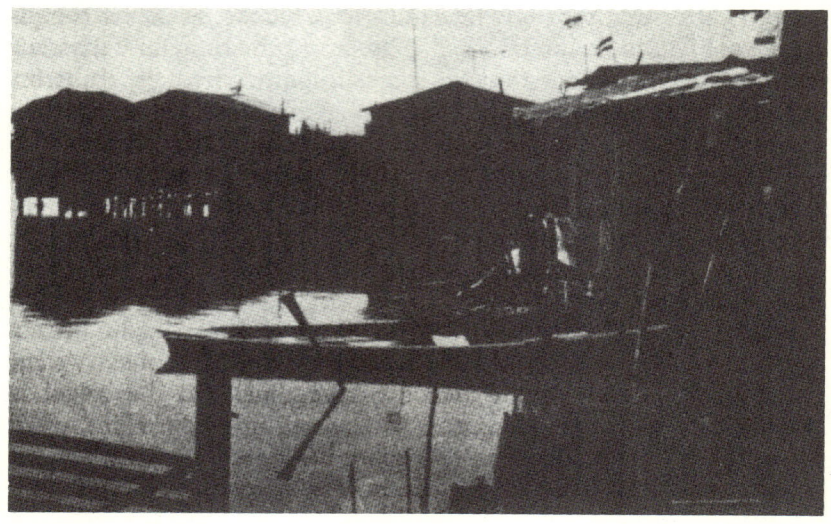

himself and his wife. During coitus with his wife he suddenly got an "electric shock" and had to stop. He began to have an affair with a neighbor's wife. He says:

> I used to get mad; yet it was my fault. I worried very much about it. I felt dissatisfied, restless, and angry. I also thought my wife would imagine I was thinking of some other woman when I was having her. She didn't openly say that she was sexually unsatisfied, but she became nervous. I worried because I thought she suspected me of having another woman. At that time we had a lot of arguments. My marital bed was a fighting ring. I wanted to build a house near my father, but my wife would not allow it. I had a lot, 1000 meters square, near my father. She wanted to live near her family, and I would have none of that. She complained about the rented house where we lived.

Mr. Tirado wanted to be able to help his family and not be helped by them, but because of his crippled hand and the many operations, it was impossible for him to work. He recalls:

> I wasn't improving very rapidly. I depended too much on my parents. I was in a bad mood. I was ashamed. I wanted to repay my parents for all the things they had done for me. It was making me a *loco*.

One night while he was lying in bed, he says he ". . . felt something hot inside of me, and then it came out of my brain. Then I became very cold and weak." He could not breathe normally. He screamed and his heart pounded; he could not stand up, he could not lie down, and his knees trembled. He thought he would die at any moment. He felt weak and faint for the rest of the night. The next day he was not able to arise from his bed. He dates his illness from that night: "I lost my love for living that night."

Mrs. Tirado was beside her husband through his pain and anxiety. All night she worked with him to alleviate his fears and make him comfortable: she heated water on the wood-burning stove for a hot water bottle for his bed; she rubbed his neck, back, and stomach with alcohol. She was very worried about his new illness. Both the Tirados thought it was a heart attack, but the doctor in the clinic who examined Mr. Tirado the next day found no evidence of a heart attack or heart difficulty of any kind.

This was an extremely difficult period for Mrs. Tirado. She was burdened with a sick, unemployed husband in addition to all the duties of the house and the care of her children. She worried over their financial needs, her husband's illness, and her children. Their debts were so large that she felt they would never be able to pay them. She lost hope of the home she had dreamed so long of owning. She grew nervous and thin; she lost her appetite; she was restless at night, and on many occasions she wept in sheer desperation.

In the 3 years that elapsed between the onset of Mr. Tirado's illness and the field work, a rainbow brightened their lives in the form of a disabled veteran's pension. Problems were created between the spouses and the neighbors, however, when, following his recovery from the psychotic episode that closed the problematic year, Mr. Tirado began to search openly for sexual satisfaction outside the home. Mrs. Tirado then had to cope with her husband's schizophrenia, his crippled arm, and his infidelity. A concomitant of this coping process is the psychophysiological neurotic difficulty summarized in the psychiatrist's assessment of her personality.

The problematic year for the Tirados began and ended with a dramatic event: the hand shattered by the rifle bullet marked the start of a year of painful convalescence; the night Mr. Tirado thought he was going to die ended the eventful year. Between the beginning and the end of that year the family experienced each of the six types of problems encompassed in our schedule. There were the illnesses of Mr. Tirado and his father. The unemployment of Mr. Tirado and of Mrs. Tirado's father placed undue stress on the nuclear and extended families. Mr. Tirado fought with his wife over sex; she became pregnant against his wishes. They could not agree on the location of the much desired home. He began to seek sexual satisfaction outside the home, but at this time his amorous behavior did not reach the point of open disrespect toward his wife that it did later. The Tirados had trouble with their neighbors over debts and his amorous behavior. Their dire poverty forced Mrs. Tirado to ask for or accept small loans from neighbors they could not repay. Mr. Tirado lost "self-respect" when he could not support his wife and children. His dream of building a house on a lot his father offered was dashed by his wife's refusal to live near his family; her dream of a house of her own was frustrated by their poverty.

Mr. Tirado believes his present "nervous" illness developed at the time he was overwhelmed by all these problems. He reiterates time after time, "They worried me and they worried my wife." He says, "All of this put me, so to speak, between two and three" (an expression which in Puerto Rico signifies between the devil and the deep blue sea).

We conclude this discussion of the Tirados with an aside from Mr. Tirado:

> Things are still that way. They have not changed. This is going to keep me isolated. It could create an inferiority complex in me.

A WIFE-SCHIZOPHRENIC FAMILY: THE PADILLAS

The Padillas are representative of the nine families in which the wife is a schizophrenic and the husband is not. The psychiatric assessment of each spouse is as follows.

Mr. Padilla. Psychiatric examination did not reveal any symptoms of importance. He is physically and mentally able to function well and in accord with his potentiality. He is liked and respected by his fellow workers. He is gregarious and free of intensive intrapsychic conflicts. He has a good system of adequate defenses.

What affects him most is illness in the family; when one of the children becomes sick he worries a lot. He is irritable when children bother him around the house. He is apprehensive about his financial situation. Persons usually do not affect him in any way unless they argue too much.

There are no pathological signs or symptoms.

Mrs. Padilla. This woman finds herself unable to do routine home chores such as pressing clothes, cooking, taking care of children. On one occasion she had a feeling that her self was separating from her body, "a very queer sensation." She feels people talk about her. She has auditory hallucinations: ". . . people knocking at my door," ". . . the steps of men around my house." She rationalizes her mental symptoms with superstitions; she projects frequently.

She has persecutory dreams of men chasing her. In her dreams the world comes to an end. She is worried excessively about the family's financial condition, the infidelity of her husband, the chores she has to do the next day. She has phobias of fire, of darkness, of health, and of her housework. She is obsessed with losing her mind. She thinks people do not like her; they say bad things about her. It takes a long time to convince herself another person is not against her, and she wishes something could be done about it.

Autistic thinking is evidenced by her marked tendency to daydream and fantasize. Other evidence of distorted thinking is observable in her excessive defenses, such as projection and rationalization; her suspicions are a secondary result of projection. Objective evidence of a thought disorder is found.

Her husband and children affect her very much. Inappropriate reactions are most prevalent in her frequent rages at her children. She becomes so angry she reaches the point of harming them physically. Alternating moods of elation and depression seize her; these alternations, however, are not frequent. Most of the time she is worried and hostile toward people. There is a marked limitation in her interpersonal relations as a result of her suspicions and mistrust of other people.

This woman is a highly tense, overtalkative individual with pronounced somatization, probably as a result of displaced unconscious hostility. Although not totally disabled, her functioning is below par because of her mental conflicts. She bites her fingernails and exhibits shortness of breath. She sits on the edge of her chair and is unable to relax. She is moderately frigid, seldom feeling sexual pleasure; orgasm is rare.

Her defenses are mainly projective. She is fighting continuous threats of ego disintegration projected in her fear of the world ending. Emotions, intense and incongruous, are frequently expressed in uncontrollable ways such as aggression against her children. Anxiety is felt as a danger signal. She prefers to stay at home, shying away from play, recreation, or group activities. Housework disgusts her. She has very much concentrated her thoughts on herself in a narcissistic way.

This woman is characterized by deveistic thinking, overwhelming anxieties, and many phobias; she has poor or no insight into her problems. She is burdened by excessive guilt over her sterilization operation. She exhibits inappropriate rage reactions during examination. Her thinking is marked by ideas of reference and she has pseudo and hallucinatory perceptions. She has strong persecutory delusions. On occasion, she shows depersonalization. She fears work and disintegration of her personality and her social situation.

This woman exhibits a clear schizophrenic pattern of a paranoid type.

The Problematic Year. During the year immediately preceding the onset of Mrs. Padilla's illness, she and her husband encountered a series of problems which she dates from the sixth month of her second pregnancy in her present marriage. She relates:

> I used to get crying spells and have arguments with my husband every day. I was upset by the fact that he was retreating from our home. He was toying around with a woman who was living in our house. He and this girl were always exchanging jokes and laughing with each other. My husband used to say to her, "You are just right!" One day I hit him over the head with a plate and it broke on his head. Then he beat me up. He hit me so hard that I had black bruises all over me. The next day I went to police headquarters. A policeman told me to go home.

Mrs. Padilla has had seven childbirths and two miscarriages; these nine pregnancies occurred between her sixteenth and twenty-fourth birthdays. At the last birth she was sterilized. Her troubles continue:

> When the birth pains began, my husband could not be found. A midwife had to be rounded up. I had a bad time. I had to be taken to the hospital in an ambulance. They examined me and sent me home because they said those were not birth pains. This was two days before the actual birth. A midwife who saw me told me the fetus was in a bad position. After the birth I suffered a hemorrhage that left me very weak. This was the worst childbirth I ever had. I couldn't even move in bed. For two days I lay in bed not being able to move. I wanted to see if lying still would cure the hemorrhage I had. My husband did not worry about this. He was calm. Two days after childbirth he wanted me to get out of bed and prepare his food. I could not get out of bed. I could not do it.

When Mrs. Padilla was 7 months pregnant her husband lost his job as an attendant in a gasoline station where he had earned $22 per week. He was unemployed for approximately 5 months. Shortly after her husband was laid off, Mrs. Padilla's stepfather lost his job, and he too was unemployed for several months. During this same time her brother also lost his job and remained unemployed for 13 months. (This interval was a time of recession in the San Juan area.) Mrs. Padilla goes on:

> At that time we did not have much money. We had to get credit. When my husband worked he gave his whole pay to the grocery and we still owed more. We lived in a one-room house with a kitchen in the same room. I worried a great deal about it. We lacked many things we needed. There was no money for medicine; we had to borrow all the time and live on credit. My husband was very worried about it. He just was not making enough money for our necessities. He was desperate.

The unemployment of Mrs. Padilla's stepfather and brother was particularly unfortunate since the mother and stepfather were supporting two children from Mrs. Padilla's first marriage whom her present husband refused to have in his home; he said they belonged to her, not him. Mrs. Padilla recalls:

> My stepfather couldn't find anything to do so he devoted himself to drinking. My mother suffered a lot, and I couldn't help her. My husband didn't worry about it at all. When I described these problems to him he did not show interest in them at all. My brother was unemployed and when he did get some money he spent it on gambling. My husband did not worry about that.

The unemployment of the stepfather coupled with his drinking and the unemployment of the brother combined with his gambling made the situation very difficult for Mrs. Padilla's mother. She was forced to do washing and ironing in the homes of other people. Mrs. Padilla says her mother was always hungry:

> She was always lacking food. She lost weight and was weak. She was so weak she could not come to see me. I could not help her either. My husband did not worry about it at all. He was not concerned with the problems in my family. I talked to him about it and he told me not to bother him about it because it was not going to do any good. He was not going to help.

Although Mrs. Padilla felt responsible for the two little girls of her previous marriage, she was unable to help her mother support them. She says:

> They suffered from weakness. They were skinny and pale and had frequent colds. They had bad coughs. I was very worried about them.

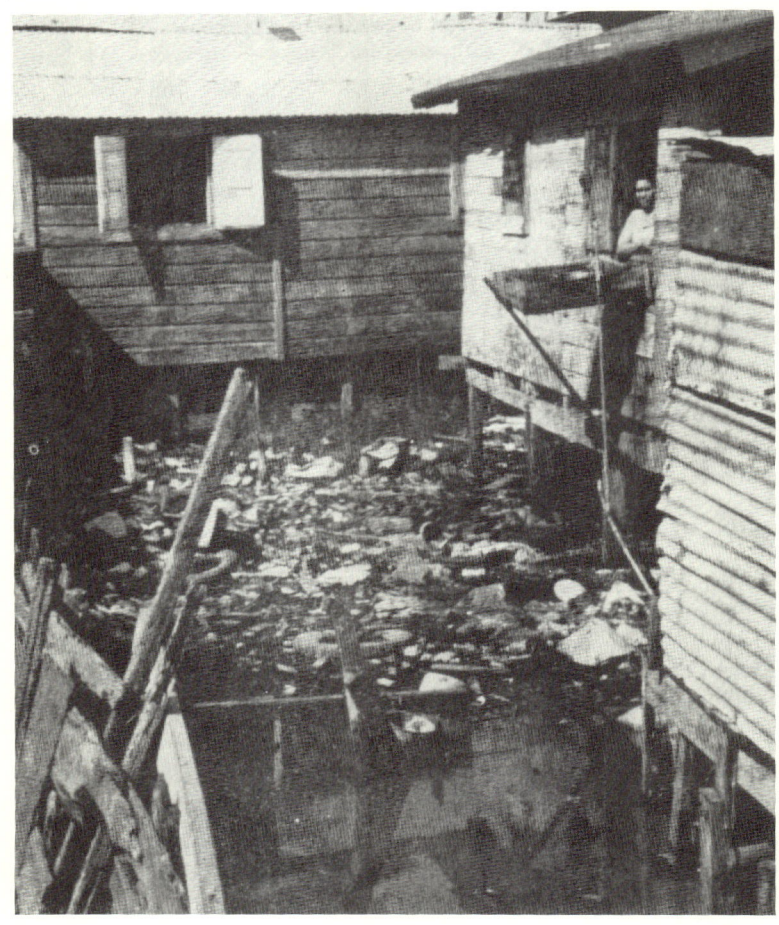

I could not even take them to the hospital. My husband would not let me. He said it was up to my mother to care for them. This upset me. I used to cry a lot about this. When I expressed a desire to take them to the hospital he fought me. At no moment did he show concern over this problem.

Two months after the difficult childbirth, Mrs. Padilla realized she was pregnant for the fifth time in 4 years. She soon developed symptoms of asthma and found it necessary to spend 2 or 3 days at a time in bed. She also suffered from a fever, headaches, and bad coughing spells during which she could not sleep. She says:

I could not do housework. I could not care for myself or my children. I could not even bathe myself. I could not go out at all.

During the worst of this period she was hospitalized for a week. Her husband found work again. His new job, which was in the government, paid him $116 a month. He began to show some interest in the family. He bought medicine and tried to make Mrs. Padilla comfortable at night by rubbing her with alcohol and herbs or by putting two pillows under her head so she could breathe more easily. This period of solicitousness for Mrs. Padilla's welfare did not last more than a few weeks; when she was in the second trimester of her pregnancy her husband began to cultivate a mistress. Mrs. Padilla was told about the affair by a friendly neighbor. She relates with scorn and anger:

> This concubine lived in the neighborhood. They could be seen together in the open, in public, and I used to spy on them. One of my husband's brothers told me that my husband has a child from this woman. I was restless, worried; I was always thinking he was with the other woman, that he was going to abandon me, that he was spending a lot of money with her. I used to fight with him over this. He used to leave the house. I went to a spiritualist to get advice. The spiritualist told me that my husband's relations with that woman had come to an end, but this did not calm me because I did not believe it. My husband did not worry at all about this. He always ate well. The only time he got mad was when I argued with him about it.

The spiritualist was right; Mr. Padilla had ended the affair, but he had entered into another one. Mrs. Padilla soon realized her husband had an infatuation with another neighbor. This time she did not need anyone to tell her about it; she watched the relationship develop. Mrs. Padilla claims this woman danced on the front porch so her husband could see her and be enticed.

> I watched through a hole in the wall. I noticed that they looked at each other and laughed. They had a little gesture that had some meaning. One night he stayed out all night. I was so upset my nerves gave way. I was screaming. I had asthma. Something inside of me wanted to burst out. I was hospitalized for five days.

While her husband was having the affair with this neighbor, Mrs. Padilla was growing heavier with her pregnancy. She was also beginning to have difficulties with her neighbors. She picked a fight with one woman who had been a friend. This woman withdrew from further contact with Mrs. Padilla. When she was about 8 months pregnant she had a fight with another neighbor who had reprimanded one of the Padilla children in the alley. Mrs. Padilla explains:

> I went to the mother of the child and I told her not to say such things. The woman looked at me and said, "If you were not pregnant you know what I would do to you!" Other neighbors heard us quarreling. When I walked toward her the neighbors held me back. I wanted to get this woman. Before this, I had not had any trouble with this neighbor. Later it worried me very much. Every time I saw this woman speaking to a neighbor afterwards, I thought she was talking about me, but at the same time when I spoke to anyone else I thought that maybe this neighbor suspected me of talking about her. I do not like to have bad relations with neighbors.

Mrs. Padilla goes on:

> ... when the birth pangs began my husband could not be found. He had put on his *guayabera* [fancy shirt] and gone out into the street. The midwife had to be rounded up. [The midwife delivered twins to Mrs. Padilla in their one-room shack.] Two days after the birth my husband went out into the street again. He was not concerned at all about my condition. In addition to having to care for four children, I was not feeling well at all.

Mr. Padilla rejected the twins, which hurt Mrs. Padilla; to complicate the situation, one of the twins was not healthy; he vomited green and black fluid. Mrs. Padilla became so distraught she took the baby to the municipal hospital. The doctor recommended that the baby be left there, and although Mrs. Padilla wanted to stay with the infant she was told she could visit the child only twice a week.

One day when she went to visit the infant she left a sister to care for the other children and to look after the house. She relates:

> When I returned from the hospital I found the house in a turmoil. My sister was sitting in the middle of the mess reading a cheap novel. I became very angry. I grabbed a broom and began to hit her. I threw her out of the house. Then I became very sleepy and I went to bed and I woke up late at night. It was only then I realized what I had done.

(Mrs. Padilla had knocked her sister unconscious and thrown her out of the house. The unconscious girl was lying in the muddy street when a neighbor revived her.)

After ten days the baby was brought home from the hospital in a city-owned ambulance, but Mrs. Padilla worried still more because he had diarrhea and continued to vomit. When ten more days passed and the child did not appear to be improving, Mr. Padilla insisted that they consult a *curandera* (folk healer) who prescribed castor oil. The parents gave the child castor oil, and shortly after, in Mrs. Padilla's words:

> ... the agony started. For twelve hours he was in horrible agony. His eyes turned in their sockets and his tongue hung out. He was gasping for breath. I cried wildly when I saw him in such agony. I asked God to take him. I could not see him suffer any longer, and when he died I felt relieved. People have told me that the laxative killed him. I did not want to give him that laxative. It was my husband who took him to the *curandera*. When the child died I began to scream and shout and cry. I hit my sister Rosa who was helping us. I began to act like a *loca*. I fell unconscious as if I were in a dream. Afterward I came out of the spell. I came to accept his death.

Mr. Padilla's infidelity was a problem throughout the year. He admits he had the affair with the young woman who lived in their home. He says, "She was ripe," meaning that she was sexually attractive and ready to have an affair with him. The second love affair involved a woman in the neighborhood. Mr. Padilla says:

> My wife threatened to abandon me. We smashed one another several times, yet I could not correct my behavior. I replied to my wife's insults with insults of my own. She had good reason to fight me, but I told her to shut her mouth. At other times she wouldn't tell me anything, just suffer in silence. She knew she was right, but she was afraid I would abandon her if she kept on fighting me. Finally, I quit this woman.

Mr. Padilla admits to the third affair, as his wife describes it. The woman also lived in the neighborhood. He says:

> I used to visit her home, but we had sexual relations elsewhere, not at her home. I did not spend the whole night with this woman. I took her out once or twice a week. My wife found out about it and she got very hot under the collar. Then she became passive about it. She suffered quietly. She was always suspecting me, especially when I returned late at night. Sometimes I was working but she thought I was with the other woman. Sometimes, I even felt sorry for my wife. She was suffering. We used to quarrel and it bothered me to hear my wife telling me the truth right to my face. She used to call me a liar and I really was a liar. She was worried that I might abandon her to live with this woman, and she felt humiliated because she loved me so much.

As Mrs. Padilla grew more distraught over her husband's behavior, he became more secretive in his relations with the female neighbors, not so much out of respect for his wife but out of fear for his own safety, as he was aware that an aggrieved husband could put a dagger in his back. To avoid this, he selected women who were separated from their husbands or women whose husbands were *atomicos* (alcoholic and drug-addicted derelicts).

Sex has been a problem in Mrs. Padilla's life since she was a child. When she was 10 years old she contracted syphilis. At the age of 16, she told her mother she would be in church, but she and a boy friend went to a room, rented by the hour, to have sex relations. The boy's mother found out, and the couple set up housekeeping in a rented room. When the girl became pregnant the couple were legally married, but after 4 years she separated from him. She then returned to her mother's house and set up the liaison with her present consensual husband, Mr. Padilla, with whom she had had sexual relations before she was divorced from her first husband.

Mr. Padilla also has a history of sex difficulties. He had premarital sex relations with a number of different women. Eventually, he married but the marriage broke up. He was not divorced from his first wife when he contracted a consensual marriage. After a while the second wife went to New York City. There were two children from the first marriage, none from the second. In due time, he set up the consensual union with his present wife.

Mr. Padilla did not expect to live with this wife for very long. She became pregnant, however, and they entered into a consensual union. From his point of view, she was one of the "flowers" he was "sampling" in his pursuit of a pleasant life. After the establishment of the consensual union and while she was pregnant, he continued to "sample" other women. The "pleasant affair of the moment" has continued for 7 years. Mrs. Padilla is resentful toward Mr. Padilla over his failure to obtain a divorce and marry her legally. He has no intention of being placed in such a position. Mrs. Padilla realizes she has "the goat but not the rope." She is convinced there is little chance of obtaining the rope, and she fears the loss of the goat unless she can gain a firm hold on him by a legal marriage. The philosophy of "pick the flowers as you go through life" has often turned Mr. Padilla's attention to other women.

In the year preceding Mrs. Padilla's psychotic break, the Padillas experienced each of the six types of problems: A complicated pregnancy was followed by the death of a baby under provocative circumstances; unemployment decimated the family's meager store of economic resources, and Mrs. Padilla's children suffered; when Mr. Padilla did find work he shared his earnings with a "concubine"; the interpersonal relations of the Padillas underwent a series of stress-provoking incidents; as Mrs. Padilla became more disturbed over her husband's behavior, she began to quarrel with the neighbors. Her dream of a legal marriage to him has never been realized—she goads him; he retaliates with infidelity.

The breaking point was reached when Mrs. Padilla returned from the hospital and found her "lazy sister" sitting in the middle of the floor reading with the house "torn to pieces," the 17-day old twin of the sick infant screaming in the basket, and food and dishes scattered over the floor by the older children. The last link connecting Mrs. Padilla with reality broke when the baby died. She, in truth, became a *loca*.

A DOUBLE SCHIZOPHRENIC FAMILY: THE GALLARDOS

The four families in which both the husband and the wife are diagnosed as schizophrenic individuals are represented by the Gallardos. The perceived onset of symptoms in the husband and in the wife occurred during an 18-month period prior to the field work. The extended problematic year and the field work overlap; thus, we are able to see the interaction between the many types of stressful experiences they faced and the onset of the symptoms in the two spouses. The psychiatrist's assessment of the mental status of each member of the spouse pair follows.

Mr. Gallardo. Situations at home affect this man most. At the onset of the disease process he was unable to work. He had to withdraw from social contacts, he was irritated by the situation at home, and he felt murderous toward his wife and children. After a few weeks he was able to adjust better and accept the demands imposed on him. He has been able to allay anxiety, partly through somatization. When his illness began he had enough strength to avert complete ego destruction.

He is harassed by negative feelings, irritation, and morbid thoughts of killing his wife and children. He expresses this also in his dreams in which he chases somebody or is fighting and is concerned that he is going to be killed. Whenever his hates are repressed, the somatization fails, and they come out in phobia or anxiety. He believes that intercourse with his wife will harm him if it is practiced more than once a week; sometimes he goes for weeks at a time without having intercourse.

His preoccupations, worries, and fantasies get him so involved in himself that he skirts the world of unreality. The disease process, though crippling, has not been so severe that his overall adjustment could be considered seriously impaired, but it is of such a degree that I would say his social and emotional efficiency has been curtailed by perhaps 50 per cent.

This man shows excessive fantasies and excessive preoccupation; he somatizes; he is afflicted with phobias; he reveals anxiety attacks. He has extreme irritations toward many things. He has ambivalent feelings toward his wife and children. His hates prevail over his love. He is impaired intellectually. He is ridden by compulsions.

These signs and symptoms lead to the conclusion that this man has decompensated into a schizophrenic reaction, pseudoneurotic undifferentiated type.

Mrs. Gallardo. The subject believes her husband's illness has caused her emotional disturbance, but she cannot see how this has happened. Putting it into her own words, her husband's illness has "caused my nervousness." She is very preoccupied with health; she is afraid that she is going crazy. She thinks she is suffering from the same type of disease as her husband. Throughout the interview she wanted assurance: "Tell me I am not going to get worse." There is capacity in the ego to see that things are not what they used to be, but it is losing its grasp. There is also an infantile attitude and wish, the magical thinking, that an adult in authority can fix things and protect her.

At the onset of her illness she had the sensation of somebody hitting her middle finger with a hammer; then it became numb and the numbness extended to her arm. She dreams, but she can recall only the dream she had the previous night: A man, not her husband, wanted to have intercourse with her; he gave her an injection which "paralyzed me completely," and she could not run away.

This woman is interested only in herself and the immediate world around her. This egocentric interest in her immediate surroundings goes so far as to affect her equilibrium, but it satisfies her own needs. I, therefore, consider her to be autistic. She is affected mostly by persons and situations: her husband, her children, her relatives, and the place she lives in. All these pressures make her "lose control" of herself and she has the desire to leave. She used to worry most about her husband's illness; now she worries about the place she lives in and that she wants to move. There is a fixed idea about moving away. She wants to leave the surroundings in which she lives. Her "mind tells me to leave." The place she lives in is bad for her; she must move out. The children and the financial situation also worry her.

Most recently, she has felt more nervous, more anxious, and as if she were waiting for bad news; her thoughts of leaving home have been stronger and less easy to shake off. Her spirit is sapped and there is no vitality in her. She feels no strength to support any emotional change. She is compulsive; she has the urge to do something and cannot rest until she does it. She has had insomnia for more than a month.

She has withdrawn from all contacts outside the family. She has no friends; she feels threatened by other people and has to withdraw. She is afraid of other people and makes no attempt to relate to others. She knows her neighbors, but she has no contact with them. She feels so threatened that she wants only to move away. Her inner feelings drive her.

There is no alternative but to consider this woman's attitude toward others and the way she relates to others as unrealistic; she is encapsulated within herself. She is aware of the world around her, but she is not able to be a part of that world and play a role in it. She says, "I feel as if I am going out; I am not the same woman." I consider that she means by this that there is no sense of sameness in relation to others; she is different from others and not a part of the whole. She is afraid of being lost in a maelstrom of nonexistence.

The subject would like to be impervious to negative feelings. She would like to be in a situation where anger or hate have no opportunity to dwell in her so she will not lose control. Her hate feelings are massively repressed. Thus, we see a mildly mannered, restrained, empty individual; even the capacity to love is affected by the repression. It appears that there is "no life" in her; she says she is "all gone out." There is no free psychic energy to be invested in things outside of her own self. She has no energy left for play and recreation. Even her home chores are done as if by an automaton; she feels if she did not do them her husband would be irritated, would argue and reprimand her; all the repressed negative feelings would come to the surface and she would lose control.

We find ideas of estrangement and depersonalization; hallucinatory experiences, obsessions, and compulsions; fixed ideas; forgetfulness, blocking, and occasional incoherence and irrelevance; autism and concretism; anxiousness; inappropriate emotional response (quantitative); restlessness, agitation, impulsiveness, and trembling; insomnia, anorexia, and withdrawal; poor relation to self, others, and things; emptiness; poor judgment and poor insight so that there is no alternative but to classify her as a personality that has decompensated into a schizophrenic way of life.

Schizophrenic reaction, simple type.

The Problematic Year. Illness, death, and physical deprivation are interwoven in the development of schizophrenia in the Gallardo family. The sequence of tangible events that led to a diagnosis of schizophrenia in both the husband and the wife began when Mrs. Gallardo, at the age of 24, gave birth to her third child, a boy. This child was delivered by Caesarean section, as were the two older children. Following the birth, Mrs. Gallardo did not recover her health as she had on previous occasions. When the baby was 4 months of age, Mrs. Gallardo was hospitalized for gynecological difficulties, and a hysterectomy was performed. Shortly after the mother's operation, the baby developed pneumonia. He recovered but was beset by asthma. Two months later, the child developed pneumonia again and was hospitalized. Three days later he died.

Mr. Gallardo tells us the exact time of the child's death, his name, and the cause of death, "double pneumonia." Then he relates:

> This had a great effect on us. We were sad for many days, and I couldn't go to work. After he died we had to move out of the apartment. There were too many things in that apartment that reminded us of him.

Mrs. Gallardo states:

> It was a bitter experience for me. When I saw him he was very sick and I knew he was going to die. They had to calm me with drugs. I was unaware of when he died. I cannot even recall having buried this child. Three days afterward I began to realize what had happened to my child.

But illness was no stranger in their household even before the problematic year. The oldest boy had suffered from tonsillitis, severe colds, and asthma since he was 3 months of age. The second child, a girl, had experienced serious illnesses from birth: she had a hernia at 15 days of age and pneumonia at 25 days; this was complicated by asthma and bronchitis. The little girl recovered from these illnesses but she was afflicted with severely inflamed tonsils at 3 months of age. Nine months of relatively good health followed her recovery from the tonsillitis. Then at 1 year she contracted pneumonia for the second time. At about this time her brother had the measles. For the next 2 years both children were relatively healthy. Near the end of this interval, the youngest child was born, suffered, and died.

Some 6 weeks after the death of the baby, the little girl who was now almost 3 years of age developed pneumonia for the third time. The father took the child to a clinic where he was covered by medical insurance through his work; this was the same clinic in which the younger boy had died. The doctors insisted that the girl be hospitalized immediately. While she was in the hospital Mr. and Mrs. Gallardo were so disturbed about the child's welfare that they felt one of them had to be at the clinic at all times. Mr. Gallardo, a stevedore on the docks, worked until two or three o'clock in the morning, which meant his wife had to stay at the clinic most of the night. On the nights when Mr. Gallardo worked late he went directly to the clinic to see his daughter before he went to the *caserío* where they lived. He was so concerned that he could hardly eat or sleep. After 3 days at the clinic, the little girl was sent home because the crisis had passed, but the child remained in bed at home for 2 or more months.

While the girl was still recuperating from the pneumonia, the boy became ill with a very bad cold and had trouble breathing. Mr. Gallardo took him to the clinic immediately, and the doctor at the clinic told him the boy's tonsils were inflamed, swollen, and covered with pus. The doctor said it would be necessary to operate, but, before this could be done, the boy would have to be given plasma and medicines so he would be strong enough to withstand the operation. The child was placed in an oxygen tent for 2 days prior to the planned operation. Mrs. Gallardo wanted to stay with the child at night, but the hospital authorities would not allow her to do this.

Early in the morning of the third day when the doctors planned to operate on the boy, the Gallardos went to the clinic. By the time they reached the hospital the boy had already been anesthetized and was on a cart being wheeled into the operating room. The parents noticed that the child, although unconscious, was vomiting; a hand lying outside the blanket was red; they rushed to the child, felt his hand, and decided he was feverish. They insisted that the nurse take the child's temperature, and, according to Mr. Gallardo, the boy had "6 degrees of fever." The parents became alarmed. In their concern for the child's welfare they demanded to see the head surgeon of the clinic.

The surgeon allegedly told them that the doctor who was to operate was an intern, not the usual doctor who performed this type of operation. This information so upset Mr. Gallardo that he would not allow the operation to take place. He wanted to take the boy home immediately, but the doctors told him he could not take the boy out of the hospital until his temperature was normal. After the temperature was reduced, Mr. Gallardo took the boy home, against the advice of the hospital authorities, and the child gradually recovered from the tonsillitis without an operation. Mr. Gallardo relates:

> We lost our confidence in the doctors at the clinic. We believe our son would have died had they operated on him in that condition. We felt terrified of losing our only son, for we had lost another son. I felt very angry at the lack of responsible behavior on the part of the authorities at the clinic. We pay for these medical services out of our salaries, and we pay for them even if we have no need to use them.

While the daughter was sick with pneumonia but before the boy developed the ulcerated tonsils, Mr. Gallardo was working on the docks all day and, when a ship had to be loaded, until three o'clock in the morning. One night after returning home late from work he was sweating freely and felt very tired. He took a bath, ate his dinner, and went to bed. The next morning when he arose and looked at himself in the mirror he was horrified: his left cheek was twisted up to his ear so that his mouth was open on the left side and his eye was staring off at an angle. He could not close his left eye; he could not even blink the eyelid. He recalls:

> The more I tried to straighten my face out the more concerned I became. I felt like leaving home without telling my wife and children and disappearing until I was cured. But then I decided to tell my wife.

Mrs. Gallardo was alarmed when she saw her husband's disfigured face. She says, "His eye was out of orbit." She rushed him to the clinic where he was told he had had a muscular spasm causing facial paralysis. The doctor said not to worry, the spasm would disappear and Mr. Gallardo would regain his former appearance. Mr. Gallardo did not believe these reassuring words. Many nights he could not sleep, especially in the first few weeks. He was convinced his facial paralysis was caused by a cerebral hemorrhage and the doctors at the clinic were keeping it from him. He thought his disfigurement would remain always. He feared that his children would become frightened of him and "even my wife would tire of me, for no one can live all her life with a monster."

The spasm in his face was not physically painful, but Mr. Gallardo was very unhappy about it. Sometimes, he says, he looked at himself in the mirror when he was alone and began to cry. His wife worried very much about it; she thought he would remain that way the rest of his life. She attempted to console him by telling him that other men were even uglier than he was. He thought she said this in jest; he knew that inside of her she wanted him to regain his normal appearance because she insisted that he not miss one appointment at the clinic where he was receiving facial massages. Mrs. Gallardo feared he might lose his head and begin to drink excessively. For this reason she tried to boost his morale, especially when she noticed that he was feeling particularly distraught.

Mr. Gallardo became so upset over his facial paralysis and his son's illness that he did not go to work for several weeks. Gradually he overcame his fear of going out in public with his twisted face and he started working again. However, he had to put up with the taunts and ribald remarks of his friends at work. One of them told him his face was twisted from sticking it into things that were none of his business; another said he had been trying to see things with his left eye that he should not see. By the end of the third month his face began to return to normal.

A short time after he went back to work there was a sympathy strike on the docks and he was out of work a month. Mr. Gallardo was very unhappy since this period without pay resulting from the San Juan local's attempt to help the stevedores' union in New York City only added to his economic woes.

> I had gone to work with my twisted face because it was necessary to have food for the children, food that they required. I had gone heavily into debt buying medicine during my daughter's illness and that of my son. When the strike started the family did not have any income and we had to go to relatives to get help. I borrowed a little money from my mother and from my stepfather. My wife's father used to bring us food and lend us money. Even with the help we were getting from relatives we experienced hunger.
>
> My wife and I did not eat so our children would have enough with the little food we were able to buy. Sometimes we bought milk and other kinds of food for the children even though we did not eat all day long. Some of our relatives bought us some groceries. They also loaned us money. We used this money to subsist.

Mr. Gallardo realized his children were undernourished, and he was fearful they might suffer a relapse of their illnesses, particularly his daughter who he knew had not regained her strength. He also was anxious about his wife. He recalls:

> She suffered quietly. We were hungry together and we had to accept that with resignation. Sometimes I felt like going out in the street to assault someone or to steal but it seemed in those moments when I was almost ready to commit some desperate act that a relative would come to help.

Mrs. Gallardo was very worried about their economic situation and the expense of the illnesses of the children. She was afraid the strike would last a long time, perhaps to the point where her relatives would be unable to aid them. Moreover, she was concerned that the little girl was still weak from her illness, and both parents were fearful that she might have another sickness.

When Mr. Gallardo returned to work after the strike, his fellow workers noticed that he was very thin. He felt weak and he thought this resulted from the lack of food he and his family had suffered while he was unemployed. Several of his friends at work commented on how pale and skinny he was. Mr. Gallardo told them he felt like "a new man"; he was working again and his facial paralysis had subsided.

A favorite brother worked with Mr. Gallardo on the docks. After the strike Mr. Gallardo noticed that this brother was very thin and pale. At first, Mr. Gallardo attributed his brother's condition to the fact that he, too, had been out of work and was probably undernourished, but as the weeks passed the brother continued to lose weight, to perspire more than the other men, and to look even paler. Mr. Gallardo noticed also that his brother was coughing a great deal on the job; he appeared to have a fever; and he trembled all over as he tried to work with the other men. As the brother grew weaker, Mr. Gallardo felt it was his responsibility to talk to him. He told his brother he had noticed the work was hard for him since he appeared weak, and he urged him to go to a doctor. The brother was affronted by Mr. Gallardo's solicitous behavior. One afternoon the brother drew a knife and threatened to kill Mr. Gallardo. He said he drew the knife so ". . . you won't fuck around with me any more like that." Later on the same day, the brother fell onto the dock unconscious. The other workmen called Mr. Gallardo who lifted his brother in his arms and carried him to a pile of sacking; he blew air into his face and fanned him with a piece of paper. After about 15 minutes the brother regained consciousness.

The next day the brother went to a clinic. He was suffering from tuberculosis in an advanced form. The doctor advised him to stop drinking and working. Instead of taking this advice, he continued to work as long as he could stand and he drank even more heavily than before. From the afternoon when the brother drew a knife on Mr. Gallardo until a few hours before the brother's death, there was no communication between the two men. Mr. Gallardo grieved because his brother was so hostile toward him and had rejected the advice that he seek medical care. He knew what his brother's children would have to undergo without a father. He believed that he should have compelled his brother to get the care he needed even though the brother rejected him. He thinks that if he had insisted the brother would not have died.

A few weeks afterward, Mr. Gallardo became obsessed with the idea that he, also, was tubercular. He felt very tired in the morning, with no desire whatsoever to go to work. He began to act differently toward his children; he would not pick them up or play with them. He made his wife separate all the objects he used to avoid exposing the rest of the family. He was extremely apprehensive of having an X-ray, thinking it would confirm that he had tuberculosis. His wife, however, talked him into going to the clinic and submitting to a medical examination.

When the X-rays were developed, there was a spot observable on one of his lungs. The doctor then examined his sputum and took samples of his gastric juices, but these yielded negative results. Further photographs were taken which still indicated a lesion on one lung. Although Mr. Gallardo had suspected for months that he had tuberculosis, he, nevertheless, found it extremely difficult to accept the fact. On the day when the third X-ray was taken, Mr. Gallardo had gone to the clinic with his wife and little daughter. As he was waiting for the results of the X-ray, the little girl came near him and spoke into his ear. At this point, the nurse who was in the waiting room told him that he should not get so close to his daughter because he might infect her. He felt like beating the nurse. As he left the clinic he thought of committing suicide.

About 3 weeks after Mr. Gallardo discovered his brother had tuberculosis, he began to drink heavily. He says:

> After I got out of work I was tired, especially when there was a lot of work on the docks at night. When I finished work at 2 or 3 o'clock in the morning, I used to go with friends to bars around the docks and drink for several hours.

Many times he did not return home until daylight; often he arrived home quite drunk. He recalls:

> My wife fought with me and she told me that I was working too hard and I had to eat better. I replied and we used to get into an argument. However, I never lifted my arm against her. Then afterwards I was sorry I had caused her problems. Yet I continued to do the same thing the next time. All this time, I could not control myself.
>
> My wife fought me for my own good, but I was blind to this and I did not pay any attention to her sermons. I told her it was none of her business. She used to cry and tell me I was irresponsible, but then we went to sleep and made peace again.
>
> My wife decided to leave me, to leave with the children and live with her father. She must have been suffering a great deal. She has always been a good wife. She loves me a great deal. I recall how much she used to cry when she had to reprimand me. I have a feeling she suffered more from having to reprimand me than I suffered from having to hear her.

At about this time trouble developed between Mr. Gallardo and his neighbors:

> I became very upset by the inconsiderate attitude of several of my neighbors. These persons knew that I had to work all night or early into the morning. Nevertheless, early in the morning they got up and made noise and I could not sleep. At first I accepted this without protest, but inside of me I felt like blowing up. This went on and I just couldn't restrain myself any longer, so I went to the administrator of the *caserío*. She said she would see what she could do but she didn't do anything at all. So I requested that I be given another apartment. There was no apartment available and I had to continue to listen to these disorders from that pack of shameless neighbors.
>
> One night the neighbors had a record player going full volume. They were screaming and yelling. I talked to them but they didn't pay any attention to me at all. Another time, I had to speak to them for they had a daughter who used to stand out on the stairs. She and her boy friend used to chew on one another. The boy used to suck on the girl's tits in the hall. It didn't look pretty at all. The mother of this girl told me that it was none of my business. I told her that she was raising her daughters to be whores, and that she, the mother, was the first whore of them all. This woman did not have a husband.

She had a lover and this man used to come and visit her some nights. The woman threatened to tell her lover on me. She must have forgotten about it because nothing happened.

The neighbors were particularly noisy on Friday and Saturday nights. At times I was afraid I would lose control of myself.

The high point of Mr. Gallardo's troubles with his neighbors occurred on Christmas Eve.

We had all gone to bed early, around 10 o'clock, for the little girl was not feeling well. She had the flu. The neighbors were having a party. The noises were so great that I decided to solve this thing right then, no matter what the consequences. I tucked a knife into my belt. At 1 o'clock I went downstairs to the apartment where the noises were coming from. I noticed broken bottles, vomit, and piss on the stairs. This annoyed me. I felt like grabbing the first neighbor I saw and slamming his head against the concrete wall. I was furious when I knocked on the door with my fist. When they opened the door I said, "Pigs, sons of the grandest whores, I shit on all of your mothers, on all of the mothers of all the persons who are here." I had the knife ready to use if one of them tried to hurt me.

The woman of the house came forward and said that I was right and they would cease partying. They did. I complained to the administration of the *caserío* again and two weeks later they got me another apartment.

I was lit up inside. I was so mad at the neighbors. I had to teach them shame. I felt an impulse to kill them all, but I tried to control it because I knew they would send me to jail. These people were not worth going to jail for. I was afraid that one day I would have to get out of bed and kill one of them. My wife was very worried. Every time I became impatient she was afraid I would commit a barbarous act and she got nervous. She knows when I am mad I can do violent things. She understands my temperament. She tries to calm me down. She is afraid they may injure me some day. She knows that one day I am going to settle accounts with the neighbors. She is afraid they will catch me some day and they will kill me.

After the Gallardos moved to a different apartment in the same *caserío*, he stopped drinking, and she agreed not to leave him. At this time Mr. Gallardo began to suffer from recurrent stomach aches and his wife developed severe pains in her abdomen. The doctor has told Mrs. Gallardo that she has abcesses in her ovary and needs an operation, but she does not want to have an operation as she has already had four; she is convinced that a woman needs her ovaries. Mrs. Gallardo says she has such severe pain in her ovary that the pain runs down her leg. She has been given medicine and hypodermic injections to alleviate the inflammation, but she is still plagued with it. She has the pain frequently. She says:

> When I have this pain I forget everything else. I have to go to bed. Sometimes I think I have cancer. This has created a great insecurity in me.

Shortly after this, the daughter was hospitalized with a high fever from inflamed tonsils. The family gave her herbs, but the fever did not come down. When she was finally taken to the clinic, she was treated with ice packs, aspirins, enemas, and alcohol rubs; eventually she was given antibiotics and she recovered. Mrs. Gallardo remembers:

> I was desperate. I ran from the hospital to home and back. The doctors did not allow me to stay there at night, but I stayed anyway.

When the child was released from the clinic she was bedridden at home. The parents were so concerned about her that Mr. Gallardo stayed at home to help care for her.

Although he had stopped drinking, Mr. Gallardo re-experienced the very bad stomach aches which had been upsetting him for several months. He began to drink again. By drinking he alleviated the pain for short periods of time, but after 3 or 4 weeks the pain became more severe. He thought he had cancer, ulcers, or tuberculosis in his stomach. When the severe pain recurred whether he was drunk or sober, he became desperate and decided to go to the clinic where the doctor prescribed "an extract made of cod-liver oil." The doctor gave him "a shot of this liquid." When he returned home and was washing his hands, he felt "electricity in my body," as if he had been shocked; he was feverish and his knees shook. He was so weak he was unable to go to work. He was ". . . hardly able to rise," and also, "I lost my affection for my wife and children."

For 4 months Mr. Gallardo did not go to the docks. He was afraid he would get a shock, fall into the water, and drown. The doctor told him not to return to work even though the family needed money. Mrs. Gallardo says, "He got the shakes; his heart almost leaped out of his chest; he had bad thoughts." One time, he grabbed a butcher knife, caught her, and told her his ideas were commanding him to cut her head off and then to cut off the heads of the children too. He got up every morning in a vicious mood. Everything bothered him. The family could not even walk about the house because the noise might upset him.

Mr. Gallardo was convinced he was dying of tuberculosis. During these weeks Mrs. Gallardo was desperate. She knew, as she said, "one doesn't raise oneself from this disease." (Tuberculosis is a death sentence.) Mrs. Gallardo talked him into going to a public health unit for treatment. She accompanied him to this unit where X-rays were taken and examinations made, all of which turned out to be negative. Mr. Gallardo told the doctor about the results of the X-rays taken at the private clinic. The doctor at the public health unit explained to him that there was a small spot revealed by the X-rays, but the spot was on his backbone, not on the lung, and was probably the result of an injury received at an earlier time in his life; it was definitely not tuberculosis. This reassurance calmed him down but he could not get over the obsession that he was afflicted with tuberculosis. Even to this day, he sometimes thinks he has tuberculosis, particularly on days when he has a pain in his back or has a cold.

During this period of economic stress, Mrs. Gallardo's father provided what groceries he could for the family. The Gallardos could not rely upon her father, however, because he had a family of his own to support, and his income was not large enough to support two families. Mrs. Gallardo states, "Whatever food we had I gave to my husband and children." She began to develop dizzy spells; a doctor at the public health clinic told her she had anemia which was making her weak. The doctor told her, "All you need is to eat." This upset Mrs. Gallardo because there was little for her to eat. She did not have the energy to take care of her husband, herself, and the children. Mr. Gallardo was so sick he was unaware of the problems she was facing. She recalls:

> I did not tell him. He simply did not know how sick I was. I had dizzy spells several times a week. I had to go to bed; otherwise I would fall down. I didn't have any energy for anything. My head ached a lot and frequently. In the morning I used to wake up and just want to stay in bed. I couldn't get up. I just didn't have anything inside of me. I went to the doctor and had some shots. He told me to eat some more, but we had no food. I am weak to this day, although my appetite is better.
>
> My husband is very sad and thoughtful. He is always crying. He is in a bad mood. I speak to him and he doesn't hear me. He has bad thoughts of killing me and the children. At times he acts like a *bobo* [foolish person]. He does not eat; he does not sleep. He has bad dreams that I am unfaithful to him. He does not feel well. He has no energy. He hardly wants to eat. He doesn't sleep developing all

those crazy ideas. He tells me he is going to die the same way his brother died. It makes me very nervous.

While Mr. and Mrs. Gallardo were coping with illness, unemployment, and malnutrition, another problem concerning her favorite sister upset Mrs. Gallardo. This sister is married to a severe alcoholic who does not provide adequately for his wife and nine children. They are frequently without food, but, nevertheless, at that time the husband acquired a mistress. The sister became ill and could not eat, even when she had food. Mrs. Gallardo says:

> Sometimes she sends her children here to beg for anything we can send. I cannot send her anything back since we don't have anything. When this occurs I cannot even eat myself thinking of my poor sister. This has had an effect on me. My husband, too, worries very much about it. When he sees those kids coming here and he cannot send anything he is unhappy. He has gone out to try to borrow something to send to them.

At this time Mrs. Gallardo's sister's daughter went to the hospital with a high fever. The doctor ordered a tonsillectomy. Mrs. Gallardo recalls:

> When I heard that she was going to be operated on, I felt very bad thinking something might happen to her. I ran right away to see her.

A few weeks later a nephew of Mrs. Gallardo who had a crossed eye was operated on. The boy's eye was straightened and Mrs. Gallardo was relieved of her anxiety that the boy might be blind from the operation.

At about this time, Mrs. Gallardo's 14-year old brother, with 3 other boys, set fire to an 11-year old boy. Her brother supplied the gasoline which was poured over the victim's head and clothing. Fortunately, the boy did not die from the severe burns; however, the group was placed under the custody of the juvenile court. The brother was paroled to his father who has to watch the boy at all times. Mrs. Gallardo explains:

> From the moment I saw that my father was desperate about this, I became desperate too. My father is the person I love most in my life. I would rather have something happen to me than to my father.

Mrs. Gallardo made an effort to help her father take care of the boy. After he was paroled to the father, she kept the boy in her home for 2 weeks to give her father a rest.

Although Mrs. Gallardo was anxious about the nervous sickness of her husband, she was becoming desperate about their economic situation. There was no food in the house; they owed 3 months' rent on the apartment, and the administration of the *caserío* had sent them a letter telling them their bill had been placed in the hands of lawyers. This confused and upset her. She did not have the money to pay the bill and she did not dare to tell her husband.

Mrs. Gallardo is terrified of the long silent periods during which her husband refuses to talk to anyone. She is particularly concerned about the hatred he has developed for her and the children. He continuously states he is going to die. He talks to her and the children about his pains and his headaches. He keeps asking God not to take him because he wants to raise his children. He sits silently with a picture of his brother in his hands, looks at it pensively, and begins to weep. Half-crying, he says not even his brother's bones are left. Mrs. Gallardo tells us:

> My husband quit work. He could not even recall where he was supposed to go to work. He just forgot all about it. I cannot go to work —I have the children. I wonder what we are going to live on. I go to bed and think only about all these problems, waiting for the new day to see if these problems will be solved. My husband does not worry about it at all; he is so foolish-like.

She uses the term *foolish* here as a descriptive adjective, not in a derogatory way; she means that he acts in a bizarre, random way. She does not understand this is the nature of his mental illness. She goes on to say, "My husband does not talk about going back to work."

Mr. Gallardo has complicated the relations of his wife with her family. An older brother of hers was joking with her son when Mr. Gallardo took offense. Mrs. Gallardo says:

> He got mad and almost beat my brother. They have not spoken to each other since. My husband does not want me to go to my father's house on account of this conflict. I wish such things would not happen. I would like to visit them. My husband does not worry at all about this. He has a grudge against my brother.

Mrs. Gallardo is concerned also about their alienation from their neighbors. She reports:

> We avoid them in order not to embroil ourselves with them. Our neighbors are gossipy; they are immoral. On the stairway you can see daughters of a neighbor kissing boys and feeling them, drinking liquor,

and so on. They have parties until late in the evening. I wish we could have good neighbors. A good neighbor is like a good brother. I don't feel right in having to avoid them. I feel inhibited and rejected. Sometimes when the neighbors are on the sidewalk I don't even dare walk by them. My husband does not worry about avoiding the neighbors. He feels like smashing them with a plank. Some day, he says, he is going to order about twenty caskets, for this is the number of the neighbors he is going to kill.

Mrs. Gallardo has been openly insulted by her neighbors. One woman said to her, "If you don't like shit and piss on the stairs, move to the *Condado*" (a high-priced residential area). According to Mrs. Gallardo, this woman had poured a slop-jar full of urine and feces over a mattress she had airing on the terrace of the apartment. Mrs. Gallardo remonstrated with her and a vicious argument took place. This woman is alleged to have dropped empty milk bottles on the Gallardos' little daughter while she was playing in the entryway to their apartment. Fortunately, she was not hit by the bottles, but the broken bits of glass covered the concrete walkway around the little girl. On another occasion, a young man walking behind Mrs. Gallardo on the sidewalk said, "I am going to kick your ass three times." This unconventional behavior symbolizes the contempt the neighbors have for her.

Mrs. Gallardo tells us her husband's nervous illness has made a tremendous change in her. She suffers from headaches; her "heart is afraid." She goes to the grocery store and forgets what she went after. She has become very fearful of her husband. She says:

> It upsets me. How can one continue to struggle? I suffer by myself. I cannot tell him things knowing he is sick. I don't bring up our problems because I do not want to upset him.

She was so nervous and distraught that when the children cried she jumped up and spanked them. She could not sleep at night for fear her husband would be calling her at any time; she was always afraid. She began to think she was afflicted with the same illness as her husband. She asked the doctor who was attending him if what her husband had was contagious. She recalls:

> I often wondered who was going to take care of all of us if we were all sick. I was very fearful I would die. Who would take care of my children then? My husband did not worry about this at all.

After school opened in the fall, Mrs. Gallardo was called to school to talk with the principal regarding the conduct of her son who repeatedly contradicted the teacher. On one occasion he picked up a chair and hit the teacher with it; another time he tripped her, causing her to fall in the classroom. The principal sent the child to the mental hygiene clinic; the doctor there told the Gallardos the boy should be cared for by a child psychiatrist. This frightens Mrs. Gallardo. She says: "Sometimes I think it might be his age. If God is willing, he will improve later on." Her husband makes fearful predictions for his son. Mrs. Gallardo relates:

> A few days ago my husband read in the newspaper of a man who was in jail for murder. This man was born by a Caesarean section. At the age of 16 he killed a girl. My husband says this could be the case with our son who was also born by Caesarean section.

A few days after Mrs. Gallardo was burdened with the problem of her son's emotional difficulty, a "hammer" hit her hand. The hammer kept pounding her and she could not make it stop. It hit her first upon the middle finger and then on the hand. Gradually, her left hand and arm became paralyzed. This imaginary beating coincided with a particularly bad spell of her husband. Urged by his wife, Mr. Gallardo went with her to a psychiatrist at the clinic for help. The psychiatrist asked him if he wanted to be sent to the psychiatric hospital. Mr. Gallardo refused, explaining he could not leave his wife and children, but Mrs. Gallardo thought it might be a good idea for him to stay there for a while.

Mr. Gallardo was the person we had originally screened for our study. We found he satisfied the criteria for inclusion in the study and he consented to be part of it. We took Mrs. Gallardo to the psychiatrist for a routine part of our mental status examination program for both spouses. The psychiatrist diagnosed her as a simple schizophrenic.

The Gallardo family are Job incarnate. They experienced more problems during the 18-month period covered by their extended problematic year than either of the other sick family types. (This is also true for the other three families in which both the husband and the wife are schizophrenic.) The Gallardos were plagued with the illness of their children and the death of a baby. Mrs. Gallardo underwent a major operation. Mr. Gallardo suffered from facial paralysis and the threat of tuberculosis. He was out of work for 3 months; then came the strike and more unemployment. As the months dragged by, he became too ill to work more than part time. After his psychotic episode, he quit work entirely. The family was almost wholly dependent on Mrs. Gallardo's father for their meager rations. Mr. Gallardo's brother died of tuberculosis. Mrs. Gallardo's sister's husband abandoned her and their nine children. Relations between the spouses became so strained that Mr. Gallardo threatened to kill his wife and children. Relations with the neighbors grew worse until the Gallardos moved from one building in the *caserío* to another, where they soon alienated their new neighbors. Both spouses were frustrated by their illnesses, their debts, their inability to help themselves, and their dependence on their relatives. The enigmatic behavior of their son was also frightening them. The onset of schizophrenic symptoms in Mr. Gallardo first, then the hallucinatory episode of the hammer by Mrs. Gallardo are sequelae to the multiplicity of problems with which they grappled through the long months of the problematic year. The tangled skein of misery that enmeshed them, whatever the cause or causes, was not unraveled by their escape into schizophrenia. They are trapped by their problems.

11
Mental Illness

Mental illness is a familiar part of life in Puerto Rico. From the time they were children, all the persons studied have seen disheveled and tattered men and women who meander purposelessly, posture, and speak to imaginary audiences. Some three-fourths of them have had to cope with the wild and irrational behavior of a relative. A person afflicted with the most familiar and stereotyped form of mentally disturbed behavior is known as a *loco*.

This chapter discusses three points, all related to the cultural definition of *loco*. The first section presents the beliefs and attitudes which sick and well persons have about and toward the *loco*. It describes how a *loco* is expected to behave. Folk theories to explain how a person becomes deranged, how he *should be* treated, and how he *is* treated are presented. The second part of the chapter outlines the sick person's experiences with mental illness which have led him to fear being labeled a *loco*. A variety of bewildering symptoms, aches, and pains torment the sick person. To understand these unpleasant experiences, the sick person classifies his illness as nervousness and develops explanations for it, but the effect of the illness is to make him believe that he is becoming a *loco*, a terrifying possibility. The third part of the chapter presents data to answer a question which is central in the thought of the schizophrenic person: How can I avoid being labeled a *loco?*

The lengthy participation of the fieldworkers in the life of the families, the neighborhoods where the families live, and the broader community enabled them to observe directly recurrent social processes centering upon the role of the *loco*. In addition, each husband and wife was asked what came into his mind when he thought of a *loco* and to describe the behavior of such a person. Finally, each was asked: "If you were single, would you marry a person such as the one you have described?" Although the question provided for answers of "yes" or "no," it was designed to provoke the person into giving rich "spill-out" information resulting from the uncomfortable intimacy of a marital union and the incongruent stigma of a deviant spouse who acts like a *loco*.

The *loco* is viewed as a dangerous person given to sudden acts of extraordinary violence. Typical comments are: "A *loco* can strike you dead quicker than a bolt of lightning." "If you turn your back, a *loco* will stick a knife into you." "If I married a *loca*, she could kill the children suddenly." "If I had one [a *loco*] in the house I would not sleep because I would have to keep my eye on him for fear he would kill me." The fury of the *loco* is different from other kinds of violence, such as fist fights which are relatively common in slum and *caserío* life. Fist fights between men and hair pulling and scratching among women are focused acts of violence provoked by insinuations, breaches of proper conduct, or a show of disrespect. Indeed, to engage an opponent bravely in a proficient display of fisticuffs is a singular mark of a *macho*. The motives of the opponents are understandable and so is the form that the violence takes, but the violence of a *loco* is disorganized, unpredictable, and directed toward persons in general, not an identifiable culprit or opponent. Since a *loco* has not been provoked deliberately, it is difficult for others to understand the motives for his violence.

Although most *locos* are violent, some are not. There is a type of "crazy" person referred to as a *loco tranquilo* (the crazy but quiet person), who is viewed not as a menace but as foolish, incapacitated, and childlike. Although his behavior is as bizarre as that of the violent *loco*, he is not considered to be a menace since he does not pose a threat of violence. The tranquil *loco* is usually accepted as a marginal participant in social groups that congregate in neighborhoods, market places, and around small bars and street corners. At times he may be the focal point of attention, particularly when he acts like a clown. One *loco tranquilo* dresses himself in a Mexican sombrero with a leather chin cord, a red bandana, cowboy boots, and a large policeman's whistle hung around his neck on a string; in holsters that dangle to his knees, tied to his thighs in the fashion of a quick-draw cowboy, he has two .44 caliber cap pistols. He often stands in the middle of a busy intersection directing heavy traffic with forceful gestures and the aid of his whistle. His performance has an air of unquestionable authority. The drivers of cars obey him good-naturedly and wave to him as they pass. This bold burlesque serves to ridicule public officials and public agencies, and it delights the friends of this *loco tranquilo;* they stand on the sidewalk and applaud his antics.

Both calm and violent *locos* are expected to perform improper and immoral acts centering around sex and excretory functions. Innumerable examples were cited from personal experiences to confirm the impropriety, immorality, and criminal behavior of the *loco*. *Locos* urinate and defecate in the streets; they play and smear themselves with feces. They masturbate openly and strut naked in public places. They have sexual intercourse with animals. They scream obscenities in public. They may sexually attack children and infants. Closely related to the theme of immorality that can be expected of *locos* is that of criminal behavior. Since *locos* lose the conception of private property, they steal; they throw rocks, falsify checks, kill children. Several persons describe struggles they have had to prevent some *loco* from setting fire to a house. Mrs. Julía claims a neighbor was made *loca* by her husband's false accusations that she was pregnant with another man's child. She meandered in the neighborhood, dressed in a nightgown. She sat on the curb, picked up her nightgown, spread her legs, opened the lips of her genitals, and screamed: "Come men, lick me like dogs! You men are dogs, so come lick." In brief, one can expect any form of outrageous behavior from a *loco*.

Locos are easily recognized: their eyes bulge in an unfocused and vague manner; they are filthy and disheveled; they have uncontrollable facial twitches. They seldom bathe; their clothes are stained and tattered and their skin is covered with mud and feces. They carry fleas and bedbugs. They swat at imaginary flies. They meander without purpose, sometimes quickening their pace as if a tormenting spirit were pursuing them. In convivial groups of persons who are joking lightheartedly, the *loco* may appear to be in deep introspective thought. At other times, he may laugh hilariously when nothing funny has occurred. *Locos* respond to the "ant hill in their minds" or the "roller skate in their brains" rather than to the surroundings.

Locos cannot assume responsibilities, are not productive, and, in fact, interfere with productive efforts since they require supervision. Some *locos* speak a strange and unknown language as if "the spirit of a foreigner had invaded their souls"; other *locos* can be understood but they say ridiculous things or refer to themselves as notable persons like Fidel Castro, Muños Marín, Adolf Hitler, or Queen Isabella.

Practically all persons raised indignant objections to marrying a *loco*. The idea is abhorred as repugnant. Compounding the danger of injury is the problem of responsibility for the criminal and immoral behavior of a fickle-tempered, deranged mate. To be married to a *loco* is to be scorned, branded, and viewed with suspicion: one must be at least partly *loco* to marry one. Seventy-seven of the 80 persons say they would not marry a *loco*; 2 of the remaining 3 quickly add that they would not marry a *loco loco* who is violent, but they might marry a *loco tranquilo* who is peaceful. According to Mr. Lebrón, the problems in marriage would be aggravated by the taunts and ridicule of men who also could seek advantage of such a wife: "If I married a *loca*, any man could come here and fuck her." Other persons replied: "That would be like putting a hangman's noose around my neck." "I would rather marry one of those horses in that pasture." "I would have to be a *loco* to marry one." "If you marry a *loco*, you don't know the difference between day and night." "If I had a *loca* in the house I would hit her over the head with a chair."

Schizophrenic persons are particularly vulnerable to being assigned the role of the *loco*. Consequently, we explored the possibility that the schizophrenic's portrayal of this role would be drawn in less harsh and more benign terms than that drawn by well people. This idea was erroneous! There is no tendency on the part of the schizophrenics to soften the portrait of the *loco*; sick and well persons describe him as violent, immoral, criminal, filthy, idiosyncratic, and worthless. Moreover, men and women do not differ in their conceptions of the *loco*. Their views are uniform and deep; perhaps they are fixed unalterably.

The *loco* has a clearly defined role in the Puerto Rican social structure. The credentials for assuming this role are easily earned if deviant behavior is visible and dramatic. Once, as a fieldworker went to interview Mrs. Aparicio, a mentally healthy woman, she noticed a crowd in front of the *caserío* where Mrs. Aparicio lives. Mrs. Aparicio, who was in the crowd, came running to inform her in an excited voice that Isabel, a next-door neighbor and intimate friend, had become a *loca*. For many hours Isabel had been weeping uncontrollably, screaming, and calling Mrs. Aparicio to come and help her. The interviewer continues:

> The number of curious persons increased. There were about 100 persons in the crowd which was composed of youngsters, teenagers, and adults. Suddenly, the door of Isabel's apartment opened, and everyone screamed wildly and fled in agitation, yelling that the *loca* was about to come out of her apartment.
> Mrs. Aparicio hurried her two children into her apartment, screaming at me to follow. I hurried into her apartment with Mrs. Aparicio.

She told me in a high-pitched voice, "She is a *loca*; I wish I could tell you how afraid I am of *locas*." She locked the windows and doors of her apartment and pushed the heavy furniture in the living room against the doors that led to the outside. She said, "Look, if Isabel comes through that door I will hide with my children in the bathroom so that you can face her in the living room." Suddenly, she thought of a better idea and said to me in a loud voice,"Run, get your car. Drive it by the back window; my children and I will get into your car and we will all go away. I don't want to be near a *loca*." Although we were standing next to each other, she shouted at me.

Her two children were calm but she told them, "Don't cry; don't be afraid. Stick close to me. This lady will take us for a ride in her car. We will go to Grandmother's house right away and we will not return even in a month unless Isabel is taken to the insane asylum." After this, she went into her room, found shoes and stockings for her children, and began to dress them, all the while commanding them not to scream, not to cry, not to run away.

I tried to calm Mrs. Aparicio by telling her that we were safer in the apartment because the doors and windows were locked, and I also told her there were many people in the yard who would not let Isabel break down the door of the apartment. She calmed down and said, "Since I was a child I have had a fear of *locos*." She opened the window slightly to see what the crowd was doing. Isabel was still screaming for her good friend Mrs. Aparicio.

Mrs. Aparicio told me that Isabel's husband, who is a baker, did not know what was going on because he had gone to work as usual. Someone had gone for him at the baker's. Three-quarters of an hour elapsed. A taxi arrived with Isabel's husband. He ran to the door of his apartment and tried to open it, but Isabel had locked herself in. Her husband was a big, powerful man. He kicked the door and beat it with his fists until finally the lock broke. We walked out to the yard when he broke in. By this time Isabel had armed herself with a knife. Her husband punched her on the chin and she fell to the floor unconscious. He picked her up, wrapped a sheet around her, and carried her to the taxi which took her to the insane asylum.

The crowd followed behind Isabel's husband. There was a lot of talk. One neighbor asked Mrs. Aparicio if she would take care of Isabel's three children. Mrs. Aparicio replied that she could not because her own were plenty of work. Later, she told me that she would not take care of Isabel's children because they belong to a *loca* and the *loca* might break out of the asylum and crash into her apartment to see her children. Mrs. Aparicio said she wanted to get out of that *caserío*. She was going to insist that her husband move to a new, private development being built on the outskirts of the town. She said, "I have seen so much of *caserío* life. Now that I have seen Isabel a *loca*, I have seen everything."

According to the psychiatrist's evaluation, Mrs. Aparicio is not an anxious person. Her fear of *locos* is shared by others who panic at the prospect of confronting such a person, but the danger seen in a *loco* often is caused by the reactions of others. Isabel's weird crying and screaming were sufficient to have the neighbors immediately label and treat her as a *loca;* once the crowd had make this identification, it reacted to Isabel as if she were dangerous. It is important to note, however, that Isabel did not arm herself with a knife until she saw the crowd milling outside her door.

The role of the *loco* may also be assigned gradually through a neighbor's observation of and gossip about idiosyncratic behavior. Whether sudden or gradual, however, the assignment of this role represents the fruition of an almost irreversible social process: that is, once the person is known as a *loco*, he will be known as such in the foreseeable future.

Considerable efforts are made to restrain or incarcerate a person who is viewed as insane. Early in the study, several families who kept mentally deranged relatives in locked rooms were discovered. One woman was kept in a small locked room by her son and daughter-in-law. To feed her, the door was opened slightly, food was put on the floor, and the door was quickly locked. Periodically, the son physically subdued his mother while his wife cleaned out the refuse which had accumulated in the room: feces, urine, ripped blankets and sheets, and remnants of rotting food. The son and daughter believe that by imprisoning her they are protecting themselves and the neighbors; nevertheless, both are fearful that the prisoner will escape or set fire to the house.

Strong reservations are expressed about the possibility of "curing" a *loco*. Several persons state that even if it were possible to "cure" a *loco* the person in question should still be treated "as if he were a *loco*." A *loco* is forever capable of exploding into wild and erratic acts of violence, and one must be prepared for this contingency. Thus, one woman notes that when she has unavoidable contact with a neighbor whose *locura* has improved considerably, she makes certain that there are avenues of escape. Although *locos* may lapse temporarily into more or less normal behavior, at any moment they may revert to outrageous behavior. The unfavorable prognosis attached to *locos* means, sociologically, that the assignment of this role pins the person into a position in the social structure from which it is difficult, if not impossible, to escape.

All persons were asked to tell us what should be done with *locos*. The tacit perspective assumed in replying to this question is not that of the *loco* but that of the person confronted with one. Thus the most common reply is that *locos* should be put in the insane asylum where they can be kept behind bars and fences under careful supervision; 80 per cent of the men and 75 per cent of the women make this recommendation. If this cannot be done, the *loco* should be kept at home by his family, confined and guarded. The harshest recommendation was made by a schizophrenic man who believes that for the benefit of society all *locos* should be summarily executed. Whereas the violent *loco* should be avoided and/or removed from the main channels of social life, different recommendations are offered for the *loco tranquilo*. Some persons believe that the *loco tranquilo* should be put in the insane asylum; most believe that he can be kept at home where he can be permitted freedom as long as some person assumes the responsibility of keeping him clean, supervising him, and answering for his foolish misdeeds.

The role of the *loco* presents a problem to nearly all schizophrenic persons but to only a few who are free of the illness. Sick persons are extraordinarily defensive about the topic of the *loco*. Time and again, they state that they are not *locos* when no such question is being asked. When asked directly, only one sick person states that he is a *loco*; only one spouse of a sick person asserts this of his mate. The remaining persons in the sick group do not admit to *locura*. Rather, after a forceful denial, they add such phrases as: "Sometimes I act like one, but I am not one." "I may eventually become one, but I am not one now." "If I don't get help, I may become a *loco*." "Perhaps I am on the road to becoming one." "Only at times do I act like a *loco*." Table 35 reports the results of the question asked of all the respondents, "Have you felt that you are becoming a *loco?*" Of the schizophrenic men, 100 per cent feel sometimes or often that they are going to become *locos*. The comparable percentage for the men who are not schizophrenic is 17. The pattern is repeated in the replies of the females. Ninety-two per cent of those who are sick think, at least sometimes, that they are becoming *locas*, and only 30 per cent of those who are not schizophrenic feel the same way. Random variation does not account for these results. Moreover, the statistical significance of the relationship is not affected by sex.

Of the 24 schizophrenic persons only Mrs. Quiromo states that she

TABLE 35 Replies to Question: "Have You Felt That You Are Becoming a *Loco?*"

	N	OFTEN OR SOMETIMES, %	NEVER, %
A. Males			
Nonschizophrenic	29	17	83
Schizophrenic	11	100	0
$p < .01$			
B. Females			
Nonschizophrenic	27	30	70
Schizophrenic	13	92	8
$p < .01$			

has never had this fear, yet she has had the label of *loca* attached to her more often and by more persons than any other schizophrenic in our study. She is engaged in a struggle against this label. Consequently, she does not admit to fears about becoming a *loca* since this would give recognition to the damaging opinions of her critics and tormentors. Mrs. Quiromo has withdrawn from social contacts. Day after day, she sits in a corner of her small shack complaining about her symptoms: she is afraid to leave her home; she is tired and confused; she has reduced her activity to a vegetable-like pace. Mrs. Quiromo's mother and her husband, who himself is a schizophrenic, have accused her of being a *loca* in the presence of other persons. Mr. Quiromo has ridiculed her in public by making gestures to indicate that his wife is a *loca*. Recently, neighbors have begun to do the same thing. Mrs. Quiromo says:

> Just to hear the word *loca* is enough to make me upset and nervous. I don't know why this is. I used to hear this word without getting nervous at all.

Mrs. Quiromo, however, is the exception. Significantly more sick than well persons fear that they are going to become *locos*. The riddles posed by schizophrenic symptoms create this fear, but at least as important as the symptoms is the fact that each sick person is behaving in some way like a *loco* and is being treated like a *loco* more frequently than are the persons not afflicted with this illness. One woman repeatedly rips her clothes and then asks her husband to repair them. Another woman no longer bathes and grooms herself, although a few months before she took great pride in her appearance. A sick husband never changes his clothes despite the fact that his wife has washed and ironed clothing for him. These persons have begun to resemble *locos* in appearance and have raised questions in the minds of their neighbors and families.

Mrs. Herrero tells us about her husband.

> A while back he came home, turned off the light, and then ran out of the house. Some friends of mine that were here pursued him, trying to catch him. They couldn't reach him. We would see him and call him, and then he would hide again. Finally, we just left him, and I went to my brother's house. I was afraid. Next day, he came to my mother's house, uncombed and with ripped clothing. My mother thought something had happened at our home. He asked about the children. My mother told him she thought they were at home. She asked him in and gave him coffee and let him sleep. I went to my mother's to tell her what happened, and my parents helped him back to our apartment. He would not eat or sleep, and he looked foolish walking all over the house without any purpose.

Mr. Gallardo cannot stand the sight of his children, even when they are behaving well. Periodically he launches into them with his fists or whips them with a belt until they are a mass of welts. Voices have told him to cut off the heads of his wife and children. Mrs. Gallardo's fear that her husband is becoming a *loco* is based on these incidents. Mr. Berríos set fire to his wooden shack, but the neighbors put the fire out before it could burn down. He cannot recall doing this although the charred interior of his home serves as a reminder to his wife of the irrational and dangerous things he is capable of doing. Mr. Santano repeatedly slices his forearm with a razor blade, adding new wounds to a mass of criss-crossed scar tissue.

Such dramatic acts are often done in the presence of spouses, relatives, friends, neighbors, or associates at work. To the observers the sick person appears to be behaving like a *loco*. The story of the deviant behavior is passed on to others who may not have been witnesses. The discrete bits of idiosyncratic behavior are pieced together into a composite portrait of the person as a *loco*; from this process the sick person's fear of *locura* emerges.

The dark imagery of the *loco* is a hard and fixed part of the social reality to which the sick person responds. Trapped between the unfolding social process which classifies him as a *loco* and the hard outlines of this stigmatized life, the sick person, nevertheless, does not view the *loco* role as more acceptable to him. A *loco* is a *loco* and few if any modifications can be made. No person, sick or well, is "out of contact" with the realities of this role.

The sick person reacts to the harsh realities of this problem by denying that he is a *loco* and by insisting that he has a "nervous condition." The term utilized most frequently by sick persons to identify their illness is "nervousness." To compare how many sick and well persons experience "nervousness," we asked each of them: "Do you suffer from nervousness?" The answers to this question, shown in Table 36, reveal a statistically significant relationship between schizophrenia and the experience of nervousness in both sexes. The overall pattern shows that all the sick persons and about one-half the well persons experience nervousness.

Schizophrenic persons have a richer, more detailed idea of the meaning of "nervousness" than the persons who are well. To the well persons, nervousness describes nothing more than occasional feelings of anxiety, but to the sick person nervousness means symptoms which are not as intense as those of the *loco*. The nervous person is angered; the *loco* becomes violent. The nervous person is worried; the *loco* is distraught. The nervous person is restless; the *loco* meanders. The nervous person does not behave in grossly improper ways; the *loco* does. Moreover, a nervous person is nervous only at certain times; the *loco* is bizarre at all times.

Moments of tranquility and security are seized on by the sick persons and their spouses to validate their case for nervousness and to invalidate the judgment of *locura*. They believe, however, that a nervous condition is the first step in the direction of becoming a *loco*, as shown by Mrs. Lebrón's statement: "I think my mind and my cere-

TABLE 36 Replies to Question: "Do You Suffer from Nervousness?"

	N	OFTEN OR SOMETIMES, %	NEVER, %
A. Males			
Nonschizophrenic	29	41	59
Schizophrenic	11	100	0
$p < .01$			
B. Females			
Nonschizophrenic	27	69	31
Schizophrenic	13	100	0
$p < .05$			

brum are on the track leading to *locura*. They are subject to nervous deviation."

Each person studied was brought to a psychiatrist for a diagnostic evaluation. The visit to the psychiatrist was an important event in their lives; they dressed and groomed themselves carefully for it. Some persons, knowing that a psychiatrist is a doctor to whom *locos* are taken, wondered if their sanity was being questioned. Their fears were alleviated when we told them they were going not to the psychiatric hospital but, by appointment, to the psychiatrist's private office where they would not have to sit in a waiting room with persons who act strangely, like *locos*.

Some weeks later, the sick persons were asked by the fieldworkers if they knew the cause or causes of their affliction. This question was followed by a number of probes which were designed to provide as complete a statement of causes as the sick person could give. *All the sick persons have ideas about the causes of their affliction.* They believe social experiences such as problems at work and in the family, worries, frustrations, and suffering due to the death or illness of a relative induced the illness. Some replies denote causes which are patently not social and psychological, such as "punishment by the spirits," "black magic," and "God's punishment due to a neglect of my religious obligations." One man attributes his illness to the effect on his brain of too much drinking. Another believes a prior illness is the cause. No sick person attributes his illness to heredity or to malformation of the brain.

We wanted to know how many sick persons rely entirely or partly upon stressful social experiences to explain the illness. To answer this question, we classified each person's explanation into one of three groups: (1) socially stressful experiences only; (2) socially stressful experiences as well as other types of causes such as bewitchment, illness, or alcohol; and (3) explanations other than social stress. The classifications are admittedly gross but, nonetheless, indicative of the dominant explanations adduced by the sick persons.

1. Sixty per cent of the sick persons based their entire explanation on life problems, worries, and frustrations. The sick men emphasize problems at work, attributing their illness to the pressing demands of dictatorial bosses, co-workers who taunt and ridicule, and the general unpleasantness of struggling for a living. The sick women focus on family life and emphasize the conflict with their husbands and other relatives; they also consider the anguish of death in the family to be a

determinant. Mrs. Urrutia's concept is typical of this first category of explanation. She says, "My condition is due to the struggle I have had with the sickness of my mother." Mrs. Urrutia and her mother live in the same household and both women experience many of the same symptoms. Mrs. Urrutia feels her husband is also a source of her nervousness.

> God only knows how I have suffered because of my husband. When I ran off with him he often got drunk. Then we fought. During those fights he tried to humiliate me by telling me that I ran off with him without being legally married. My husband dislikes my mother and many times is disrespectful toward her. One night I went to look for him and found him in a bar, drinking with another woman. I beat this woman, but my husband left the bar and did not return for several hours. After this incident, I always followed him when he went out. I thought he had another woman. Incidents like this have made me sick.

2. Twenty-five per cent of the sick persons believe the illness has emerged from social as well as nonsocial causes. Mr. Santano believes his illness is the result of the incessant battle he has with his demanding, hostile, and aggressive wife, who also suffers from schizophrenia, the noise at the electric plant where he worked, and the weakness he felt from undernourishment. The prime culprit, however, is his mother-in-law. According to Mr. Santano, his mother-in-law has bewitched other members of the family, even causing her former husband to become completely bald; he says:

> My mother-in-law has me bewitched. When my wife and I fight, my mother-in-law allies herself with my wife. She has also bewitched her own brother. She is the type of person who enjoys pulling out two eyes instead of one.

3. The remaining 15 per cent of the sick persons explain their illness by referring only to the world of spirits, to the actions of God, to bewitchments, and to physical weakness resulting from a prior illness. Although these persons also report having experienced many personal and family problems, they are not considered to be causes of the affliction.

Most schizophrenic persons seek explanations for the illness in the personal problems and conflicts they have had in their lives. Since the illness is complex and the symptoms pervasive and vacillating, a number of causes, not just one, are cited in each explanation. Were the illness specific and confined to one part of the body, the explanations adduced would perhaps also be simple. Sick persons believe the bewildering onrush of many fickle but tormenting symptoms must have been preceded by a set of causes.

The sick persons do not uniquely and individually formulate explanations to account for their nervousness. Explanations are developed in interaction with their spouses and by talking to relatives, friends, neighbors, and associates. The husbands and wives of the afflicted persons have explanations for the illness similar to those of the sick persons, one-half viewing social experiences as the source of the illness.

The culture provides the same set of explanations for the symptoms of the schizophrenic as for the extraordinary actions of the *loco*. Mrs. Núñez believes:

> *Locura* is caused by problems in life and worries. The mind is invaded by these things. Suffering causes *locura* also. If one is frightened suddenly or hears bad news, one can become a *loco*. Hunger also causes it since the moment comes when one is so weak that the mind is lost.

Compounding the dilemma of the sick person who wants to avoid the stigma of the *loco* is the belief that the causes of schizophrenia and *locura* are the same. Underlying the common explanations for the nervousness of the schizophrenic and the bizarreness of the *loco*, there is a moral logic which stipulates that the causes are all evil. The axiom that bad effects must have bad causes is rooted firmly in the culture. Nowhere do we find acts of kindness, a benevolent spouse, or moderation in drink or habit cited as causes. Unpleasant events and arguments at home or at work are believed to be important. Illness is not the work of a good God but of a thundering punitive one. It is a bad spirit or a bad person availing himself of the instrument of bewitchment who is responsible.

The sick persons believe their nervousness was ushered in by an invasion of symptoms that was sudden, not gradual. Suddenly, they experienced fever, chills, pain in the heart and stomach, headaches, trembling hands, fears, itchy skin, swollen varicose veins, loss of breath, and hot fluids and gasses in their stomachs. They also began to hear voices and have visions, changing moods, and nightmares; they spoke incoherently, exploded into fits, withdrew from other persons, could not sleep, and were weary.

The sudden advent of this variety of symptoms leads each person to believe that his nervousness began at one specific point in his past. Three of the twenty-four schizophrenic persons believe the illness began before their present marriage, antedating it by a mean of 3 years. Twenty-one of the schizophrenic persons, or 88 per cent, believe that the onset of the nervousness occurred during the present marriage, a mean of 6 years having elapsed from the time of the marriage to the time they believe their nervous illness to have started.

The date of the onset is embedded firmly in the minds of the sick persons. When the question of date of onset was raised in many different forms and at many different times during the interviews, the same date of onset was always given. Most spouses agree with the sick person on the dating of the first symptoms, but there is, of course, no way of knowing if the date of the perceived onset coincides with the actual beginning of the schizophrenic process. All sick persons have detailed recollections of the first experience of the symptoms.

Mr. Ramos says:

> Suddenly I became forgetful, and when I looked at things they seemed to be going around. I had bad, wrong dreams, and I could not sleep. I became fearful, even of little things. I felt like a person full of problems without being able to do anything about them. I thought I was going to die and would be put in a casket. My heart beat faster and I felt so afraid. My side hurt. I couldn't drive a car because my legs shook. My hands trembled. I couldn't control myself. I was in a bad mood for no reason. When my boss reprimanded me for being forgetful I told him to go to hell. I started to drink liquor and come home late. I wanted to lie down in my bed, lock myself in my room, and not see anyone.

All the sick persons resemble Mr. Ramos in having experienced an acute onrush of symptoms, but, unlike Mr. Ramos, some believe that specific events initiated the nervous condition. Mr. Gallardo reports that he went to a clinic because he was very tired and was given a "shot of cod-liver oil," after which he went home and drank a bottle of milk of magnesia, three Alka-Seltzers, and half a bottle of Pepto-Bismol—then, suddenly, his nervous symptoms began.

An unexpected traumatic event is seen by some sick persons to have initiated the nervous illness. Mr. Cardona became distraught when his 4-year old son had a violent reaction to a small-pox vaccination. Tormented by the idea that his son would die, the father immediately succumbed to a nervous illness. Drunken sprees, prolonged labor in childbirth, and fights with neighbors and associates at work are also believed to have started the nervous afflictions, but, regardless of what the precipitants are thought to be, the illness brings, in the words of one man, "an explosion" of physical and mental disturbances which overwhelm the person with a feeling of malaise.

The sick persons and their spouses believe that the nervousness of the sick person requires the control of the environment in the setting of the home and the neighborhood rather than the control of the person through confinement, as is recommended for the *loco*. Since turmoil in the social scene is believed to be responsible for the nervous condition, tranquility and rest are recommended. Conflicts should be avoided and recreation provided. These recommendations are logically related to what the sick person and his spouse consider to be the causes of the illness.

They believe that good care and adequate medical attention can prevent the nervous person from becoming a *loco*; the most important way is to provide a tranquil environment. Thus, 60 per cent of the sick persons and the same percentage of their spouses state, without being given a choice of answers, that they or their spouses need rest and tranquility to alleviate their nervousness. The nervous person should receive medical attention, consisting of thorough physical examinations and laboratory tests; X-rays should be used to look into their heads to find out what is going on. Vitamins should be prescribed and drugs should be given to alleviate anxiety. They also want shots to be given, although they do not specify what the contents should be. (The air of therapeutic mystery that surrounds the syringe and needle is also important.) These persons want a direct and forceful medical penetration to get them off the road leading to *locura*, since strong reservations are expressed about curing a *loco*. Although social experiences are emphasized as much to explain *locura* as to explain nervousness, such recommendations are rarely offered for the treatment of a *loco*.

Before they received psychiatric care, several schizophrenic persons were of the opinion that the type of psychiatric care received by nervous persons and *locos* differs. They thought *locos* were interned at the insane asylum whereas nervous persons receive ambulatory care. They no longer believe that this is the case, however, because many of the persons receiving out-patient care, with whom they sat in the waiting room, were, from their point of view, *locos*. This was an upsetting experience to the sick persons, and now they do not make the distinction between in-patient and out-patient psychiatric care.

In brief, the schizophrenic persons' description of symptoms is designed in such a way as *to differentiate nervousness from locura*. Indeed, the manner in which the concept of nervousness is elaborately defined represents an effort to separate it from the imagery of the *loco*. Otherwise subtle distinctions important to the sick person are sharpened; in effect, to challenge them is to question the boundaries of his sanity.

The experience of multiple attacks on the body, the overwhelming malaise, continues to be present. Table 37 shows that proportionately more sick than well persons feel that they have all sorts of ailments in different parts of their bodies. This difference is statistically significant among the men and the women. Those persons who have multiple ailments *but who are not schizophrenic* do not point to a time in their lives when they experienced a sudden and violent onrush of symptoms. The multiple ailments are composed of aches and pains and symptoms which vary in intensity from day to day, even disappearing on some days: trembling hands do not tremble on some days; headaches come and go. Some days even bring a complete remission of symptoms, but they disappear only to be replaced by equally distressing ones: headaches no longer occur, but joints begin to ache; nausea is replaced by nightmares; fainting spells give way to a painful gaseous stomach. In the vernacular, "If it isn't one thing, it's another."

Table 38 shows that, irrespective of sex, proportionately more afflicted persons report having aches and pains that come and go than those who are not afflicted with schizophrenia.

Nervousness has brought a deep and persistent fear. Anxieties make the sick person act as if he were under threat even though there are no external dangers; bad news, insults, injuries, and attacks are awaited with trepidation. Ordinary experiences become imbued with extraor-

TABLE 37 Replies to Question: "Do You Feel That You Have All Sorts of Ailments in Different Parts of Your Body?"

	N	OFTEN AND SOMETIMES, %	NEVER, %
A. Males			
Nonschizophrenic	29	41	59
Schizophrenic	11	82	18
$p < .05$			
B. Females			
Nonschizophrenic	27	33	67
Schizophrenic	13	92	8
$p < .01$			

TABLE 38 Replies to Question: "Do You Have Aches and Pains That Seem to Come and Go?"

	N	OFTEN AND SOMETIMES, %	NEVER, %
A. Males			
Nonschizophrenic	29	55	45
Schizophrenic	11	91	9
$p < .05$			
B. Females			
Nonschizophrenic	27	41	59
Schizophrenic	13	92	8
$p < .01$			

dinary threats: "I keep my children in the house because they will get killed outside." Mr. Herrero refuses to enter his house until his wife makes sure that nobody is inside who wants to kill him; despite his wife's assurance that no one is in the house, he continues to sleep with a machete under his pillow.

The sick persons' fears are centered upon a number of identifiable events, objects, and situations, the major ones being their wretchedness and the fear of the future. When distressed, they feel that they "fall apart" or lose control of themselves. They are unable to tolerate the usual noises of *caserío* and slum life. They are haunted by the question, "*Will I become a loco?*" The sick men are anxious about their inability to provide for their families and, even more, about the difficulty of presenting themselves "in a normal way" to other persons. The subtle nuances of interaction, performed routinely and acceptably by husbands who are not ill, are problematical to the sick. The usual routine of seeing and speaking to other persons is thrown into question, and doubts emerge. Fears of doing things incorrectly pervade the day-to-day activities. Mr. Espinosa says:

> I don't feel satisfaction in talking to other people. I have been robbed of my personality. I am not the same person. I feel desperate. I don't want to go out. I would like to go on errands and do things correctly, but I can't do them correctly.

Sick women fear that a relative may die or be injured. Whenever Mrs. Iglesias hears a child cry she immediately runs out of her shanty to scan the lagoon in fear that one of her children has drowned. To hear a child cry upsets her whole day. Another sick woman has nightmares in which Catholic nuns parade by, chanting funeral orations over caskets with the bodies of her relatives.

Although angered by her husband, the sick wife is fearful of him. Her fear of his rough commands often borders on panic, as evidenced by her trembling and stuttering when her husband comes home. Mrs. Lebrón says:

> When my husband comes home and opens his mouth I cannot do anything. Do you know what it is like to live with a man who comes home only to fight?

The sexual demands of the husband also create anxieties in the sick wife. If she denies her husband sexual access, he is angered and seeks other sexual outlets; if she submits she feels ill because of her deep repugnance toward sexual intercourse. Mrs. Padilla states:

> How tired and weary I am from my husband wanting to have me every night. My husband has halitosis, putrid teeth, and stinks. I can't stand his trying to kiss me. It upsets me.

To describe the unpleasantness of their inner life, sick persons often use metaphors: "a churning inside of me"; "a restless spirit inside of me"; "a machine inside of me that goes faster and faster"; and more often, "an electrical charge that goes through my body." Anxiety expresses itself also in a number of somatic reactions and complaints. Each person was asked several questions pertaining to his experience with symptoms of anxiety. The analysis of the replies shows that when sex is controlled and the sick and the well compared, consistently more sick than well persons experience the following: [1]

1. Trembling hands that upset them
2. Very hard beating of the heart
3. Dizzy spells
4. Shortness of breath while not exercising
5. Cold sweats
6. Throbbing of pulse in the neck
7. Tight chest

The sick and well persons among the husbands and among the wives differ significantly in each of these seven symptoms; proportionately more sick than well persons have these symptoms. The pattern is uniform and clear. Physically, the sick persons are reacting as if they

---
[1] See Appendix 3 for these tabulations.

TABLE 39 Replies to Question: "Do You Have Periods of Fatigue or General Weakness?"

	N	OFTEN OR SOMETIMES, %	NEVER, %
A. Males			
Nonschizophrenic	29	45	55
Schizophrenic	11	100	0
$p < .01$			
B. Females			
Nonschizophrenic	27	59	41
Schizophrenic	13	100	0
$p < .01$			

were exposed to objective dangers. They brace themselves incessantly for an attack. Understandably, they all suffer from periods of fatigue or general weakness. Table 39 shows that when sex is controlled, proportionately more sick than well persons report the experience of fatigue. The overwhelming sense of weariness experienced by the schizophrenics is expressed by Mr. Espinosa.

> It is somehow as if the spirit has been lifted out of me, and my material self has been left without a spirit, or as if the spirit of an old man has come into my physical self and I do not feel like doing anything. When I do not have problems, I feel calm and relieved, but when I have problems then I become as heavy as a truck.

In arriving at a diagnosis of the sick persons, the psychiatrist who made the mental health evaluation took into account withdrawn behavior. The examining psychiatrist frequently notes that the sick persons are "isolating themselves from other persons," "secluding themselves," and "avoiding the world of friends and associates." Table 40 is based on the reports from the psychiatrists. This table shows that a disproportionately large number of schizophrenics, men and women, have withdrawn from interpersonal relations. The inference to be drawn is that symptoms of withdrawal are relevant to the psychiatrist's diagnosis of schizophrenia.

To understand the settings from which sick persons withdraw, it is important to recognize that husbands and wives have quite different patterns of social participation. Women are sharply restricted to their homes and immediate neighborhoods, but the men are not. Women see mostly their relatives and friends in the neighborhood; the men

234 Becoming a Schizophrenic

TABLE 40 Psychiatrists' Reports of Withdrawal

	N	NOT WITHDRAWN, %	WITHDRAWN, %
A. Males			
Nonschizophrenic	29	100	0
Schizophrenic	11	18	82
$p < .01$			
B. Females			
Nonschizophrenic	27	96	4
Schizophrenic	13	8	92
$p < .01$			

roam widely in pursuing their jobs or seeking entertainment. The entertainment of the women consists primarily of gossiping with relatives and neighbors, listening to the radio, watching television, and occasionally attending a spiritualist's session, a baptism, wedding, or funeral. Women spend the largest portion of their day attending to the needs of the children and cooking, washing, ironing, and cleaning their homes. Thus, relationships in the neighborhood are of much greater relevance to women than to men. Table 41 indicates that 96 per cent of the well women report having friends in the neighbor-

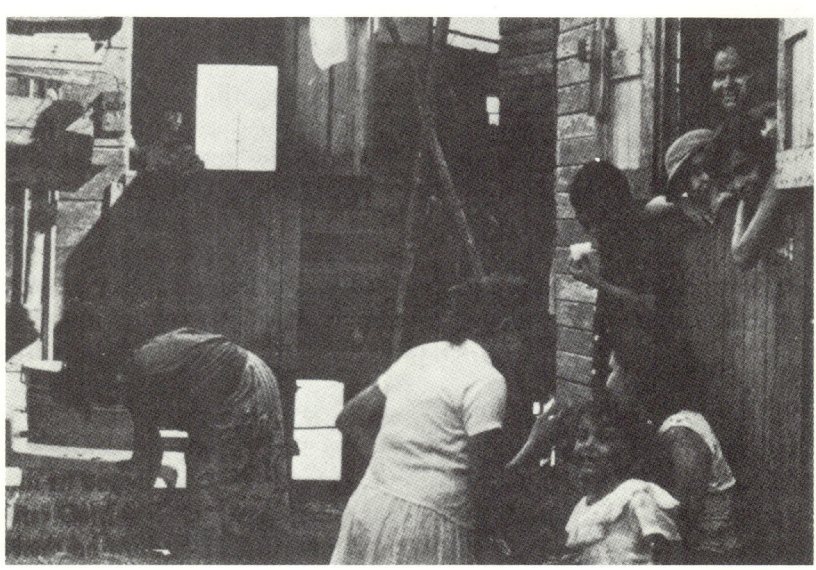

TABLE 41 Replies to Question: "How Many of Your Friends Live in This Neighborhood?"

	N	FEW TO ALL, %	NONE, %
A. Males			
Nonschizophrenic	29	79	21
Schizophrenic	11	91	9
$p > .05$			
B. Females			
Nonschizophrenic	27	96	4
Schizophrenic	13	38	62
$p < .01$			

hood, whereas the comparable percentage for the schizophrenic women is 38. This relationship is significant. In contrast, there is no significant difference among the sick and well husbands in the number of friends who live in their neighborhoods.

The alienation of sick women from their neighborhoods is reflected also in their comments and those of their husbands. Mr. Nieves states that his sick wife

> . . . does not want to make friends with our neighbors because she believes in keeping them at a distance. She says that this way she can avoid problems and lead a calm life.

Similarly, Mrs. Iglesias says,

> I do not like to have relations with my neighbors, to be involved in their affairs. I like to live according to the saying, "One is better off in one's own house than in another person's house."

Another sick woman, Mrs. Padilla, has a recurrent daydream in which she is a bathing beauty dressed in a bikini. In this fantasy she romps gaily on the white sands of a beach that adjoins an expensive tourist hotel in the Condado section of San Juan; she is surrounded by handsome men who comment on her beauty. The reality of obscene and vulgar neighbors rudely contradicts this dream. She states her case for complete isolation:

> When I am alone or locked up in my room I feel smooth and rejoiceful. My heart does not ache; my chest feels no pain. I can hardly wait until my daughter is 3 years old. Then she can go out to play and I will be left alone. Life is thinking more than living.

236 Becoming a Schizophrenic

The sick husband's withdrawal is more noticeable than the wife's, as he has never been confined to the immediate vicinity of his home. Men spend many hours in *cafetines* which are their centers of communal activities. A typical *cafetin* sells refrigerated, canned, and fresh foods as well as rum and beer. There are several serving tables and chairs and a juke box. During the late afternoon and evening, men of the neighborhood congregate inside the *cafetin* or immediately outside. Some sit on small wooden boxes playing dominoes; others stand quietly sipping beer and occasionally exchanging a joke with their companions. Another group of men stand in rapt attention listening to a friend orating about politics. Sports and recent sexual conquests are under discussion by other groups. Several men are listening to a baseball game or a horse race over the radio. A *cafetin* is a central meeting place, a convivial setting comprised of small cliques of men.

All the husbands and wives were asked how often they went to *cafetines* for entertainment. Only one wife reports that she goes to *cafetines* for entertainment; she goes at least once a week. Table 42 shows that 60 per cent of the men go to *cafetines* for entertainment at least once a week. Of direct relevance to the process of withdrawal, however, is the more frequent participation of well men than sick men in *cafetin* life; 72 per cent of the well men and 27 per cent of the sick men go to *cafetines* at least once a week for entertainment. By not participating in *cafetin* life, the sick men sever themselves from one of the main roots of the masculine world. This withdrawal is accompanied by a more general retreat from the role of the *macho*, the he-man in the Puerto Rican culture.

When did the sick persons begin to withdraw from friends and associates? To answer this question, we asked each sick person a series of questions about his participation in social groups before and after he believes the illness began. In practically all cases, evidence of pro-

TABLE 42 Replies to Question: "How Often Do You Go to *Cafetines* for Entertainment?"

	N	AT LEAST ONCE A WEEK, %	LESS THAN ONCE A WEEK, %
Nonschizophrenic husbands	29	72	28
Schizophrenic husbands	11	27	73

$p < .05$

nounced withdrawal begin at the time the illness is perceived to have started. Mrs. Quiromo is the only schizophrenic person, out of the twenty-four, who was clearly withdrawn prior to her acknowledged experience with the illness. Mr. Nieves' description of his wife's withdrawal is typical.

> Before my wife got sick, the neighbors liked her a lot, helped her, visited her. Now she avoids them.

Mrs. Herrero says of her husband:

> His friends used to invite him out, but since he rejected the invitations they no longer invite him. Some of them visit us sometimes and he doesn't seem to like it. I don't know why, for they haven't done anything against him. He presents a dog's face to them when they come in. Sometimes they come in the door, look at him, and walk out the door. I notice that the neighbors try to speak to him as infrequently as possible, and when they know he is here they do not come to visit me. When one goes to visit some place and one notices there is a coolness present, one is not likely to return.

Similarly, many sick persons state that now, in contrast to before the illness, "I am no longer interested in seeing friends"; "I don't see my friends any more because I don't trust them"; "I am indifferent toward them"; and, "I no longer share things with my friends." In brief, the pattern of recently emerging symptoms has been accompanied by the attrition of social relations culminating in withdrawal.

Undoubtedly, the lassitude experienced by the sick person robs him of energy he could expend on social relations, but withdrawal appears also to be a response to the horror of being identified as a *loco*. That the behavior of the sick person is often interpreted as *locura* is indicated by experiences such as that of Mrs. Gallardo who, one day, asked a neighbor to stay with her husband while she went on a brief errand. The neighbor replied that he would not because he did not want to fool around with *locos*. Mrs. Gallardo concludes: "I learned from this that the kind of illness my husband has is not the kind you tell anyone about." Or, as Mr. Espinosa says,

> People say that one is a *loco* because of the way that one comports oneself. One is not the same; one's hands shake; one's head feels droopy and one's eyes tend to pop out. I cannot sit still. I have to be moving all the time.

At the least, the sick persons are viewed with suspicion; some are clearly identified as *locos* and treated accordingly. As one fieldworker was trying to locate the home of Mr. Berríos, he observed a group of teenagers throwing rocks at a man who jumped in the air to avoid being hit. The boys were calling: "Look at the *loco*. We make him jump like a goat." The *loco* was Mr. Berríos. Such punishment hastens the retreat of the sick person from social relations and symbolizes at the same time the withdrawal of society from him.

Moreover, the sick person has learned that to speak fully and indiscriminately about the illness with friends and associates exacts the heavy price of the charge of *locura*. To guard against this threat, the sick person confides only in selected persons and avoids describing the symptoms that make him appear to be a *loco*. Two considerations guide his choice of a person in whom to confide the problem of his illness. First, the confidant must be sympathetic and have special knowledge, qualifications, or resources which empower him to give advice, direct therapeutic assistance such as prescriptions, massages, or the like, and perhaps some form of material aid. Second, the confidant must neither view him as a *loco* nor encourage others to do so. Spouses and blood relatives are ready confidants as they are unlikely to hurl a charge of *locura*; moreover, they have a familial obligation to help the sick person. Mrs. Quiromo is the only schizophrenic who has suffered open stigmatization from immediate family members, her husband and her mother.

Affinal relatives are not likely confidants for the sick person. The obligation to help is diluted as it crosses in-law lines. The help provided by affinal relatives is designed to enable the spouse of the sick person to cope with the illness, particularly if it poses a danger of physical harm. Sometimes, in fact, the solidarity of blood relations may threaten the marriage of the sick person and his spouse when the spouse is drawn into an alliance against the schizophrenic. The formation of such an alliance is premised on the threat of the *loco*-like behavior of the sick person. For the person or his spouse to divulge information about the illness may be the first step in the development of such an alliance.

Forty-five per cent of the sick persons state that they have never spoken to friends about the illness for the following reasons:

> I do not speak to my friends about my illness, for around here you cannot trust anyone. If one were to tell them about it, they would repeat it and exaggerate it.

> If I were crazy I wouldn't tell them because they would avoid me. I would never come close to being a *loco*, so why should I tell them anything?

The spouses of the sick persons state similar reasons for withholding information about the illness.

> I don't want to spread the news that my wife is sick of the nerves because then people would exaggerate.
>
> I don't speak to people about my husband's illness because there are some people who instead of helping you will ridicule you. Why tell them if they cannot help you?

Fifty-five per cent of the sick persons state that they speak to their friends about the illness, but some admit to feeling uneasy and anxious about it. Mr. Ramos says:

> I am afraid when I speak to my friends about it because if I tell them one thing they may think it is another. I am afraid they will laugh at me. They wouldn't trust me the way they used to. I am afraid if I tell them how I feel they will avoid me.

Those who speak to friends insist that these are intimate friends, confidants, persons to whom they can divulge their innermost secrets without fear that the illness will become a matter of gossip. The relief experienced in having a confidant with whom one can "undrown" is weighed against the potential danger of an unreliable confidant.

Mr. Aponte and Mr. Espinosa are friends and speak to each other about their symptoms which they have found to be almost identical; they are companions in misery. To Mr. Espinosa, Mr. Aponte is a true friend unlike others he once had. "When I used to tell my other friends about my illness they thought of me as inferior and lost respect for me." Neither sick man feels inferior when he speaks to the other; neither is in a position to foist the stigma of the *loco* on the other since both are equally vulnerable to this charge.

The sick persons choose judiciously to speak about certain symptoms but not others. Mrs. Quiromo, whose mother calls her a *loca*, avoids describing some features of her illness to her mother: "If I were to describe my condition fully to my mother, she would not understand." Mr. Espinosa says:

> When I speak to my friends I do not bring up the question of my nerves. What I do is talk to them about the problems I have because I feel tired all the time.

Visits to the psychiatric hospital are not discussed indiscriminately. A regrettable mistake early in the field work brought this point to our attention. A fieldworker was discussing the visits to the psychiatric hospital with the wife of a sick man when she was overheard by the wife's relatives. A period of pronounced silence and embarrassment followed. The relatives had not known that her husband was undergoing psychiatric treatment; they had been told that the interviewer was there concerning some matters of social security.

Some sick persons try to control their telltale behavior in the presence of other persons. Mr. Espinosa reports,

> My neighbors don't know that I am not feeling well because I have hidden it from them. I try to control myself a lot. If they call me to come downstairs to talk with them, I put my hands inside my pockets so they will not see them tremble.

The problem of comportment is well stated by Mr. Dávila, a schizophrenic. "If I were a *loco*," he says, "I would try to walk straight and pretend that I was not a *loco* so that people would not notice it." Mr. Dávila has not been successful in following his own prescription, however. Once while he and his wife were visiting her relatives, he burst out of the house in wild flight, screaming that evil apparitions were pursuing him. Other sick persons also act like *locos* when their "minds leave" their bodies, meaning that they lose awareness of themselves and of other persons. Afterward they are unable to recall the events that transpired during such a period. When sick persons have such lapses they erupt into uncontrollable violence against their spouses and children, friends and associates, or relatives, or they meander randomly in their homes or in the neighborhood. During these periods they may remain relatively articulate or become incoherent.

Sick persons often avoid doing things they know will exacerbate their *loco*-like behavior. Mr. Berríos notes that when he drinks he explodes into violence. His neighbors have begun to identify him as a *loco*. Now Mr. Berríos refuses to drink rum and beer, hoping to appease his neighbors; during his sober moments he fears the punishment he receives for drinking and acting like a *loco*. Excessive sexual intercourse makes Mr. Cardona shake; his knees tremble, fatigue overwhelms him, and his affinal relatives begin to gossip. As a result, the Cardonas have decided to restrict sexual intercourse.

The withdrawal of the sick person from friends and associates is ironic in view of the fact that he, more than the well person, wants and needs companionship. He wants to speak about his illness almost to the exclusion of other topics; the interviewers noted that questions unrelated to the illness served as points of departure for the sick person to discuss his illness. Afterward, he felt "undrowned," having experienced a genuine sense of relief. Many times the interviewers were thanked for being patient listeners and reliable confidants.

SUMMARY

In this culture the role of the *loco* is a sharply defined stigma. To become a *loco* is to be viewed as having lost virtually all socially valued attributes. The repugnance felt toward the *loco* indirectly reflects many basic values in the culture: the *loco* behaves in ways contrary to everything considered good, desirable, and attractive. To the public it appears as if the *loco* has entered a supernatural conspiracy with the Devil against the ethical and aesthetic norms of Puerto Rican life. It is no easy matter to make amends after such outrageous behavior; the public's confidence is not easily restored. Once a person is viewed as a *loco* he will be treated as such in the foreseeable future.

A normal social role such as friend, father, or husband applies to a person's behavior in specific social situations, but the role of the *loco* is comprehensive and dominant; it infects the entire web of interpersonal relations which enmeshes the person. To be a *loco* is to be imprisoned within an all-enveloping role. The illness has not blurred the sick person's conception of the role of the *loco*, nor has it dimmed his awareness of the condemnation and suffering which it entails. To circumvent the sting of this role the sick person differentiates between the possibility and the actuality of being a *loco*, insists that he is not a *loco*, and identifies his illness as nervousness. He takes great pains to distinguish elaborately between nervousness and *locura*.

The sick persons believe their illness began at a specific time in the recent past. Suddenly they were overwhelmed by a variety of symptoms, some of which come and go, and others which disappear only to be replaced by equally tormenting ones. Life problems, social tensions, and conflict are the most common explanations adduced for the illness by the sick person. They want rest and tranquility to allay their overwhelming fatigue and anxiety.

Although the sick person is deeply absorbed in his illness and yearns to speak about it, confidants are carefully selected. The illness is suppressed as a topic of conversation with friends and associates. Efforts are made to pretend that he is not a *loco*. He controls activities which exacerbate his *loco*-like behavior. These efforts are relatively futile, however, as the symptoms of the illness are strong and readily visible in the crowded social setting in which he lives. In point of fact, the sick person has begun to be viewed and treated as a *loco*. He withdraws from society out of fear that he will be stigmatized as a *loco*; in turn, the rejection by his friends and associates pushes him to withdraw. The stigma attached to this role is so strong that the withdrawal of the sick person from participation in all types of social groups appears to be a natural sequel to the condemnation he suffers.

12
Coping Behaviors

Twenty of the twenty-four schizophrenic persons in this study were brought to our attention either through their referral to public psychiatric agencies in the community or their solicitation of service from these agencies. The remaining four were diagnosed as schizophrenic when we took them to a psychiatrist for the mental status examination. We followed all the sick persons for 20 months. At the end of this period we searched the clinical records of all psychiatric agencies in the community to determine the course of their illnesses insofar as they were reflected in the records of these agencies. We found that none of the schizophrenics had been hospitalized: 42 per cent had never seen a psychiatrist other than when we had them examined for this study; 58 per cent had seen a psychiatrist at least one other time, but the median number of visits was only 2. Five persons, 21 per cent, saw a psychiatrist more than five times. The therapy administered by the clinics where these patients were treated is primarily organic in orientation; tranquilizers are often prescribed, and electroshock treatment is given sometimes. One man received psychotherapy. Mr. Cardona, a spiritualistic medium, was of interest to a psychiatric resident who treated him while collecting life history material from him for teaching purposes.

The medical records of the sick persons show that, although severely psychiatrically ill persons may be referred to a psychiatric agency, a significant number do not, in fact, receive care, and the treatment received by those who do is limited in amount and kind. Despite the prestige associated with the medical profession, in the lower class of San Juan psychiatrists are infused with stigma. The persons who have had treatment went to the psychiatric agencies with trepidation. Mr. Tirado agreed to go to an out-patient clinic only to discover that it was the old insane asylum, well known throughout the Island as the place where *locos* go and are kept. He says, "This upset me very much because I am not a *loco*." Mrs. Quiromo was deceived by her relatives who told her she was being taken to a vocational school in Río Piedras. She says,

> If I had known that they were going to take me to the insane asylum I would not have gone. They were trying to deceive me. They were trying to tell me that I am a *loca*, and they were trying to hide from me where they were taking me.

Mrs. Quiromo never returned for treatment.

The social role of being a patient in a psychiatric clinic is new, unfamiliar, and accepted reluctantly with, at least some, alarm. Coping with mental illness is primarily a family problem. Outside the family, it is dealt with by spiritualists and members of other religious groups. We now review the ways in which nonmedical institutions provide therapeutic outlets for sick and well persons.

Early in this study we learned that persons afflicted with a mental illness frequently come into contact with spiritualistic mediums before, during, and after their visits to psychiatrists. Local psychiatrists are aware of these folk therapists, and spiritualistic mediums have some understanding of the functions of psychiatrists. In some cases a psychiatrist and a medium may come in contact with the same patient. One psychiatrist told us of a recent experience he had with relatives of a patient brought to him for a special purpose. The relatives wanted the patient's aggressiveness calmed so that he could be taken to a "genuine" therapist—a spiritualistic medium. Adding insult to injury, mediums are known to have used psychiatric clinics in the San Juan area surreptitiously to treat ambulatory patients, and outpatients at one psychiatric clinic commonly refer to psychotherapy as *pases* (the symbolic gestures performed by mediums in order to cure).

To follow up these observations we asked the sick and well persons a series of questions about their beliefs in spiritualism, the frequency with which they attend spiritualistic sessions, the practice of spiritualism in the family, and their willingness to communicate their problems to a medium. Some questions focused on the experiences the persons had at such sessions, the treatment they received, and their belief in the effectiveness of the treatment. In addition, we directly observed the actions and reactions of the sick and the well persons to numerous spiritualistic sessions in which we participated.

The ideology of spiritualism is elaborate, complex, and only partially codified. Spiritualism involves the belief that the visible world is surrounded by an invisible universe populated with spirits who have moral qualities of goodness or evil.[1] They have the power to penetrate the visible world and to attach themselves to humans; they may manifest themselves as a reincarnation of some other person or thing. As metaphysical beings they are able to coerce and influence human affairs, oftentimes in a very dramatic manner. Spiritualistic doctrine also asserts that persons may develop *facultades* (psychic faculties or mystical antennae) which enable the individual to communicate with spirits. In this sense, the person with *facultades* has gained a measure of control over the spirits; consequently, an individual with *facultades* may exercise influence over human affairs by commanding the obedience or favor of the spirits.

For some persons, belief in spiritualism means more than these metaphysical assumptions indicate. Belief in spiritualism may also connote an implicit judgment of the positive or negative moral force in the community of spiritualism as it is practiced in Puerto Rico. A person can believe in the validity of these propositions and assert, nevertheless, that spiritualism may be used for evil purposes. The underlying assumption is that persons with *facultades* can control the visible world by operating through the universe of spirits. Such control is analogous to possession of an instrument that can be used, depending upon the designs of the user, for evil or beneficial purposes.

The beliefs in and practices of spiritualism are distributed throughout the society with perhaps a relatively pronounced tendency toward concentration in the lower classes.[2] In the higher classes, however, spiritualists and their followers are careful to distinguish the type of spiritualism they embrace from that of lower-class spiritualism. Higher-class spiritualists energetically assert the scientific and experimental character of their beliefs; they argue that lower-class spiritualism is irrational, superstitious, and not based on the philosophical doctrines of Allan Kardec, who is considered to be the foremost codifier of spiritualistic doctrine.[3] The persons whom we studied are not familiar

---

[1] For a discussion of the moral qualities of the spirits from the point of view of the spiritualist, see Allan Kardec, *El Libro De Los Espiritus*, Editorial Orion, Mexico, 1951, pp. 147–180.

[2] The type of survey data required to determine the prevalence of spiritualism and its differential distribution across the class structure are not available. It is obvious that, to assess the broader societal significance of spiritualism in Puerto Rico, survey data of a descriptive nature are a minimal requirement.

[3] Allan Kardec's writings are referred to very often in spiritualistic sessions. For an official biography of Kardec, see Henri Sausse, *Biografia de Allan Kardec*, Editorial

with the many distinctions, classifications, and subtleties in Kardec's works; the logical consistency of the metaphysics of spiritualism are of little or no concern to these persons.

The social setting in which contacts between the medium and a solicitant for help takes place varies from a private consultation to a session involving a group of fifteen or twenty participants. These meetings are organized explicitly to serve the participants; consequently, social action is channeled toward the solution of problems stated by the participants.

A typical room where a session is held is decorated with banners proclaiming "Charity and Humility" and with portraits of Franklin D. Roosevelt and Mahatma Gandhi. A sober-faced, almost life-sized figure of a cigar-store Indian, looking ominously at the ceiling, stands with arms crossed before the congregation. The odor of burning incense pervades the room. The head medium [4] opens the session with a long prayer from one of Allan Kardec's works, directs herself to the auxiliary mediums, and asks them to concentrate—preparations designed to develop the correct mood to welcome the spirits. As the session develops, the head medium directs her attention to the participants in terms of the order of their seating as they face the table where she and the auxiliary medium(s) sit. The head medium then proceeds to probe, interpret, treat, and prescribe for the ills and maladies afflicting the individuals. The medium's prescriptions include a variety of herbs, ointments, medicated hot baths, and massages that have symbolic meanings. Spiritualistic prayers presumed to have curative effects are recommended. Advice and orientation are given. Since the session generally requires intense participation by the members, the medium frequently relieves moments of tension by joking.

Participants who have developed *facultades* show through contortions, spasms, screeching, babbling, and deep breathing that they have been possessed. The behavior manifested varies in accordance with the kind of spirit that has communicated with the possessed person. Participants with and without psychic faculties provide the human problems around which the session revolves.

The group meeting is structured around four types of social roles: (1) the head medium, (2) auxiliary medium(s), (3) followers with *facul-*

Victor Hugo, Buenos Aires, 1952. This biography contains its own review (pp. 138–139) allegedly provided by the spirit of Allan Kardec which spoke through one of the participants in a session attended by the author of the biography.

[4] Joseph Bram, "Spirits, Mediums, and Believers in Contemporary Puerto Rico," *Trans. N.Y. Acad. Sci.*, 20 (1958), 340–347.

tades, and (4) followers without *facultades*. It is interesting to note that the four roles are arranged in a hierarchy of leadership and power according to the participants' alleged degree of influence over spirits. These roles are differentiated and coordinated by the degree of charisma imputed to the incumbents. We have observed individuals diagnosed by psychiatrists as schizophrenics effectively play each of the aforementioned roles.[5] Moreover, their role performance was validated strongly by the enthusiastic aceptance of others in the session.

Spiritualism acquires its leaders through informal primary group processes, not professional education or training. A person becomes a head medium by establishing a reputation for competence in dealing with the supernatural and in effecting cures. The reputation develops among a circle of friends and associates by word of mouth. The spiritualistic groups in the slums and *caseríos* of Puerto Rico have no formal bureaucratic relationship to each other. Although mediums form friendships and visit other spiritualistic sessions, no central hierarchy integrates the activities of the many small spiritualistic groups which abound in the subculture of the lower class.

In 80 per cent of our families at least one spouse believes in spiritualism; in 48 per cent both spouses believe in spiritualism. In 40 per cent of the families at least one spouse sees mediums; in 20 per cent of the families both spouses communicate with mediums. Beyond going to séances, 45 per cent of the families perform a variety of spiritualistic acts at home: Water containing ingredients prescribed by mediums is used to scrub the house and purify it spiritually, or water consecrated by symbolic gestures is drunk for its therapeutic effect. Baths are are taken in water containing aromatic herbs. Concoctions are burned to drive evil spirits out of the household. Spiritualistic prayers taken from one of Allan Kardec's books are recited.

The figures on the proportions of persons and families who (1) believe in spiritualism, (2) attend sessions, (3) take their problems to a medium, and (4) practice spiritualism at home show that it is not a woman's religion any more than it is a man's—both sexes are equally devout; the proportion of husbands and wives involved is about the

---

[5] Lee R. Steiner has made the same kind of observations on the American scene. She says, "I've encountered psychopathic personalities with Jehova complexes, at the lowest rung in both integrity and knowledge, who have effected emotional cures. It is my very definite impression that there is very much correlation between validated knowledge and emotional cures. And I feel that this same condition obtains, at the moment, in professional therapy as well as in the occult." "Why Do People Consult the Occult?" *The Humanist*, **XIX** (1959), 19–30.

same. In point of fact, when a person believes in spiritualism, attends sessions, is disposed to communicate problems to the medium, or practices spiritualism at home, the same is usually true of his spouse. Thus, involvement in spiritualism is organized according to the family, not the individual. Women, however, are more active in persuading their husbands of the value of spiritualism than are the men in persuading their wives.

Although spiritualism provides detailed and meaningful explanations for the symptoms of the schizophrenic, it does not attract *only* persons who are so afflicted. Proportionately more sick than well persons believe in spiritualism, attend and have attended sessions, practice it at home, and go to mediums when they have problems, but none of these differences is statistically significant. Almost as many well as sick persons are attracted to this type of religious help for dealing with meaningful problems of daily life.

Mrs. Badillo, a 37-year old woman who, according to the psychiatrist in the project, was subject to hysterical hyperkinetic seizures was also diagnosed by a practicing spiritualistic medium. Mrs. Badillo relates,

> Yes, I went to consult a spiritualist to see what the attacks meant. The medium told me that there was a young man who was in love with me. The mother-in-law of this young man bewitched me through an evil spirit. This evil spirit takes me over in a violent way.
>
> Do I believe the medium? Of course I do! She described many events in my life that were true. When I see the mother-in-law of this young man I get an attack. This proves that she [the medium] is right.

Spiritualism actively provides and shapes social meaning for its troubled participants. In the lower class, spiritualism is coterminous with the fabric of social life. It is woven into the intimate trials, strife, and interpersonal turmoil that enmesh the members of the socially and economically deprived stratum. Spiritualism is institutionalized to discharge the tensions and anxieties generated in other areas of social life. For example, in spiritualists' sessions, a problem frequently brought up by married women is the suspected infidelity of their husbands. In such circumstances the medium may call upon the spirit of the rival woman, assume her role, and interact with the troubled wife. The medium indicates this change in her personality by gesticulating, altering the quality of her voice, and in general acting *como una mujer de la calle* (like a woman of the street) who is assumed to be the kind of woman that would lure married men from their spouses. The troubled wife then attempts to convince the spirit of her rival that she should leave her husband alone, on the grounds that she (the spirit) is causing untold suffering. The net effect of such a dramatic exchange appears to be that the wife is left with a feeling of coping with her problem.

The medium is perceived to be competent in managing a wide spectrum of human problems. She is not a specialist, for she is expected to be a healer, an expert in social relations, and knowledgeable in explaining the paradoxes and ironies of a life that is in many ways bewildering. Mediums are consulted about such physical symptoms as headaches, loss of weight, chest pains, rashes, insomnia, and hallucinations. Problems which stem from interpersonal friction also are taken to the medium: men report arguments and fights with coworkers and bosses; mothers report problems the children have with teachers and fellow students; wives often report the infidelity of their husbands. In addition, premonitions are validated by the medium, and problems beyond everyday expectancy are brought to the medium for solution: the miscarriage of a fetus lacking human characteristics, rashes of bad luck, nightmares.

Medical doctors, on the other hand, are not credited with the priestly omniscience required to interpret the riddles of experiences, nor are medical doctors expected to preempt the area of illness. According to Mr. Cardona,

> Mediums understand things that the doctor-psychiatrist does not, that is if the doctor is not a spiritualist. If psychiatrists were to know about spiritualistic matters they would be doctors in the broadest sense of the word. When the doctor does not know about spiritualistic matters, he should consult with a spiritualist, and in this way they could come to an agreement. Spiritualists would treat the spiritualistic part of the problem and thereby rid the individual of possible evil spirits. Psychiatrists could treat the nervous system, if this were affected. There would be much success then.

The basis for the medium's claims of competence stems from the assumption, in spiritualistic ideology, that all individual problems are material or spiritual, or a combination of both material and spiritual things. Such a dichotomy may have little or nothing to do with the outstanding complaint presented by the subject. Rather, it is a classification of the source of the problem, and, as we mentioned before, spiritualistic ideology imputes power to the inhabitants of the metaphysical world. Consequently, if the etiological roots of the problem can be traced to the invisible world, it is a spiritual problem. Such problems, therefore, are within the control of the medium. Material problems, in contrast, have their causes in the visible world of hard facts. These, consequently, fall within the competence of doctors, druggists, nurses, and other professionals devoted to therapeutic activities.

Few behavioral or medical problems have a conspicuous material cause immediately apparent to the subject, the medium, or others; therefore, problems are invariably classified as spiritualistic by the medium who is consulted. Thus the medium effects a rough division of labor, relegating to herself therapeutic competence to deal with a vast range of problems, many of which are disorders of personality in the broad, nontechnical sense of the term. One-half the persons interviewed are willing to take any or all of their problems to a medium. It is important to note that many persons professing doubts and reservations about the efficacy of spiritualism hasten to consult a particular medium who becomes known for dramatic cures.

We have selected the Ubarri family to illustrate how spiritualism affects the lives of men and women who are free of schizophrenia. In this family, spiritualism serves to rationalize interpersonal problems. Our staff psychiatrist diagnosed Mr. Ubarri as an inadequate personality in the technical sense of the term. In the psychiatric report, attention is called to a persistent and general characteristic of this subject: he is intellectually aware of his responsibilities, but he does not make an effort to fulfill them. Although Mr. Ubarri recognizes the need to earn money for his family, he has built up a pattern of unconscious justifications in order to avoid work. The psychiatrist and the fieldworkers report that Mr. Ubarri fails to fulfill a basic part of his role as head of the household. Mrs. Ubarri realizes that the capacity to provide for the family depends on the job market, but she complains that her husband does not even try to seek employment.

Mrs. Ubarri was diagnosed by the psychiatrist as having a psychoneurotic conversion reaction. As a wife who is *conforme,* she is not expected to express feelings of anger caused by her husband's failures, and the psychiatrist reports that her symptoms are attributable to her inability to express such feelings. Despite her suppressed anger and disgust, her patience and forbearance are recognized even by her husband; he says,

> She is very good to me. If she had been another woman she would have left me. What other woman would live with a man who does not support his family as he should? God knows if she had been

another woman, she would have abandoned the children and run off with another man. My wife suffers silently and seldom says anything.

Mr. Ubarri is quite satisfied with his wife. If he had to do it all over again, he would marry the same person. Mrs. Ubarri reports:

> I knew about him before I had actually met him. He had a reputation in that neighborhood. He was known for his gambling with dice and cards. He used to stroll around with prostitutes. He couldn't hold a job. He used to carry a dagger tucked under his belt. He was a drunkard. He was a fighter. He had served a prison term for cutting a man.

Mrs. Ubarri says her husband's behavior now is basically the same. She admits, however, that he sometimes shows her kindness; without sarcasm, she relates that he saves his cigarette butts for her.

The spiritualistic medium Mrs. Ubarri consults says that her husband is possessed by an evil spirit, whose purpose is to torment her. If she can withstand the suffering produced by this evil spirit, it means that she is made of the correct moral fiber. In effect, she is undergoing a *prueba* (moral test). Mr. Ubarri agrees that bad spirits have a lot to do with his inadequacies, but by attending spiritualistic sessions he has gained some control over his evil impulses. He reports:

> Whenever anybody says anything that I do not like, the blood goes to my head. I tremble all over and feel that I have to fight to get even. During a session they worked on me, they performed *pases* on me, and they gave me prescriptions. I have felt better since then. I don't fight as much. I don't drink as much.

Mrs. Ubarri also believes that spiritualism has foretold the future. At one session, Mr. Ubarri was told by the medium, "Get away from rum! If you do not get away from rum you will have a serious problem." The prediction came true. A few weeks after this advice was given, Mr. Ubarri was arrested for bootlegging rum. During his trial, Mrs. Ubarri continued to attend spiritualistic sessions in the belief that a medium with the correct spiritualistic contacts could influence the outcome of the trial. Mr. Ubarri was convicted, however, and sentenced to serve 8 months in jail. We completed our study of this family while he was serving the sentence.

After we finished the interviewing, we continued to visit Mrs. Ubarri and found her bad luck persisting. A physician she consulted about some annoying physical symptoms diagnosed tuberculosis. She comments:

> I do not believe what the doctor tells me. I believe what my uncle [a spiritualistic medium] tells me. He says the chest X-rays are a manifestation of the spirit of my brother who died of tuberculosis. Since my brother was very fond of me, his spirit does not want to leave me. This spirit is the cause of my fevers, chest pain, headaches, coughing spells, and loss of appetite.

We lack direct evidence bearing on the therapeutic impact on mental illness of participation in spiritualistic sessions, but we have abundant information on the manner in which participation serves as a method of coping with the specific problems generated by the mental illness. Mrs. Cardona, the wife of a paranoid schizophrenic, described to us the disrupting effect her husband's incessant and pervasive suspicions were having on the performance of her role in the family. Any time that she was not within the radius of her husband's vision, he accused her of infidelity. She says,

> Then I decided to take him to see a spiritualistic medium since his suspicions had created an impossible situation. She [the medium] and the other people in the session advised him. He has not been suspicious since then. They explained that it was a test he was undergoing since he was in the process of developing *facultades*. They told him that he should devote himself to charity and to the good and that he should concentrate on the development of his *facultades*. My husband is now a medium, and when he does not feel well he performs *pases* on himself in front of the mirror. He feels better afterwards.

Mr. Espinosa, another schizophrenic, reports that when he feels restless and fearful inside, dissatisfied with himself and others, and not wanting to see anyone, he turns to the spiritualist for help.

> I go to sessions because they make me feel good and rested inside. They bring me peace. I go to them because the medium is the maximum authority in knowing how to rid one of those evil spirits and demons that upset one inside.

Mr. Aponte who also suffers from a severe psychotic illness reports:

> Before I go to a session I feel unhappy. When I get to the group I talk to the medium and the others and I feel good. When the others begin to talk about their problems I feel as if I am not alone. They [the group] make me feel sure of myself.

Such reports come from the mentally afflicted individuals in our study with sufficient frequency to indicate that attending group sessions serves, at least, to ease and alleviate intra- and interpersonal strains.

We do not have the research design to test the proposition that spiritualistic group sessions alter the personality structure of mentally ill individuals in the direction of mental health. We believe, however, that spiritualistic sessions have many of the therapeutic advantages of group psychotherapy.[6] In addition to the presumed advantages of group psychotherapy as practiced in clinical settings, spiritualistic sessions are coterminous with the fabric of values, beliefs, aspirations, and problems of the participants, as little social distance separates the afflicted person from the medium. (By way of contrast, psychiatric treatment at this class level involves bringing together persons who are separated by a vast social gulf; to the lower-class person the psychiatrist is a distant symbol.) The other participants in the session are often neighbors, so that the session is characterized by face-to-face contacts and interpersonal intimacy. The spiritualist and her followers form a primary group in which problems are discussed in a convivial setting. Problems expressed in this setting are classified, interpreted, and rendered understandable within the compass of a belief system that is widely accepted even by those who profess not to believe in spiritualism.[7]

When a mentally afflicted person is experiencing alienation from his social groups because of his deviant and enigmatic behavior, he finds in the spiritualistic sessions a group that accepts his behavior as credentials for full participation. Persistent hallucinations, for example, are not symptoms of a deranged mind experiencing things unperceived by others—an interpretation which serves to isolate the sick; rather, hallucinations indicate the development of psychic faculties that may eventually serve to put the lucky person in more permanent contact

---

[6] For a statement of the therapeutic advantages of group therapy, see Marvin K. Opler, "Values in Group Psychotherapy," *Int. J. Social Psychiat.*, IV (1959), 296–298.

[7] "If you ever talk to a Puerto Rican who says he doesn't believe in spirits, you know what that means? It means you haven't talked to him long enough." This statement is attributed to a Puerto Rican in Dan Wakefield's *Island in the City: A World of Spanish Harlem*, Houghton-Mifflin, Boston, The Riverside Press, Cambridge, 1959. Even though this quotation represents an exaggerated notion of the prevalence of spiritualism among Puerto Ricans, it holds a very valuable hint to the interviewer collecting data on spiritualism. Oftentimes, respondents will deny their belief in spiritualism when first questioned. Once the interviewer has established a warm and secure relationship with the respondent, however, the latter may not only admit his belief in spiritualism but may provide descriptions of numerous incidents that dramatically substantiate the belief. It is our impression that members of the higher levels of the class structure are more reluctant to express such beliefs than are lower-class individuals.

with the invisible world. Relatives, friends, and associates are encouraged to cooperate with the sick person so that he will fully develop *facultades*. Participation in a spiritualistic group serves to structure, define, and render institutionally meaningful behavior that is otherwise perceived as aberrant. The behavior of the mentally ill at a spiritualistic meeting is within the folkways and mores of that cult; outgroup vices become ingroup virtues.

In Chapter 11 we point out that mental illness has a cultural meaning beyond the psychiatrist's frame of reference. To go to a psychiatric clinic or to the insane asylum can be the first step in assuming the role of the *loco*. The spiritualist, as believer and participant, offers an afflicted person an alternative role that encompasses and sanctions his idiosyncratic symptoms, and, moreover, one that does not impose on him the burden of stigma. The spiritualist may announce to the sick person, his family, and friends that the afflicted person is endowed with *facultades*, a matter of prestige at this level of the social structure. Thus, the institution of spiritualism is a form of folk psychiatry, serving its believers without their paying the penalty of community stigma associated with psychiatric agencies.

Spiritualism claims competence in the interpretation and treatment of what are, in psychiatric terms, pathological symptoms. If an individual reports hallucinations, it clearly indicates to the believer in spiritualism that he is being visited by spirits who manifest themselves visually and audibly.[8] If he has delusions he is told that evil spirits are deceiving him about himself as well as about others; his thoughts are being distorted by interfering bad spirits, or through the development of his psychic faculties spirits have informed him of the true enemies in his environment. Incoherent, rambling, and cryptic verbalizations indicate that he is undergoing a test, an experiment engineered by the spirits. If he wanders aimlessly through the neighborhood, he is being pursued by ambulatory spirits who are tormenting him unmercifully. To the usual person living in a slum or *caserío*, these explanations are more credible than those theories premised upon the intricate functions of the id, ego, and superego, all of which are concepts far removed from common experience and belief.

In our study, 75 per cent of the husbands and 80 per cent of the wives (77 per cent of all) are Roman Catholic. Proportionately as

---

[8] Allan Kardec discusses the different ways in which the spirits may communicate and the corresponding *facultades* that spiritualists may have in *El Libro De Los Mediums*, Editorial Orion, Mexico, 1951, pp. 183–224.

many sick as well persons are Catholic. Of the 18 persons who are not Catholic, 2, both men, have no religious affiliation. The religious identifications of the remainder are: Pentecostal, 7; United Evangelical, 3; Mita, 2; Disciples of Christ, 1; Evangelical Baptist, 1; Presbyterian, 1; and Church of God (Mr. Quiromo's personal religion), 1.

There is no overlap in membership between religions. A person is either a Catholic or a Protestant, but not both. Moreover, if he belongs to one Protestant denomination, he does not belong to another, but the pattern of mutual exclusion does not apply to spiritualism; 63 per cent of the persons affiliated with one of the foregoing religions also affirm a belief in spiritualism. Overlap between spiritualism, on the one hand, and Catholicism and Protestantism, on the other, is the pattern, not the exception. No person, sick or well, expresses discomfort about believing in both spiritualism and some other religion despite the fact that Catholic and Protestant clergymen often inveigh against spiritualism as a pagan faith.

Believers in spiritualism are found disproportionately among Catholics (68 per cent) in comparison to Protestants (50 per cent). Although the unequal concentration of spiritualists in the Catholic group can be explained by the operation of chance, the direction of the difference is what we would expect. Protestantism is a minority religion composed of tightly knit denominations which proselytize energetically. Whereas nominal affiliation in a Protestant denomination is unusual, it is the rule rather than the exception in the Catholic group. Protestantism in the slum and *caserío* culture enmeshes the lives of its followers to an extent seldom experienced by a Catholic.

Beyond baptism and perhaps the marriage ceremony, Catholicism as a faith is irrelevant to most of the persons we studied, of casual interest to some, and a matter of weekly involvement to only two persons, both women. Catholic churches are not found in the depths of the slum areas where our families live. Irrespective of location, they are seldom, if ever, communal meeting places for slum- and *caserío*-dwellers. During the 3-year period of pretesting and interviewing for the study, no member of the Catholic clergy ever visited one of our families; indeed, only rarely is a priest or nun seen in the areas in which we worked. Church attendance is infrequent, for out of the eighty persons studied only two go to services at least once a week. The remainder go irregularly, for special occasions such as Holy Week, or never.

Mrs. Quiromo and Mrs. Urrutia, who are both afflicted with schizophrenia, are the most devout Catholics in our study. Mrs. Urrutia goes to Mass every Sunday morning before her husband and daughters have awakened. Unlike most persons who are prone to exaggerate the frequency with which they go to church, she seldom speaks about it. She does not try to persuade her husband to go to church. Even though Mr. Urrutia is a Catholic, he views religion as *cosas de mujer* (habits of women). Nor does Mrs. Urrutia insist that her three daughters go to church except during Holy Week. To Mrs. Urrutia, religion is a personal matter strictly between herself and the Church; she uses the confessional at church to "undrown" herself of anguish, confusion, and guilt. Although she wants to talk about the symptoms of her illness and the baffling experiences it has brought, neither her husband nor her mother, who is afflicted with identical symptoms, wants to listen. Thus she tells the priest about the drop of water she feels rolling around in her head, the brusque treatment she receives from her husband, and the hostility she harbors toward her mother, but she is reluctant to tell him about the lover who visits her often in her dreams. Mrs. Urrutia is overwhelmed by erotic pleasure in these dreams which are vivid and real to her; with her husband she is frigid, recalcitrant, and never achieves orgasm, but after such a dream she often awakens to an orgasm. Overcome by her confusion and guilt feelings, she recently threw caution to the winds and described the dream to the priest. The priest who interpreted the dream as a wish to be unfaithful reprimanded her and instructed her to pray. Mrs. Urrutia has decided now that it is best to confess only the "usual sins."

Mrs. Quiromo is unlike Mrs. Urrutia in that Catholicism affects almost her entire life. Upon marriage, she exacted promises from her husband that he would convert to Catholicism and that the children would be brought up in this faith. During the day, Mrs. Quiromo sits in a corner of her home, withdrawn from her environment, and fantasizes that she is a nun in a convent surrounded by other sisters in prayerful meditation. Mr. Quiromo, who is also a schizophrenic, considers himself a prophet, a prime interpreter of the Bible, and a leader of his own congregation. After marriage, his halfhearted efforts to become a Catholic ended abruptly when a priest told him he would have to pray to be converted. Mr. Quiromo immediately dropped to his knees and began a noisy recitation of prayers that he himself had written. The priest reprimanded him severely for what he regarded as an act of mockery and ridicule. Because of a series of revelations that came to him, Mr. Quiromo views himself as the prophet through whom Christ will visit Puerto Rico; he sees the Catholic Church as riddled with morally wrong assumptions.

Mr. Quiromo suffers from his wife's disinterest, from his in-laws' acid comments about his infidelities, and from the ridicule of neighbors about his singing of original hymns. As he relates the wretched treatment he receives from an ungrateful world, he finds solace in the idea that Jesus also suffered the scorn and punishment of his fellow men and that he, much like Jesus, must bear the pain of stigma.

Another double schizophrenic couple, the Gallardos, have recently converted from Catholicism to the Disciples of Christ. After the first onrush of schizophrenic symptoms, Mr. Gallardo developed a hatred toward his co-workers, friends, and neighbors until only the next-door neighbors were viewed as friends. These neighbors took the Gallardos to a meeting of the Disciples of Christ. At first, Mr. Gallardo was suspicious, but when the minister came to visit him, took him to the hospital for treatment, and gave him money to buy milk for his children, both he and his wife were converted. Now the Gallardos go to meetings of the Disciples twice a week and are often visited by other members of the congregation. At the services the Gallardos listen to the problems of the followers and, in turn, recite their own. All are bound together in a cooperative effort to give each other material and spiritual help. Although Mr. Gallardo doubts much of what he hears at the services, he says,

> I feel better each time I attend. Everyone likes us, respects us, and wants us to return. This makes me want to attend more services.

One family, the Aparicios, belong to the Mita religion which is native to Puerto Rico. It began 23 years ago when a woman member of the Pentecostal Church in Arecibo broke with the minister, was inspired to form a new church, adopted through divine revelation the name Mita, and began to call on the people to redeem themselves of sin. Mita's followers are estimated to number in the thousands (according to the Aparicios, 5000), practically all of whom live in the San Juan area.[9] The Church subsists from voluntary donations and from a number of small shops and restaurants located in the vicinity of Mita's home. As an active enterprise, the Church helps its followers to weather the vicissitudes of their impoverished life. Food and clothing are distributed to the members, many of whom believe that physical and mental illness can be cured by their belief. Mita's followers wear

---

[9] San Juan *Star*, January 5, 1964.

white clothing during services. The faith glorifies devoutness, charity, and humility—qualities attributed to Jesus—and proscribes cursing, drinking, and adultery. There is no such thing as nominal affiliation in the Mita faith; one is either a fervent believer and practitioner of the faith or not of the Church.

The Aparicios, both of whom were diagnosed by the psychiatrists as mentally healthy, are ruled by their involvement in this Church. On Tuesdays, Thursdays, and Sundays, the mother, father, and two children don white clothing to go to services. Usually, they meet other members as they walk to church, often making up an informal procession on the sidewalks of the busy thoroughfare on which it is located. Mr. Aparicio reports:

> At church, I forget my material problems. I communicate with God, and I am the happiest man on earth. My wife feels the same thing.

The Aparicios were Catholics until 10 years ago. Mrs. Aparicio explains that her older sister was suffering from a long-lasting rash of blisters and sores.

> The good Lord told her to go to Mita, that this was her solution. She made a promise to God that if Mita cured her, then she and the family would become Mitas. She was cured. That is why I am a Mita.

Mrs. Aparicio converted her husband to the Mita religion, but she would now prefer to be married to a nonbeliever, which would allow her the opportunity to convert another soul to Mita. Also her misunderstanding of the bonds of religious brotherhood creates tension between the spouses; Mrs. Aparicio now rejects her husband's sexual requests as incestuous. Although the psychiatrist saw no serious symptoms of psychopathology, he describes Mrs. Aparicio as a religious fanatic. Her neighbors avoid her because she proselytizes at every possible moment. The fieldworkers were able to adapt to her religious zeal with patience and forbearance but not without strain. After her mental health examination, she told the fieldworker that she had almost converted the doctor.

Mr. Aparicio was also a believer in spiritualism when he got married, but his attitude has changed drastically.

> The spirits of the dead people cannot communicate with the living. Once a person has died he passes to the throne of God. From there he never leaves. Spiritualism is a thing of the devil because it confuses people and claims their souls. It is a deception. Spiritualists

are people with diabolical ideas, which instead of doing good for humanity are leading to its damnation. They are people who cheat and work with infernal books.

This vehemence against spiritualism is understandable. To reiterate a point stated earlier, strong involvement in a recognized religion removes a person from the powerful attraction of spiritualism.

The sum and substance of the participation in formal associations of the forty families are small. Although 25 per cent of the men belong to labor organizations, the union movement has only now begun to achieve power, and its hold over the husbands in our study is erratic and tenuous. None of the husbands attends union meetings regularly. Two received unemployment benefits when their unions were on strike; a third, Mr. Gallardo, took advantage of his union's medical plan by going to a local clinic. Three men have borrowed money from cooperative groups composed of fellow employees of the agencies for which they work. Two persons have attended Parent-Teacher Association meetings; one man belongs to a local civil defense group. Participation in formal organizations associated with the life of the higher classes is largely outside the purview of the lower class.

SUMMARY

Voluntary associations play a negligible role in the lives of the sick and well persons. Outside the nuclear and extended family, religious beliefs and practices are the most important source of social support. Although most persons identify themselves as Catholic, the affiliation is primarily nominal, far removed from the daily life of all but two women in the study. Two-thirds of the Catholics and one-half of the Protestants believe in spiritualism. Belief in spiritualism assumes an invisible world of good and bad spirits who intrude in human affairs and can be employed by persons who have developed *facultades* to cure illnesses, arbitrate personal disputes, and explain events incongruous with common sense.

The small but energetic Protestant denominations, which affect the lives of one out of every five persons, are directly interwoven into the trials and tribulations of persons living in slums and *caseríos*, much as is spiritualism, but spiritualism derives its support from informal, primary group processes without organized efforts to proselytize. The spiritualistic interpretations for the symptoms of the mentally ill are simple, credible, and given in a setting free of the stigma associated with psychiatric treatment at the insane asylum.

Spiritualism is the most prevalent form of social organization outside the family which helps the schizophrenic person cope with his illness. Viewed more broadly, spiritualism is the one institution to which the people turn for help in their hours of need. They know it will have an answer to their plaintive questions. The medium understands their subculture; she knows how to placate the troubled by plausible interpretations of their troubles. She provides social support to an emotionally disturbed person.

PART V THE IMPACT OF SCHIZOPHRENIA ON THE FAMILY

The seven chapters in Part V examine important dimensions of family structure and processes as they are related to the presence or absence of schizophrenia in the four family diagnostic groups: control families (both spouses free of schizophrenia), husband-schizophrenic families, wife-schizophrenic families, and double-schizophrenic families (both spouses schizophrenic). Chapter 13 describes what the spouses expected from their marriages and outlines the major disillusionments they have experienced in marriage. Chapter 14 focuses on the economic condition of the family and discusses the effect of schizophrenia on the role of the husband as a provider for the family. Data are presented on the financial needs of the family as perceived by sick and well men and on the efforts made by the wife to cope with the economic problems created by the husband's impairment. Chapters 15 and 16 examine the ways in which the different family groups are related to the larger network of the kinship system.

Chapter 17 discusses sexual problems; the central question of this chapter is: Are tensions surrounding sexual intercourse between the spouses interwoven with the presence or absence of schizophrenia? Schizophrenic persons behave in idiosyncratic and deviant ways. Chapter 18 and Chapter 19 deal with social control in the family. Does the illness exempt the person from normal responsibilities? What influence, if any, is brought to bear on him to correct his behavior? Or is the illness accepted and are efforts made to compensate for the failures of the sick person?

By the use of case material, diverse dimensions of family life are pieced together to form a composite portrait of families in the four diagnostic groups.

13
Family Structure and Process

From the beginning of the field work we observed differences between the families in the ways husbands and wives interact with each other. In some families the husband and wife engage in animated and friendly conversation, often expressing affection through good-natured jokes; each spouse admires and respects the other. In other families the spouses are estranged from each other, living in a state of repressed, sullen hostility; they go to bed at different times and arise at different times to avoid speaking to one another; tension is deep and pervasive. In still other families, the spouses are embroiled in incessant conflict; they communicate with one another in special ways: favorable or complimentary words are never exchanged; curses, alternating between direct and indirect insults, are hurled; arguments explode into physical violence as husband and wife kick or beat each other with their fists or any object that is handy.

To illustrate that the quality of interspouse relations is evident to an observer, we quote from a fieldworker's report.

> From the way each spouse talks about the other, I can feel that there is a mutual understanding, tolerance, consideration, respect, and admiration. Both feel that they have selected the perfect mate, even though they do not say this in so many words. One can see that the house is clean and the arrangement of the furniture is in good taste. On the other hand, when I visit a disorganized home for the first time, I feel upset by the lack of cleanliness of the household as well as of the people living there. The children are dirty, ragged, and fearful of their parents and of strangers who come into their houses. The wife complains about the behavior of the husband—his drinking, gambling, and pursuing of other women. They quarrel bitterly.

After all the interviews with each family were completed, a staff conference was held to discuss the role relations of the spouses, patterns of social support, issues and tensions, points of consensus and disagreement, and amount of communication in the family. These several dimensions of family life are summarized by the term *cohesion*. The fieldworkers who interviewed the family presented data and led the discussion. At the end of the conference, each member of the staff was asked to disregard the psychiatric status of the spouses and assign a numerical rating to the family in terms of a five-point scale of cohesion. A family with maximum cohesion was given a rating of 1, with minimum cohesion a rating of 5; ratings of 2, 3, or 4 were given to a family according to how closely it approximated either extreme. Although each staff member without consultation assigned the rating to the family which had been discussed, there was little disagreement among the staff. The most frequent rating assigned to a family was taken to represent the degree of its cohesion.

To examine the relationship between the cohesion and schizophrenia, the forty families are divided into the four diagnostic groups used throughout the book. Table 43 presents data on the ways the fieldworkers evaluated cohesion in each of the four diagnostic family groups.

Family unity decreases from control families to husband-schizophrenic families, to wife-schizophrenic families, and on to the double schizophrenic families. The rank order of the four diagnostic family

TABLE 43 Staff Ratings of Family Cohesion by Diagnostic Family Group

	N	MODE *	MEAN *
Control families	20	1	1.9
Husband-schizophrenic families	7	2	2.3
Wife-schizophrenic families	9	3	2.8
Double schizophrenic families	4	4	4.0
All families	40	1	2.4

* To illustrate the meaning of the modes and means, the ratings of the families in the control groups are described: In this group, the mode of the staff's rating is 1 for 10 families, 2 for 4 families, 3 for 5 families, and 4 for 1 family. Since the rating of 1 is the most frequent, it is taken to represent the control group. The mean is computed by multiplying the number of families which received the same rating by the value of the rating, adding the results, and dividing by the total number of families in each diagnostic group as shown by the N column.

groups is the same whether the mean or the mode is followed. The structure of social relations between husbands and wives appears to be related to two factors: schizophrenia, and the sex of the spouse (or spouses) afflicted with a psychotic disorder.

The rank order of cohesion for the four diagnostic family groups given in Table 43 *suggests* a relationship between schizophrenia and the structure of social relations in the family. We present these data with caution because the judgments of the members of the staff are subjective, as they knew the psychiatric status of the spouses when they rated a family. This knowledge may have influenced their judgments regarding the degree of cohesion between husband and wife. Each fieldworker recorded his judgment of a family on a secret ballot, however, and there was general consensus among the fieldworkers on the level of cohesion in a family.

The point of view adopted to examine both expectations and disillusionments in marriage is that of the person who was interviewed; we examine his evaluation of his marriage by employing standards which he, himself, believes and feels are important. So that we could collect the relevant data, each person was asked, "What did you expect of marriage at the time of your marriage?" He then was asked to compare his experiences in marriage to his initial expectations.

What do men expect of marriage? Both sick and well men expect that marriage will bring into their lives a sense of order which is lacking in the life of a single person. "When one is single, one jumps from one place to another, depending upon one's friends," comments Mr. Berríos. Mr. Medina claims, "In marriage one can have an orderly life, a formulated life." Even men who reminisce nostalgically about the freedom of a single life, of carousing in *cafetines*, or enjoyable affairs with a variety of women emphasize the value of having a stable home that routinizes and organizes their everyday lives. To a man, marriage does not mean that the joys of a single life have to be relinquished entirely; order and freedom can be combined.

Order is achieved by having a "good" wife who willingly performs the tasks of homemaker by sewing, washing, ironing, cooking, cleaning, and taking care of the children. She does not visit her neighbors too often or for too long a period; a "gadabout" who embroils herself in neighborhood gossip can never be an ideal wife. Before she visits a friend or goes shopping, a good wife consults her husband, making sure to inform him of her whereabouts at all times; she is sexually faithful and does not speak to men who are not relatives so that her fidelity is never in doubt. She is not expected to make a financial contribution to the family; to the contrary, the husband does not want his wife to work and, upon marriage, if she is employed, he insists that she quit her job: "A woman's place is at home." From his point of view, it is important that a wife be *conforme*, accepting of the status quo. She does not pressure him to provide more for the family. She restricts her curiosity about his activities away from home. She does not try to control him by arguments and fights. The husband values an attitude of passive acceptance in his wife because it allows him a greater margin of freedom: "A man is married only at home."

What do women expect in marriage? Both sick and well women look on marriage as a means of escaping the controls of their parents. They want to be the *ama de la casa* (mistress of the home). Because of the desire to achieve independence from their parents they are only dimly aware of the new controls that will be imposed upon them in marriage. Even women who during childhood and adolescence were conscious of the restrictions suffered by their mothers in meeting the demands of their husbands, being confined to the household, and guarding themselves against gossip in the neighborhood view marriage as a way of achieving a large measure of freedom.

An ideal husband provides for his family, is faithful to his wife, and is loving and considerate. He is aware that his wife has few opportunities for entertainment; to give her relief from the monotony of daily household work he takes her on walks, to the movies, and to visit relatives, but a "good" husband never takes his wife to dance halls or bars where women of the "happy life" congregate. To do this would be to treat her as a common woman of the "low life," as morally cheap. This would also expose her to the sexual advances of other men, and the husband, as a man of dignity and respect, would be called upon to fight in defense of his wife.

Dignity and respect are two important concepts in the structuring of expectations in the family and the ordering of interpersonal relations. Dignity (*dignidad*) is a self-concept. A man who has dignity has inner coherence; his self-concept is accepted by his associates. He neither transgresses against the dignity of others nor does he permit disrespectful people to impinge on his dignity. *Dignidad* is related to *respeto*, but the former refers to an individual's conception of himself, whereas the latter is expressed in overt behavior.

The value of respect is often mentioned by husbands and wives as they describe ideal family life. No adequate translation of the term *respeto*, with all its rich connotations of sentiment and emotion, can be found in English. The situational meaning of *respeto* is most apparent in social contacts between the sexes, between young and old persons, and between persons of noticeably different socioeconomic status. Personal and social differences are recognized clearly by the use of *usted, señor, señora, don,* and *doña,* in contrast to the familiar *tú* which is an informal address. The proper behavior that accompanies the formal usage is reserved and cordial; to engage in inappropriate familiarity or intimacy is a mark of disrespect because it blurs important personal and social differences. Generally, to disregard or disdain a person's legitimate rights, his justifiable desires or requests, and his personal sense of worth and esteem is to be disrespectful. A child who raises his hand in anger against his father or mother is disrespectful. A man who touches another's face or buttocks deliberately is extraordinarily disrespectful since this is a taunt designed to express contempt.

Respect is considered to be of paramount importance in relations between a husband and wife. If a choice has to be made, 73 per cent of the wives and 70 per cent of the husbands prefer respect over love from their mates. A majority of persons, irrespective of their mental diagnoses, choose respect over love in marital relationships. A wife shows respect by obeying her husband and a husband by being faithful to his wife, in particular by not parading other women before her. When a person chooses respect over love he does not mean that love is unimportant. Rather, he means that respect is a necessary precondition for love; that without respect love is impossible; that love grows out of respect. Thus, an obedient wife and a faithful husband contribute to the development of loving relationships in the family.

To secure further information about the family ideals, we asked each person to describe a "good" husband and a "good" wife. Following his description of the ideal roles, the person was asked to tell us how well he and his spouse perform their respective roles. The interviewer went on to a series of questions to uncover those aspects of family roles that were or were not being fulfilled. The values associated with marriage and the family and the extent to which the values are being realized can be inferred from the answers to these questions. Husbands and wives, regardless of mental status, agree substantially on the characteristics of an ideal spouse; slight differences in emphasis by sex are apparent, with the husbands advocating an accepting, or *conforme,* wife and the wives accentuating the importance of a faithful husband. Overriding the difference in emphasis is the fact that husbands and wives share values which prescribe desirable behavior in the family. Consensus in family values stems from cultural norms that are a part of lower-class life. These ideal norms are verbalized by men and women irrespective of their mental status.

A question that brought us a copious "spill-out" of information was, "If you could live your life again, would you marry the same person to whom you are married, a different person, or would you never get married?" Almost all persons replied with a lengthy description of their spouse, the marital situation, and their feelings toward both. The reply, "That question fits like a ring on my finger," was typical. Others said, "If you only knew how often I have asked myself that same question."

Table 44 shows the percentage of persons who would choose to remarry the same spouse if life could be relived. The differences between the percentages in the table are not statistically significant, but the direction of the differences is consistently from the control families toward the double schizophrenic families. The percentages suggest two inferences: first, the well women married to sick men are experiencing gratifications in marriage despite the many incapacities of their husbands who are bedeviled by a variety of disturbing symptoms; second, the families in which the wives are schizophrenic represent a "special group." To pursue this point a step further, the families with schizophrenic wives were compared to the remaining families in terms of the husband's choice, the wife's choice, and the mutual choice of husband and wife. Each of the three comparisons yields a statistically significant difference beyond the .05 level of chance. Significant differences, therefore, can be observed when the forty families are di-

TABLE 44 Percentage by Diagnostic Family Group Who Would Remarry the Same Person

		THOSE WHO WOULD REMARRY THE SAME PERSON		
	N	HUSBANDS, %	WIVES, %	BOTH SPOUSES, %
Control families	20	75	55	50
Husband-schizophrenic families	7	71	71	71
Wife-schizophrenic families	9	22	11	11
Double schizophrenic families	4	0	50	0

TABLE 45 Fulfillment of Marital Expectations

	N	MARITAL EXPECTATIONS FULFILLED	
		HUSBANDS, %	WIVES, %
Control families	20	95	75
Husband-schizophrenic families	7	86	71
Wife-schizophrenic families	9	78	33
Double schizophrenic families	4	25	0

vided into two groups—families with schizophrenic wives and families with well wives. Persons who would choose not to remarry their spouses are concentrated disproportionately in the families with sick wives.

How many persons feel that, in general, their marital expectations have been fulfilled? Seventy per cent of the eighty husbands and wives report that their experiences in marriage have been about what they expected. Table 45 shows the percentage of husbands and wives in each diagnostic family group who report that, in general, their expectations have been fulfilled. The percentages indicate that the families are arranged in descending order from control families to husband-schizophrenic families, to wife-schizophrenic families, and then to double schizophrenic families. The same order is found among the husbands as among the wives, but the differences in percentages in the diagnostic family groups, either among the husbands or among the wives, are not statistically significant. On the other hand, when the thirteen families with schizophrenic wives are compared to the remaining families with wives who are not sick, significantly fewer sick wives state that their marital expectations have been fulfilled ($p < .01$). Presently, we shall see that the sick women are strongly disillusioned with most aspects of their marriages.

In each of the four diagnostic family groups, expectations have been fulfilled in marriage for fewer wives than husbands. Husbands are more often satisfied with the outcome of their marriages than are wives. Many persons who state that their expectations have, in general, been fulfilled still cite a variety of problems, unfavorable experiences, and points of disillusionment in marriage which they did not anticipate.

Four points of disillusionment recur repeatedly: the demand for order in the home, the retention of the husband's freedom, the loss of the wife's freedom, and the deprivations forced on the family by economic considerations. In succeeding paragraphs we discuss the first three themes of disillusionment. The issue of poverty is covered in Chapter 14.

The typical husband, regardless of his mental condition, views marriage as an arrangement which will bring "order"; it provides a "formulated life" in which things are as they should be. The husband emphasizes the importance of peaceful routines in marriage. The achievement of these ends rests largely on the extent to which the wife performs her duties reliably by creating order and tranquility in the home and in working for her husband, children, and her relatives. As the following statements demonstrate, a husband gives credit to his wife when he feels that she is doing her part.

> My wife is a good houseworker and this is what one needs in a woman. She cleans the house and she sends the children to school clean. She is good, and for that reason I have not had to worry about getting another woman.
>
> My wife takes good care of the children. When I return from work I know that my food will be ready and my clothes washed and ironed when I need them.

Many husbands state the same point, but Mr. Iriarte is the most enthusiastic in calling attention to his wife's devotion to duty. (Neither husband nor wife in this family is schizophrenic.) To substantiate his point, Mr. Iriarte tells how his wife managed the birth of their last child. Late in the afternoon when Mr. Iriarte returns from a hard day's work in an automobile shop, he likes to eat his dinner in peace. As he sits to eat, his wife ushers the children away, then stands at his side ready to serve and help him. On the afternoon she began to feel the initial pains of childbirth, she continued to cook the evening meal for her husband. By the time he returned from work she was sure the contractions were a prelude to childbirth, but she served her husband, and as he ate she went to the bedroom and delivered the baby.

Mr. Julía says:

> A single man is worth a thousand married men. I am married, but I live like a free man because I do what comes out of my balls. I come home at the hour I want.

Mr. Padilla dreams of the freedom enjoyed by Mr. Julía:

I would like to stay away from home later than 9:00 at night. I would like to leave home, stay away two or three days, and then be received well, without arguments or fights, when I return home.

A wife does not approve of such behavior, however, and even her desire to be *conforme* does not encompass passive acceptance of her husband's infidelity. Mrs. Badillo says,

I have been happy with him for he is a wonderful man and a hard worker. We are poor but he provides everything he can. Oh, but how he made me suffer when we were first married! He was in love all the time and promised marriage to some girls during my first pregnancy. He came home with lipstick stains. When I talked to him about it he used to leave the house to eat out in the street. He encouraged me to visit my family in the country. When I returned several persons told me what he was doing. He had about fifty girl friends.

Upon marriage, the typical man continues to center much of his life "in the street" with his friends and in *cafetines*. Freedom to roam the streets is consistent with the life the husband led as a single man, but his wife expects him to come home after work, to show an interest and commitment to family affairs, and to be an ideal husband. The prevailing role of the *macho*, however, conflicts with the prescriptions entailed in being a good husband. Thus, to the husband, marriage poses a dilemma. With the passing of years it appears that the husband resolves the dilemma in favor of his family. Then he is no longer bothered by the ridicule of his co-workers who tell him that he has been tied, shackled, and made to "sit upon a trunk" like a ventriloquist's dummy. Mr. Badillo has been married to the same woman for 18 years, longer than any other husband in the study group. To the delight of his wife and in contrast to his early marital life, Mr. Badillo is now a home-centered husband who employs his skills as an upholsterer to embellish and repair the furniture in his home. Mrs. Badillo boasts:

My husband has never beaten me, nor has he abandoned me. He knows how to repair furniture, and the inside of my apartment looks nice, doesn't it?

The hypothesis that the problem of masculine freedom is felt most acutely early in marriage cannot be tested, however, because the persons in this study group are only between 20 and 39 years of age, and the mean number of years the spouses have been married to one another is 8.7 years.

The schizophrenic husband married to a well woman renounces social activities which remove him from his family. Mrs. Cardona tells us, "My husband has all the qualifications I wanted in a man. He is not a wise guy; he does not have the vices of rum and gambling." Of more relevance is Mrs. Espinosa's comment: "My husband takes me out when he can. Compared to other husbands who are never in their homes with their children, he is just wonderful." In comparison with the well man, the sick man seldom leaves his home, and when he does it is for short excursions or in the company of his wife. Home to him is a protective nest, governed by a doting wife who is extremely concerned with his aches and ailments. His wife does not suffer the disillusionment of the wife in the control family who must wait for many years before her husband develops a deep commitment to his family.

The schizophrenic wife married to a well husband is disillusioned by the many hours her husband spends away from home. For instance, Mrs. Janer complains that she seldom sees her husband. After work he meets his friends to play billiards. He comes home late in the evening and insists that his dinner be served promptly. Early in the morning he leaves for work. Several times he has promised to take his wife and the children on a *paseo* (Sunday afternoon walk), but each time, after Mrs. Janer and the children have bathed and dressed, her husband fails to come home. To Mrs. Janer the incident that best illustrates her husband's lack of concern for the family occurred when she had her last child, a daughter. Many hours after the child was born, Mr. Janer finally appeared at the hospital and according to his wife:

> When they showed him our daughter, he said that he did not want her, that he did not want to bring a piece of dog meat to his house, nor did he want a pair of slippers [symbolic of daughters]. Then he brought me home and the stitches broke and I had a bad infection. My husband was not around.

Mr. Janer centers his activities away from the family, as do most of the well men married to schizophrenic women. By way of contrast, the schizophrenic man married to an afflicted woman vacillates between his family and the outside world, unable to stabilize his life in either setting. Consequently, the double schizophrenic families are riven by conflict.

The typical well woman married to a well husband is greatly involved in her home duties. Sometimes she feels that marriage has robbed her of freedom and, even though she continues to work diligently, she may occasionally feel enslaved or exploited.

> If I were single, I would be free. When one gets married, one becomes a slave. One gives one's whole life to the home and cannot go out.
>
> When one is single one has more freedom and less problems. Life is easier because you don't have as many obligations.
>
> Men, from what I have seen, are bothersome. They use their women as servants. They are only good to boss others around. At times they see you are busy doing something, but they make you stop to take care of them.

The well woman married to a schizophrenic man has additional burdens, but she seldom complains; over and above the usual routine of work, she must keep an unusually quiet household because her husband is easily upset by the normal noises in the slums and *caseríos*. If the children are "acting up" or if the neighbors create a disturbance, he explodes furiously; it is her duty to pacify the children or request quiet from the neighbors. In spite of added problems, all except one of the well women married to schizophrenic men have found compensating values in the marriages. They shoulder their burdens with few complaints.

The loss of freedom the sick woman feels is compounded by her husband's demanding and disrespectful behavior. Unlike her husband, she does not have a well-delineated role that would serve to remove her from the everyday disenchantment of her marital life. The sick wife, regardless of her husband's mental condition, is hard put to provide the orderly household desired by her husband. Meals are not served on time; laundry is not washed and ironed as it should be; then, in the words of Mrs. Janer, "He comes home to scold me and it is terrible. . . . If only he were easier on me." In brief, the schizophrenic woman is profoundly disgruntled with marriage, more so than the well woman, the sick man, or the well man.

Out of anger, frustration, and a sense of oppression, the sick woman develops a utopian world into which she sometimes projects herself. Although the sick man does not have a comparable dream world and, therefore, cannot retreat into the soothing comfort of an organized pleasurable fantasy, he does not confront the ugly discrepancy between the unreal world and the grim social reality that envelops all persons. In the fantasy world of the sick woman, no obligations, demands, or expectations are imposed on her. She comes and goes as she pleases because neither husband nor parents impose restrictions on her; children do not cry for her care; there is no housework; the husband does not pester her for sexual relations; fatigue disappears, and she can rest as long as she desires. In this ideal dream world a woman is free from physical and emotional strain. Harsh words are never spoken; inner turmoil and fear disappear as she is enveloped in benevolent human associations. The utopian world abounds with fun and entertainment. It resembles television advertisements which show clean, smiling, and cheerful persons who romp with abandon on the white sand and stop only to light each other's cigarettes, all to the background music of a gay tune.

The sick woman *knows* she does not live in such a world. Her real world is too different: it demands much and gives little. When she compares the real to the unreal world, she sees herself as a person experiencing untold suffering like a martyr; but she lacks the religious cause and the philosophical resignation of the martyr. The many exigencies of family life in the lower class allow her only fleeting visits to her utopian world.

SUMMARY

There is firm agreement about the values and ideals associated with marriage and the family. Expectations in marriage have, in general, been fulfilled; the proportion of persons who believe this decreases from the control group to the husband-schizophrenic families, to the wife-schizophrenic families, and finally to the families with both spouses schizophrenic.

Ideally, the wife is home-centered, devoted to her duties, accepting responsibilities, absolutely faithful, and careful not to have unnecessary social contacts with men. In addition to being a provider, the ideal husband is considerate of his wife and faithful to her. The man looks upon marriage as a way of stabilizing his life; the woman as a means of achieving the freedom she desires but lacked while living with her parents.

Husbands and wives agree in their definitions of ideal conjugal partners, ideal parents, and ideal offspring. Of central importance in their definition of ideal family roles is the value of respect. Husbands and wives consistently choose respect over love from each other. Respect, they believe, creates order and tranquility in family life. Respect also creates love and affection.

Family values, however, are only a part of the scheme of values in

Puerto Rican society. There are other values that compete and conflict with the family values that have been described in this chapter. *Machismo*, for example, the creed of the *macho*, represents a set of masculine values that outlines the ideal activities for men which typically are centered outside family life and are inconsistent with the idea of a "good" husband. The effect of these mutually exclusive values creates recurrent and widespread disruptions in family life, centering around the issue of infidelity.

The tendency of the husband to be drawn away from the family into masculine social activities disillusions the wife in the control group. The sick husband does not have many social relationships outside the family, which delights his well wife. The sick woman, particularly if she is married to a well man, inveighs against her husband because of his excessive absence from home and his lack of interest in the family. The control family wife, as well as the well wife married to a sick man, is deeply immersed in her family, although periodically she bemoans her lack of freedom. To the sick woman, the housework required to keep an orderly household is an extraordinary hardship. Out of a sense of oppression she fantasies a utopian world composed of persons who are kind and permissive to her.

The findings based on the question, "If you could live your life again, would you marry the same person, a different person, or never get married?" reinforces the inference that the sick wives are a disgruntled group. Moreover, proportionately fewer husbands would choose their sick wives than would husbands not married to sick women. These data suggest that the impact schizophrenia has on a family depends on the sex of the afflicted person.

14

Economic Dimensions of Family Life

Each family lives in the urbanized area of the San Juan metropolitan community. More specifically, 65 per cent of the families live in slum areas and 35 per cent live in *caseríos*. No family derives its income from subsistence crops; all live in a complex, money-dominated society and are dependent on a cash income. The economic level at which the families live is a prime source of activity and discontent. These husbands and wives expected marriage to bring them relief from the poverty they knew as children; actually marriage has multiplied their problems.

The economic level of living of a minority of husbands and wives coincides with what they expected in life; indeed, only a few persons cite evidence of progress. The fortunate few tell us:

> I no longer have to ask my relatives for help. I have a house, a television set, a radio, and now we are buying other things. I have a life ahead of me in which to acquire many things.

To Mr. Nieves, the most striking symbol of his affluence is that he no longer has to drink warm water; he points with pride to his new pink refrigerator which now cools the drinking water. He has a new $200 high-fidelity record player, new mahogany living-room and bedroom sets, a new gas stove, a console television set, and an $80 oriental lamp hanging from the ceiling of the living room; all these items were bought on credit. The Nieves family lives in a 4-bedroom apartment in a *caserío* for which he pays $14.50 per month. In addition to his wife, Mr. Nieves has to support 8 children on the $30 a week he earns as an assistant cook in one of the San Juan hotels. Mr. Nieves' new-found affluence is as much a function of the prevailing system of installment buying (buy now—pay later with a minimum down payment, *pronto*), as it is of his earning power. Installment buying is a common practice among the few persons who have temporarily achieved their economic expectations.

Unlike Mr. Nieves, the majority of husbands and wives are overwhelmed by their impoverishment. Marriage, somehow, was supposed to bring an "undrowned" life, that is relief from poverty. This large majority voice their frustrations in familiar terms:

> We live in misery. I have few comforts.
>
> I have a houseful of children on whom I have to spend every cent I make. I can't save anything.
>
> Oh, if I were to tell you everything I expected! I wanted to own a house. I wanted to help my poor relatives. I wanted to travel. But nothing has been as I expected.
>
> Instead of taking me to a home, he [her husband] brought me to live with his sisters. I wanted to have a few things I did not have before—a house and some furniture.
>
> Our life has been a disaster. We live in water and mud. In some inexplicable way, something to eat always turns up.

Mrs. Janer summarizes the typical feeling: "I wanted to have the things I needed, but it has not been that way."

Marriage lays bare the raw edges of poverty and creates a renewed awareness of privation primarily because, in the words of Mr. Medina,

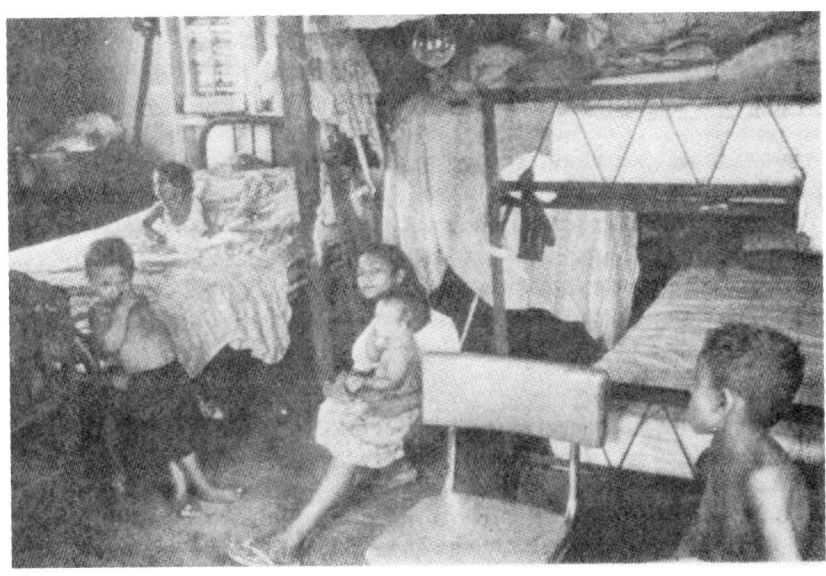

"The heavy load of marriage comes from having children." Mr. Iglesias states: "Because the children suffer too much when a person is poor and can't buy the necessary things for them." Mrs. Domínguez' statement is more poignant:

> God should not let poor people have children! Only those who own houses should have them. When so many children are born to poor people, it makes more suffering for the necessities of life.

Most persons in each of the four diagnostic family groups feel an economic strain. When a man marries he is no longer the recipient of support but the source of it. The onus is placed on him in a family situation that multiplies needs and desires. In addition to the expense of establishing a neolocal home, new dependents have to be fed, clothed, and cared for. Regardless of the wife's mental status, the family with a schizophrenic husband experiences most sharply the tribulations of a marginal economic life. The sick husband is either unemployed, underemployed, or in the process of withdrawing from work. He and his wife are disillusioned by his incapacity to provide for his family.

Despite the prevailing disillusionment which results from abundant needs and scarce resources in family life, husbands and wives quarrel over this point in only 20 per cent of the families. This percentage is based on an examination of the manifest content of the issues about which husbands and wives argue. The typical wife does not openly blame her husband for his failure to provide better. She realizes that jobs are few, often irregular, and wages are low. Moreover, she is *conforme*; although being *conforme* allows wide latitude to the expression of diffuse grievances, it proscribes criticizing the husband's efforts to provide.

Arguments over financial matters are confined mostly to the thirteen families with schizophrenic wives and either well or sick husbands. The stench of open sewers, the swarming mosquitos, the sweat-stained, rotting mattress, and the thin legs of the children—the many conspiracies of poverty—all converge upon the distraught schizophrenic wife. Her anger erupts because she believes that her husband is spending money for things outside the family's needs. Mr. Iglesias comments:

> We fight because once in a while she brings up things I can't afford, such as television, refrigerators, and baby cribs. I suffer because what I earn is not enough to buy these things. I explain to her that I can't buy them and she fights me, saying that I probably have another woman whom I support and for that reason I can't give her

Economic Dimensions of Family Life 279

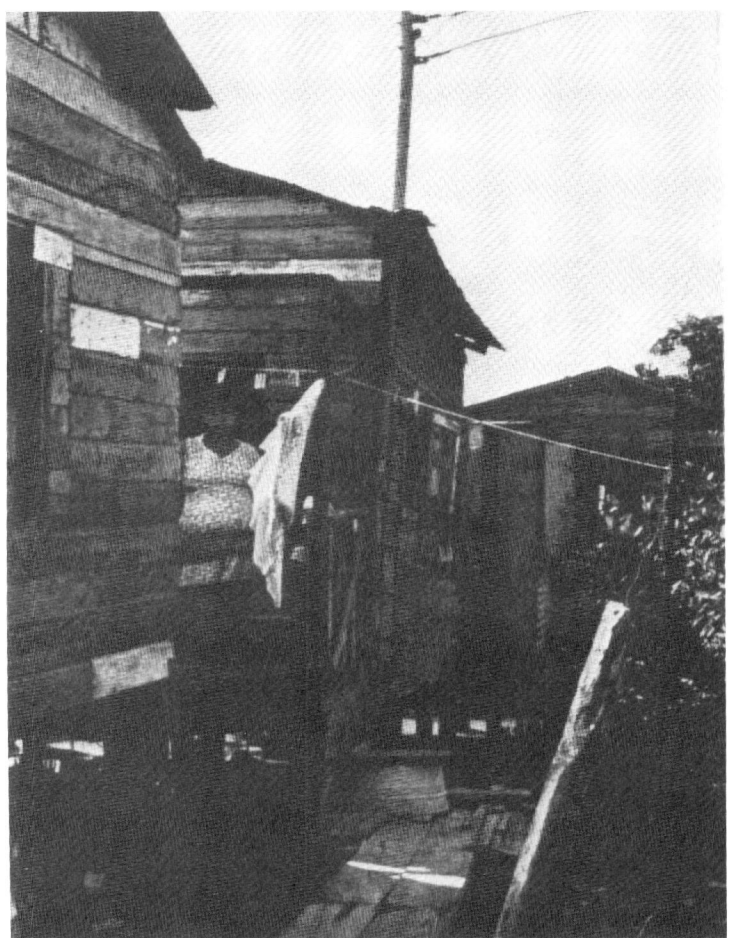

the luxuries she asks for. I explain to her that the money I make is not enough for one woman, let alone for another woman, but she does not accept this explanation. She is jealous and fights me. I'll never get married again.

The Urrutias illustrate how a family tries to bridge the gap between scarce resources and abundant needs. Mrs. Urrutia's maneuvers to raise the family's level of living beyond the earnings of her husband typify the actions of schizophrenic wives. This household is composed of Mr. and Mrs. Urrutia, their three daughters, aged 12, 9, and 7, Mrs.

280 *The Impact of Schizophrenia on the Family*

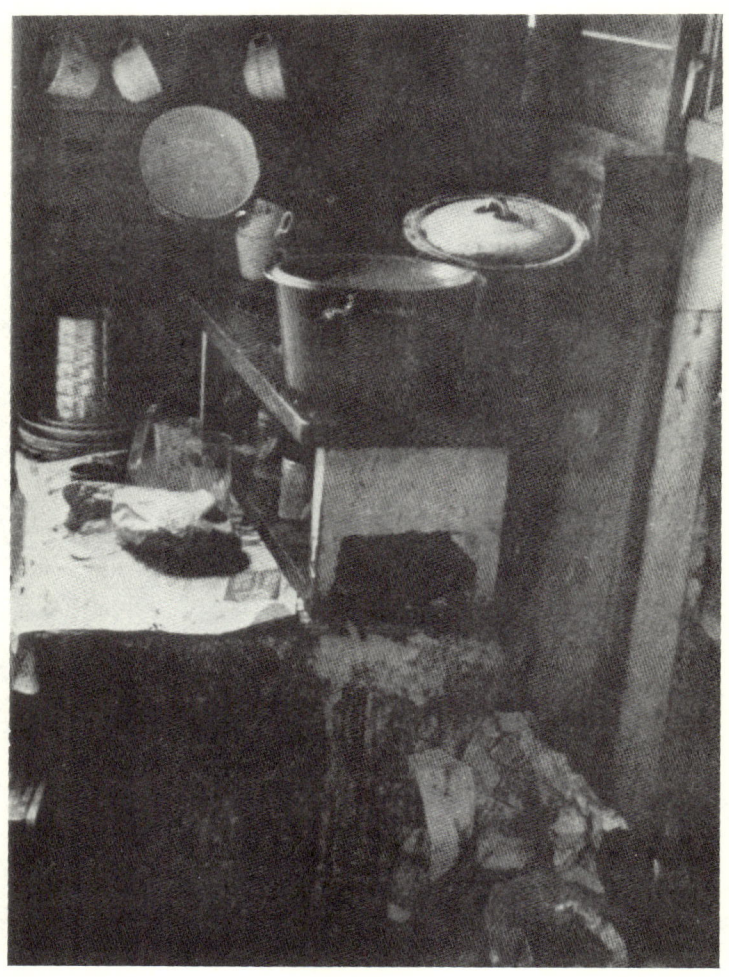

Urrutia's widowed mother, and a half-sister. Mrs. Urrutia is 36 years of age, finished the fifth grade in school, and is afflicted with schizophrenia. Mr. Urrutia, who is 39 years old, was diagnosed by the psychiatrist as mentally healthy. He attended school 1 year but he did not complete the first grade.

Mrs. Urrutia's father visits the family and helps them out periodically. Her mother, who was separated from her father, married again and was widowed when her second husband became staggering drunk, imagined he was Jesus, and drowned trying to walk on the waters of the lagoon. The mother now receives $13 a month from public welfare.

When the field work began, Mr. Urrutia was employed as an unskilled construction laborer, bending steel rods and placing them in reinforcing frames for concrete buildings. If he is not working with the steel rods, he is hauling cement, pushing a wheelbarrow, or doing other unskilled manual work for which he is paid an hourly wage. When a building is completed he is unemployed until construction starts on another one. Once construction is under way, he never misses a day irrespective of the weather or his health. When Mr. Urrutia is employed and Mrs. Urrutia's mother receives the $13 relief check, the family income approximates $150 per month. These funds support the seven members of the household with a per capita income per day of 73 cents; this is close to the median figure of 71 cents per day for class V families in the metropolitan area.

The Urrutias rent their lot from the Urban Renewal Corporation for $1 per month and are 6 months behind in the payment of the rental. Mr. Urrutia built their home himself. He procured materials for it by scrounging from a dump, carrying home lumber from the construction firm which employs him, and, when necessary, by buying some pieces. The house is frame and covered with boards. The roof is made of corrugated-iron sheets. The one interior wall is made of cardboard. Mr. Urrutia also built a one-room shack in the front yard for his mother-in-law and her daughter. The lot is surrounded by a fence made of boards, rusty barbed wire, and corrugated-iron sheets. The family lives inside of this compound with a flock of chickens and five dogs. The chickens are maintained for their eggs, although occasionally the family kills one for a meal. The large, vicious dogs are kept to protect the family.

To enter the Urrutias' compound, a visitor has to shout from the gate. Usually Mrs. Urrutia's mother answers the call by arriving at the gate with a heavy club 3 to 4 feet long. The dogs snarl, bare their teeth, or lunge at her as she escorts the visitor; she then whacks one on the head, sometimes shredding its ear from the blow. Mrs. Urrutia's mother castrated these dogs with a rusty razor blade because she did not want them "doing ugly things" to the bitches in front of her granddaughters.

All the furniture in the house has been purchased on credit except a print of Christ with a crown of thorns on his head which the family owns fully. The specific items in the shack are an electric refrigerator,

282 *The Impact of Schizophrenia on the Family*

a television set, a wrought-iron living-room set consisting of a sofa and two chairs, a chromium dining table and chairs, three beds with iron posts, a bureau, and a gas stove. All their clothing is kept in the bureau.

The Urrutias eat rice and beans every day; once or twice a week they have boiled codfish. Some days they buy a tin of Norwegian sardines, mash them into the oil in which they are preserved, and spread them on the rice. Occasionally, Mrs. Urrutia's father, who makes his living by peddling fresh fish from a small pushcart, exchanges his unsold

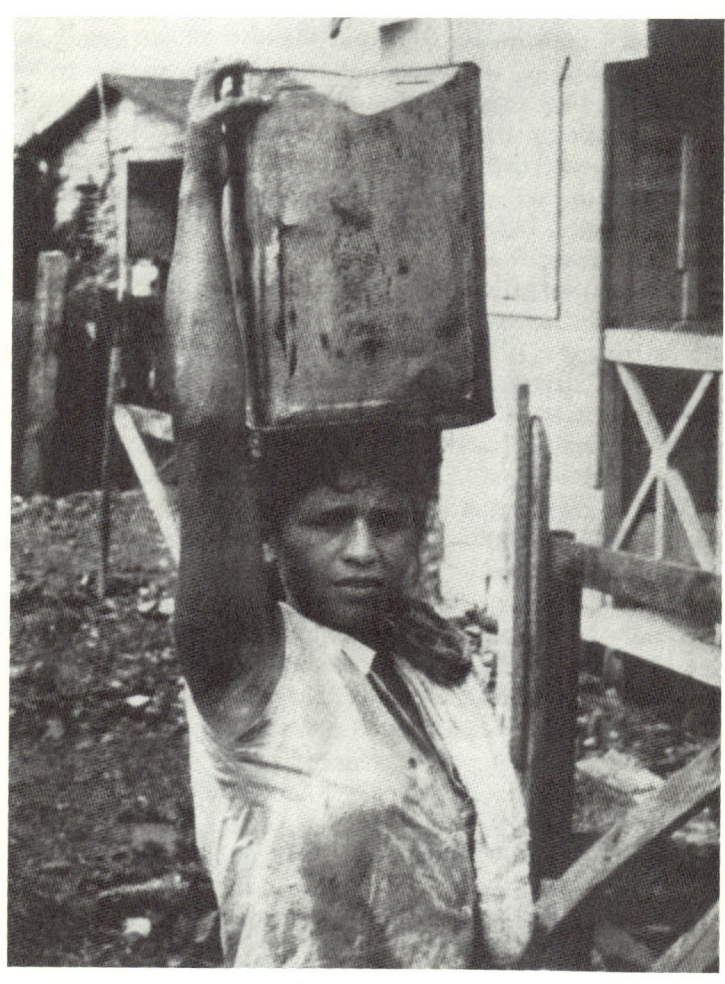

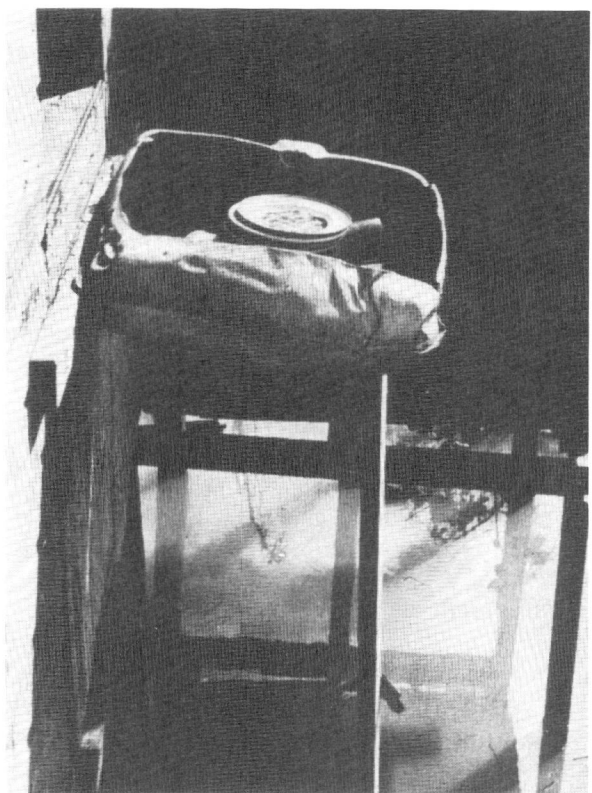

fish for a bunch of green bananas; he then brings the fruit to his daughter who boils them for her family.

Before going to work in the morning, Mr. Urrutia gathers the eggs his hens have laid and takes them to his mother who lives nearby; he also gives her the loose change from his pocket. In addition, he had been sending $3 a week to a brother in New York City whom he was told was unemployed. Recently, the brother sent a picture of himself dressed in a suit, sporting a wide smile, and embracing an American Negro girl from Harlem. Mr. Urrutia was angered by this display of affluence and gaiety and immediately discontinued sending money to the brother.

Mr. Urrutia does not allow his wife to get a job, despite her desire to work and his periodic unemployment. He says, "My wife's place is at home." About 5 years ago, however, when the family was destitute, he allowed her to take a job in a factory that made insect repellents. Mrs. Urrutia was unhappy at work and under tension because of a rumor that her boss had seduced three girls on the job. One day when she was feeling "nervous," another worker spilled insect repellent on her. Mrs. Urrutia felt this was an insult to her dignity and respect; enraged by the woman's behavior, she yelled: "If they turned you loose in the pasture, you would eat the grass." She then left the factory and never returned to work.

Mrs. Urrutia was saving money to have her broken false teeth repaired. Recently, a sanitation inspector told the family they had to build a new latrine because the old one was overflowing into the yard and had become a health menace. The inspector also ordered them to dispose of the chickens. Mr. Urrutia bought lumber with the money his wife had been saving and built a new latrine, but he thinks the inspector has no right to make him get rid of the chickens; he says, "The chickens will stay." Mrs. Urrutia was not distressed by having to chew food with her gums as she could eat boiled bananas and beans. However, she did miss eating the *pegao* (crunchy rice at the bottom of the pot) which she liked, so after several weeks she talked a dentist into repairing her false teeth on credit.

At about this time she went to the neighborhood grocer and asked him to write a note stating that her credit was good. Since the Urrutias had not paid their bill, the grocer was surly and reluctant. As Mrs. Urrutia describes it, he gave her a "dirty look." She says, "I don't care if he gives me dirty looks. I have the expression of a cobbler" (a bland and imperturbable look). This grocer is a small-business owner, a lower-class slum-dweller, and little better off economically than the Urrutias; he cannot afford to antagonize his customers lest they disregard their debts to him. When Mrs. Urrutia stared him down, he gave her a statement to the effect that her credit was reliable. Armed with the statement she went to another store selling garments and yard goods and established credit. She then charged clothing and yard goods until the owner refused her any more credit.

Although the Urrutias owe money to many people in their neighborhood, payments are not made on a regular basis. Bill collectors who threaten to repossess the items they sold to the Urrutias are given a token payment. One month, irate bill collectors forced them to pay $100 on the different bills they owed. In spite of their indebtedness at this time, the Urrutias planned an elaborate celebration for the graduation of their oldest daughter from the sixth grade. The family discontinued eating until they could save $20. The graduation dress, a must for the occasion, was made by the girl's godmother from many yards of lace and embroidery which had to be purchased. On the morning of the graduation, the daughter was sent to the beauty parlor for a haircut and permanent wave. After the ceremonies, the entire class went on a picnic to the beach. Mrs. Urrutia was satisfied that she had fulfilled her obligations to her daughter and to the class. She says with pride, "One eats every day, but one graduates from the sixth grade only once in a lifetime."

The Urrutia family is very proud of their oldest daughter's achievement in graduating from the sixth grade. The celebration of this achievement fits into the pattern of other ceremonies and holidays. Families make extraordinary sacrifices to participate in such events. Baptisms, weddings, funerals, Christmas, the coming of the three kings after Christmas, and Holy Week are not occasions for counting pennies and curtailing expenditures. These are moments of gaiety in an otherwise incessant struggle to live. During these moments of relief, primary group ties between friends, coparents, near relatives, and distant relatives are renewed. Empty stomachs often accompany efforts to participate with splendor and affluence on these gala days and attest to their importance in the society.

After we completed the field work, Mr. Urrutia was unemployed for several months. During this interval, all their furnishings were repossessed by their creditors, the grocer did not allow them to charge any groceries, and food for the family had to be provided by relatives and from the $13 monthly check from public welfare received by Mrs. Urrutia's mother. Even Mr. Urrutia's treasured chickens were eaten by the family. As one member of the family put it: "The wheels go around; sometimes you are on top and sometimes you are on the bottom."

The debts of the Urrutias are typical of lower-class families. Furniture is purchased on credit. Payments are met on a catch-as-catch-can basis. Creditors make dire threats to repossess or to take the case to court to get payment. If threats do not work, the seller repossesses the furniture and sells it again on credit. When a family loses furniture due to repossession, they often regain it by establishing credit elsewhere. One merchant may be used as a means to establish credit in another store, as the Urrutias used their grocer despite their precarious relationship to him. Usually these families do not know the extent of their debts, and efforts are made to meet only the most immediate and pressing expenses.

Money earned from employment is the most important source of income for the family. Seventy-three per cent of the husbands have full-time jobs, 12 per cent part-time jobs, and the remaining 15 per cent are unemployed. Twelve per cent of those employed are skilled workers, 50 per cent are semiskilled, and 38 per cent are unskilled laborers. They work as janitors, kitchen assistants, construction hands, ambulatory barbers, mechanics, bus drivers, handy men, and so on. One man sells fruit and vegetables.

In addition to earnings, some families receive disability pensions, public welfare payments, room rentals, and, in one case, the Veterans Administration gives allotments to a veteran of the Korean War who is going to school. Relatives who live with families and are employed make financial contributions to the family, but some families also receive weekly, bimonthly, and monthly donations from relatives who do not live with them. Table 46 shows the amount of income that results from these combined sources classified by diagnostic family group; it does not include occasional and irregular gifts of money or loans from friends, relatives, and neighbors, as these are not stable sources of income and are, therefore, difficult, if not impossible, to estimate. Nor are material gifts such as furniture and medicines included in the table, as their value in dollars and cents cannot be clearly determined. Thus, Table 46 includes only the relatively stable income that the household of the family receives every month from all sources.

Table 46 shows that the mean of the gross income for *all households* is $150 per month. Each household has a mean of 5.8 persons. Therefore, the per capita income which is available to each member of the household per month is about $26, slightly less than a dollar a day. In determining the actual per capita income, however, which would include irregular gifts of money from other persons, usually relatives, the amount would have to be modified either upward or downward because the families are deeply enmeshed in a pattern of reciprocal help with

TABLE 46 Mean Gross Incomes of the Households

	N	GROSS MONTHLY INCOME
Control families	20	$169.45
Husband-schizophrenic families	7	115.12
Wife-schizophrenic families	9	155.55
Double schizophrenic families	4	100.79
All households	40	150.00

TABLE 47 Employment According to Mental Status of Husband

	HUSBANDS SCHIZOPHRENIC, %	HUSBANDS NOT SCHIZOPHRENIC, %
A. Employment of Husbands		
Full time	27	90
Part time or unemployed	73	10
$N =$	11	29
$p < .01$		
B. Employment of Wives		
Full time	45	3
Part time or unemployed	55	97
$N =$	11	29
$p < .01$		

relatives who do not live with them. Gifts of money are exchanged as needs and problems arise. Thus the economic level of a family at a particular time depends both on its regular income and on its role as beneficiary or donor of familial help.

The differences between the means in Table 46 are not significant at the .05 level. The table shows, however, that the husband-schizophrenic and the double schizophrenic families receive less gross income than the control or wife-schizophrenic families. This difference reflects the reduced earnings of the sick man. Whereas the husbands who are not afflicted with schizophrenia earn $146 per month from their labors, the sick men earn $50. The difference is significant beyond the .01 level.

Data on the employment status of the men indicate also the economic impairment that results from schizophrenia. Section A of Table 47 shows that schizophrenia exacts a heavy price. To compensate for the economic impairment of the sick husband, a number of wives have secured employment. Section B of Table 47 shows that a larger proportion of wives with sick husbands are employed than are those with well husbands. Table 46, nonetheless, shows that the economic level of these families remains below that of the families with the well husbands. At this level of life, small differences in family income make large differences in family affairs. "Will we meet the payment on the refrigerator?" "Can the children have new shoes?" "Are my son's clothes presentable for school?" Families with sick husbands can seldom answer such questions in the affirmative.

Closely related to these harsh questions is the idea the husbands, as breadwinners, have of the financial needs of the family. To uncover data on this point, we asked each husband how much money he would need every month for his family to have the things they desire and need to live comfortably. The mean monthly income that all the men state in reply to this question is $245. The mean income that the schizophrenic men state, however, is $196, whereas the mean income that the nonschizophrenic men state is $264. The mean for the schizophrenic men is significantly smaller than that of the other men ($p < .01$). Schizophrenic husbands think their families can live comfortably on a reduced income. To test the possibility that these husbands perceive their family's financial needs in more modest terms than other men as a result of the reduced family income, the relevant data are analyzed in two ways. First, the income of the family is subtracted from the income men believe is required for their families to live comfortably. This subtraction yields the difference between realized family income and income the men believe is required for the comfort of their families. The mean of this difference is $87 for the sick men and $99 for the well men. These means are not significantly different.

The second approach involves the computing of Pearson's product moment correlation coefficient between family income and the income the men believe their families require to live comfortably. The correlation between the two variables is $+.55$, taking as the N the entire group of 40 husbands. The 95 per cent confidence limits of this correlation, determined by the use of Fisher's "Z Transformation," are $+.29$ and $+.74$. Of direct relevance to the explanation advanced for differences in perceived financial needs between schizophrenic and nonschizophrenic husbands are the correlations *within* the two diagnostic groups of husbands. In the group of schizophrenic husbands, the correlation is $+.63$ with 95 per cent confidence limits of $+.05$ and $+.89$; in the well group, the correlation is $+.49$ with 95 per cent confidence limits of $+.15$ and $+.93$. Exactly the same procedures were applied to the data from each group. The difference between the correlations in the sick and well group is not statistically significant.

What do these statistical results mean? First, the income that would satisfy the desires and the comfort of the family is thought to be greater by the well than by the sick men. Second, this difference results in part from the fact that sick men have lower incomes and that, relative to what they have, the sick men do not require significantly less than other husbands for the comfort of their families. The third point underlies the first two points: there is a correlation between family income and the income the men believe their families require. This correlation applies to the entire group of families, to the families in which the husband is schizophrenic and to the families with husbands who are not afflicted with a psychotic disorder. Thus, the correlation is stable since it is not affected by the presence or absence of schizophrenia.

Even within the restricted lower-income bracket into which these families fall, the husbands as heads of households adjust their ideas about the needs of income to the reality of their economic status. Schizophrenia is a profoundly disturbing illness; the men who suffer from it may be "out of contact" with much of the sociocultural world which envelops them, but they are not out of contact with the grim business of formulating the income needs of their families, at least no more or no less than are the mentally healthier men.

We have seen that the schizophrenic men are employed full time less often than the well men. Does this reflect a long history of erratic employment, of inability to hold down a job, and of prolonged periods of unemployment? Have the schizophrenic men *always* suffered difficulties in employment?

Many kinds of data can be brought to bear on this question. First, both sick and well men started to work at about 14 years of age. Since they entered the job market at the same age, neither sick nor well men had an initial advantage in employment. Second, the sick men have had a mean number of 6.3 jobs from the first to the last time that they were employed; the comparable figure for the well men is 8 jobs. Statistical significance cannot be attached to the difference between these means. Third, the mean tenure in each job for the sick men is 2.8 years; for the well men it is 2.4 years; this difference is not statistically significant. From the first job to the last, there is no difference in diagnostic groups in the total number of years of employment or of unemployment. Thus, sick and well men do not differ in terms of *when* they started to work, the *number of jobs* they have had, the *length of employment* in each job, and the *number of years* that they have been employed or unemployed.

Despite the similarity of the occupational history of the sick and well men, there is one noticeable and statistically significant difference between them: the mean income that the sick men have received for all their jobs is $86.53 per month; for the well men it is $114.96. Inspection of the occupational history of the sick men indicates that a relatively abrupt reduction in earnings is associated with the date at which they perceive the illness to have started. This reduction is attributable to unemployment, to an increased rate of absenteeism, and to an inability to qualify for normal salary increases immediately prior to the date of the perceived advent of the illness. This is a point of frustration voiced recurrently in the stories told about occupational experiences during the problematic year.

In point of fact, only three of the eleven sick men have been able to sustain full-time employment since the time of the perceived onset of the illness. To focus more fully on the employment problems of the schizophrenic men, we asked all husbands to tell us about their employment, past and present—the kind of work, their attitudes toward their jobs, the quality of relationships with their companions and superiors at work. The employed men were directly observed at work since our fieldworkers sought to interview at all places and at all times of the day and night.

The problems that confront the sick men at work are more dramatic, more profound, and more agonizing than those of the well men. They stem from impairment, both perceived and actual, brought on by the illness and from conflict with their work mates and superiors. The sick man becomes a ready scapegoat for his associates and bosses. He is too anxious, too doubt ridden, too inept in the verbal repartee, which is an admired skill among his associates, to have anything more than peripheral membership in his work group. He is vulnerable and defenseless except in situations in which he is trapped by the taunts and ridicule of other men; then he strikes back with whatever weapons he can.

Four problems at work are most conspicuous.

1. The schizophrenic man's annoyances are magnified many times. Annoyances which are unbearable at work are also the object of unpleasant auditory and olfactory hallucinations away from the job. A sick man who has long aspired to become a skilled carpenter, got a job as assistant to a carpenter, but the noise of pounding hammers upset him and soon he became distraught; day and night, at home and at work, the noise of the real and imaginary hammers torment him. A man who works as a janitor in a hospital is about to quit his job because of the intolerable odor of the disinfectants which he must use to mop the floors; his wife, the food she prepares for him, his clothing, his body, and his bed, all seem to reek of the pungent disinfectant.

2. The schizophrenic man has imperfect motor skills. Often, trembling hands and feet impair his ability to work. The assistant car-

penter just mentioned often smashes his fingers. A waiter in a glamorous tourist hotel in San Juan quit his job out of fear that he would spill the trays of food on the elegant diners. A spray-gun operator with erratic aim finally quit his job painting furniture. The driver of a *carro publico* (a jitney) could not control the brake pedals and was fired from work after a rash of automobile accidents.

3. The schizophrenic man's "disorganized mind" is a cause of inefficiency and confusion at work. One man is employed as a clerk in a small street-corner grocery store catering to the residents of nearby slums and *caseríos*. He searches aimlessly among the wares, often coming back with items not ordered by the customer. He plans to quit his job; "My mind," he confesses, "is disorganized."

4. The sick man has problems with his boss and co-workers. His many peculiarities of behavior are observed by his work mates and superiors. They think he is unreliable, absurd, and unmanly. Suspicions begin to grow that there is a *loco* working with them. One man was identified as a clown by his associates and his boss in the paint factory where he worked. The boss in a playful mood pushed this man's head into a barrel filled with ammonia; the fumes caused him to be hospitalized for 2 weeks and he never returned to work. Another man was the butt of jokes by his associates at work. To worry him they told him with expressions of urgency and concern that the boss was angry at him and was looking for him; when the man sought out the boss, he discovered that his associates had been joking. As a result the boss began to view him with a jaundiced eye, baffled by his eccentricities. Eventually, the sick man armed himself with a knife and engaged one of his tormentors in a fight, after which he quit work.

The three sick men who still work full time are accumulating serious absentee records and have expressed their plans to quit work. They will either be fired or quit their jobs, but more likely they will gradually withdraw from work and eventually be unemployed. The impairments experienced by the schizophrenic man combined with the punishment addressed to him by persons at work lead him to retreat from work and into his family of procreation.

SUMMARY

Marriage multiplies needs, and each spouse experiences a renewed awareness of economic privation. A husband is expected to provide sustenance for the family. The level of living of the family depends primarily on his being employed and on the amount of money he earns.

Schizophrenia impairs a husband's capacity to provide for his family. The loss of his earnings reduces the overall income received by the family, even though the wife tries to earn a living. Sick and well husbands adjust their ideas of the income needs of the family according to the amount of income received by the family.

The schizophrenic wife complains bitterly to her sick or well husband about the economic problems the family experiences. Conflict between the spouses over economic hardships does not occur in the families with well wives regardless of the psychiatric status of the husband. The Urrutia family illustrates the strategies the sick wife employs to fulfill the material needs she believes are necessary.

15
Social Control in Marriage. I

Chapter 13 reported the emphasis that is placed on *respeto* in the family. Respect is relied on to regulate the distribution of influence among the members of the family. Neither the sex nor the mental condition of a person affects the commonly held idea that a woman should defer to her husband who is viewed as the legitimate head of the household. Both are enmeshed, however, in a set of reciprocal rights and obligations. A person's willingness and capacity to assume the rights and to fulfill the obligations of his role(s) in the family are important parts of social control. Social control depends, moreover, on the effectiveness of the rewards and punishments employed to maintain the desired, or to correct the undesired, behavior of a member of the family. Of relevance to social control is the process of changing role relationships which result from departures from the normal, culturally established roles. As one spouse fails to perform an obligation, the other may not be able to reestablish normal performance; consequently, the spouse changes his own role to compensate for the failure of his mate to perform the culturally prescribed role.

This chapter and the next demonstrate that schizophrenia is related to the various facets of social control in marriage. The patterns of social control in the families with spouses who are both well (control families) are described first. Then the husband-schizophrenic families are presented. The following chapter continues the presentation of findings on social control by turning to wife-schizophrenic families and to families in which both spouses are schizophrenic (double schizophrenic families).

CONTROL FAMILIES

The division of labor between the sexes restricts the wife to her home and the immediate neighborhood but frees the husband to spend long hours away from home. Patterns of entertainment also remove the husband from his home and his wife. It is common for a man to stop in bars here and there on his way home from work. Moreover, he often returns home only to eat his dinner, shave, bathe, and change into freshly laundered pants and shirt before going out for an evening of fun.

The work and play activities of the husband are carried out in settings in which the wife does not participate. Some wives do not even know the specific nature of the work performed by their husbands; others are doubtful about where their husbands work. The cultural expectation that a "good" wife does not pry into her husband's efforts to make a living limits her understanding of what her husband does away from home. In contrast, the husband can easily observe how well his wife carries out her tasks as a homemaker; he can infer how diligently his wife has cleaned the house or apartment, washed and ironed the clothes, bathed the children, and prepared the meals. These differences between the sex roles give the husband an advantage over his wife; he can evaluate her habits of work but, since so much of what he does is out of her sight, she cannot evaluate his.

Some wives do not know how much their husbands earn. When asked to estimate their earnings, the wives are uncertain and tend to underestimate. Typically, the husband gives his wife a portion of his earnings for family expenses. He keeps the remainder to spend on his own entertainment. He does not account to his wife for the money he spends on himself. Although the wife would like to know how much he earns and what proportion he "throws away" drinking, gambling, or on other women, she suppresses her curiosity in deference to the norm to be *conforme* or accepting. The husband is not bound by a comparable norm. He can probe as he wishes and as he sees fit into all aspects of what his wife does.

Early in the field work we observed that wives became fidgety and nervous during the afternoon hours when they were supposed to be cooking and preparing the home for the arrival of their husbands. It was not wise to conduct an interview at that time of the day; also, it was inappropriate for the interviewer to be present in the respondent's home as her husband arrived. After work a man expects to relax. He expects his family, particularly his wife, to acknowledge his presence by giving him the undivided attention that befits a head of the household. In recognition of this fact, neighbors who may be visiting the wife scurry away.

A majority of wives in the control group greet their husbands with special efforts to make them comfortable. Such gestures serve to ease the strains of the day's labors which the husband undergoes. A good illustration of this point is Mrs. Aparicio's behavior when her husband returns home from work. She does not permit the children to bother their father. Within the limits of her budget she prepares the foods that he enjoys. She serves his dinner with plates, glasses, and silverware kept immaculately clean; a freshly laundered tablecloth is spread on the table. Through such efforts, Mrs. Aparicio honors her husband and expresses her gratitude to him for being a good provider.

A husband who comes home to a disheveled house with noisy and dirty children and a wife who is oblivious to him will ask his wife: "Did you spend the day gossiping with neighbors? Why aren't the children clean? Why isn't dinner prepared?" He has the right to demand answers to these questions. On the other hand, a man will view as a malcontent a wife who demands that he account for *his* activities during the day. To avoid such a charge, a woman seldom questions her husband even in cases where he barely supports the family.

Mr. Ubarri is a self-styled carpenter, unemployed for 6 months, who does not make a consistent effort to secure a job. Friends occasionally tell him of a job opening, to which Mr. Ubarri responds by making feeble inquiries at his own convenience. Periodically, when he realizes that his family is eating only handouts provided by neighbors and friends, he is overwhelmed by guilt. He then thinks of breaking into a store to steal merchandise, or he contemplates suicide by jumping into the black waters of the lagoon under his shack home. He does not alter his usual daily activities, however, which consist of walking the slum neighborhood, mooching drinks from friends, and helping a widow repair her shack for which he is paid in sexual relations. Mrs. Ubarri considers her husband a careless and indifferent provider, but she does not prod him to seek employment. Her stoic patience, her habit of being *conforme*, inhibits her from expressing anger toward him. Such overt acceptance of her husband's indolent ways is characteristic of the typical wife in the control group who rarely pressures her husband to explain the management of his finances, although the typical husband in the control group is a much more reliable provider than Mr. Ubarri.

At present, only one wife, Mrs. Guerrero, earns money by working, although 80 per cent of the wives in the control group would like to be employed. The desire to work is not a romantic illusion but one based on experience, for 7 out of 10 women in this diagnostic group were once employed. Since they are experienced and willing to work, why are more wives not employed? Primarily, because of the husband's outright prohibition, as he believes that woman's place is in the home. Women who were working were forced by their husbands to leave their jobs at the time of marriage or had to quit shortly thereafter when they became pregnant. Wives tell their husbands how much greater the family income would be if they were allowed to work; their husbands are adamant in denying this request.

Mrs. Guerrero sews and irons at home, earning from $6 to $12 a week. Although her income is reliable and does not require her leaving home to earn it, her husband disapproves and several times has threatened to throw the sewing machine out the window. When he returns from work Mr. Guerrero often finds his home in disarray because his wife spends the day doing someone else's work. He is robbed of a dignified homecoming and the recognition that should be bestowed on the head of the household.

The husband's authority is based on norms and values that rationalize the image of a dominant male. Moreover, the fact that the family subsists on his earnings enables him to wield an influence disproportionate to that of his wife. A husband sometimes withholds money from his wife to force her to behave in a more acceptable manner, but when a woman earns an income her husband loses a measure of control in the family. Mr. Guerrero opposes his wife's earning money. He notes that since she started to sew and iron clothes for others she is "uppity" and thinks she "wears the pants in the family."

The husband in the control group typically gives his wife a portion of his earnings so that she can buy for the family. Few decisions have to be made about how to spend the portion of earnings he gives his wife, as the needs of the family are compelling. Although a husband sometimes brings home groceries or clothing for the family, his wife usually attends to such matters. The purchase of food exhausts most of her funds; the little that remains is spent immediately on shoes, clothing, and other items that she and her children have long awaited. The husband usually purchases his own clothing.

The decision to buy an expensive commodity, a television set, furniture, or a refrigerator, is made jointly by the husband and wife. We observed many families in a local sewing machine store to see how they made the decision to buy. Although a sewing machine is for the use of the wife, the husband is involved in its purchase and, more often than not, he reserves the right to veto her choice. The wife examines the sewing machine, asks questions, and tests the machine; the husband stands by, less active than his wife, but occasionally asks questions about technical features of the machine, its price, and the manner in which payment can be arranged. The wife checks her opinion and preferences with her husband's. If he approves, an agreement is reached. The husband then begins to bargain with the clerk or owner of the store. (Bargaining is very typical of Puerto Rican business.) If the husband is not present, the wife waits until he can go to the store to inspect the machine, to approve the purchase, and to make arrangements for payment.

Another mark of the husband's authority is the wife's conformance to the expectation that she stay either at home or in the immediate vicinity. When her husband is at home, a woman always asks his permission to go shopping or to visit a friend or relative, and ordinarily it is granted. The wife's departure from home is justified if she goes on an errand or if she is called upon to discharge an obligation to a member of the nuclear or extended family. If the wife is absent when her husband comes home, he is angry. Unless she can explain her absence in terms that are acceptable to him, he reprimands her sharply. An unexpected illness or accident to a child or relative is an acceptable reason for being absent. If she leaves without a fixed destination, her husband suspects her of having an extramarital affair. Such rambling is the prerogative of man, not woman.

A man does not like to have other men visit during his absence from home. The belief that sexual opportunities invariably lead to sexual relations underlies this attitude. Some husbands were hostile when a male fieldworker was found waiting at their homes to interview them. One husband finally told us that he did not like to have *any* man visit his wife; it was embarrassing for him to express this attitude since in every other respect he had extended to us the hospitality characteristic of the families we studied. A few men do not approve even of blood and affinal male relatives visiting during hours of work. It is not unusual for a husband to prohibit his wife from having casual social contacts with men, but conflict seldom occurs over this point since the wife avoids situations that might cause her husband to suspect her of infidelity.

When a husband disapproves of his wife's behavior, he chastizes her; he becomes sullen and taciturn; he may reduce the amount of expense money he gives her or deny her what she wishes. Not infrequently, he beats her, but this usually occurs only if the wife continues to defy his orders or if she retaliates with insults or ridicule. Only an unusual wife initiates physical violence against her husband, because then he beats her all the more severely. Although the husband does not have a monopoly on punishment, he is quick to employ it. Rarely does he reward his wife to bring her back into line.

A wife is by no means powerless in her marital relationship. The punishments she directs against her husband are seen most clearly when she believes that he is being unfaithful. Then she is no longer an accepting, *conforme* wife. She erupts with scathing insults; she refuses to cook for him. She does not launder his pants and shirts, particularly if they are lipstick stained or reek of perfume. She threatens to leave with the children. She recalls incidents with a former boyfriend or husband to taunt him that she has not always been his sexual property. She vigorously denies him sexual relations.

A husband, confronted with such an outburst, often leaves home. His departure is symbolic of an important control he wields over his wife: the threat to abandon her. This threat acts as a restraint on the wife who, in general, has deeper social and emotional commitments to the stability of her marriage. Moreover, there are avenues available for the husband to escape both the chastisement of an irate wife and an unsatisfactory family life. These are found in the groups and patterns of social activities so important a part of the masculine world in slum and *caserío* life. A test of the wife's influence on her husband is the extent to which she can make her husband's life more home-centered and draw him away from the opportunities to escape responsibilities of the family. This influence is premised firmly on her family-centered skills. The husband, to the extent that he relinquishes his street-centered activities, correlatively loses a sense of power in his family. His freedom is being curtailed and, from the point of view of his friends at the *cafetin* or his associates at work, he concedes to his wife on a point that is central to the creed of the *macho*.

In most control families, however, the pervading tone of marriage is not one of an overbearing, dictatorial husband who shouts commands in order to exact blind obedience from his wife. Although the balance of power is in favor of the husband, the wife is punished only when she defaults in her obligations or trespasses grossly upon his masculine prerogatives. All but a few wives are reliable, deferential, consistently hard workers devoted to their families. They provide their husbands with an orderly family life. Consequently, few husbands need to resort habitually to punishment.

Moreover, since the husband is absent from home during the day and on some evenings, the wife has some independence in managing the affairs of the family. In particular, the day-by-day decisions that concern the upbringing and socialization of the children are largely in her hands. Even while at home, the husband tends to remain aloof from mundane household decisions and activities which, often, he views as matters that are of relevance only to his wife.

Husbands and wives have an interest in each other's welfare and in that of their children. Although the husband does not tell his wife very much about his experiences at work or elsewhere unless they are troublesome, the couple shares hopes, dreams, and aspirations. They discuss the education they would like their children to have. They speak about the concrete house they would like to own. They classify neighbors as *gente decente* (decent people) or *gente de mala fé* (people of bad will). From their points of view few neighbors are *decente*, and thus the couple yearns all the more for a dream house in a higher-status residential area so that their children can have friends of better quality. Some couples watch television or listen to the radio together. One husband reads the newspaper every day to his illiterate wife.

A woman listens sympathetically to her husband's problems. She is often more concerned with his health than he himself; when he is ill she urges him to stay home to rest. Many husbands describe their wives as motherly because they offer nurtural support as well as *consejos* (advice). The men appreciate and often follow such advice. In addition, a wife is deeply involved in the lives of her blood and affinal relatives. She, more than her husband, addresses herself to the preservation of affective familial ties, to the solution of internal problems in the broader family, and to the giving of nurtural support to needy relatives. A wife's deep and pervasive involvement in the broader family makes her valuable to her husband. Insofar as she maintains vital and active family relations, she makes available to him the emotional, economic, and social benefits that accrue from belonging to a coherent kinship system. The usefulness of the broader family is most apparent when husband and wife experience an economic crisis, illness, or serious accident.

It is instructive to discuss the Domínguez family because it represents *a clear-cut exception to the usual pattern of male dominance in the control group*. Mrs. Domínguez, a narcissistic, hysteroid, and mentally deficient but not schizophrenic person according to the psychiatrist, wields inordinate influence over her husband who has no symptoms of psychopathology.

Mrs. Domínguez spends from 60 to 70 hours a week listening to the radio and watching television, mostly daytime serials. During the evening hours, she watches musical programs that present local singers and dancers. In the living room of her *caserío* apartment, prominently displayed alongside her radio and television set, is a large, colored photograph of her taken a number of years previously. The photograph bears little resemblance to its subject whom the psychiatrist describes as "ugly, skinny, and prematurely old." Whereas Mrs. Domínguez is dark skinned, with hair that is, in the vernacular, *pelo de pasa* (kinky), and lacks upper and lower teeth, the photograph depicts a person of white complexion, with flowing, wavy hair, and white, even teeth. A closer look at the photograph shows that it has been assiduously retouched. Nevertheless, to Mrs. Domínguez the photograph is an accurate portrait.

The fantasy embodied in the photograph is reflected in Mrs. Domínguez' presentation of herself to men other than her husband. The psychiatrist reports her attempts to be alluring, provocative, and seductive during the diagnostic interview. When Mrs. Domínguez goes for walks with her husband, she paints her face heavily with rouge, wears a multicolored dress and flamboyant necklace, and wiggles her hips invitingly. The innumerable compliments (*piropos, hechando flores*) that her appearance and manner elicit from the groups of casual men who stand about the streets infuriate her husband.

Mrs. Domínguez calls her husband a worthless drifter because he moves from one job to another; he feels that she forces him to take unacceptable jobs, such as greasing cars. When they watch television, she determines the program they view; she sits on an easy chair, he on the floor. Mr. Domínguez is no longer an *aficionado* of sports, nor does he drink with friends as he once did. He also does most of the housework. "Soon," his wife boasts, "he will do all of it because I am going to get a job as a seamstress."

For several years Mrs. Domínguez rejected her husband sexually, ostensibly because she feared becoming pregnant. When he asked her to undergo sterilization, she argued that the operation would cause her to have a heart attack. As a result of his wife's insistence, Mr. Domínguez was sterilized,[1] but she continues to deny him sexual access. In a relaxed moment, Mr. Domínguez confesses that he is not the *macho* he once was.

Mr. Domínguez is haunted by the suspicion that his wife is unfaithful. A few weeks before the interview, when she berated him for being a worn-out old man (he is 13 years her senior) and accused him of being nothing but an inconsequential pubic hair, he grabbed a knife and chased her through the neighborhood. After his anger had subsided and he returned to the apartment to go to bed, Mrs. Domínguez

---

[1] Mr. Domínguez is the only male in the study who has been sterilized.

returned, mixed cockroach poison with water, drank it, and staggered into the bedroom screeching that she was dying. He took her to a public hospital to have her stomach pumped.

Mrs. Domínguez states that she married her husband out of pity: "He was an old man and had a child from a former marriage for whom he was unable to care." She claims she also wanted to escape from her father who beat her every day. Now, she no longer pities her husband; she slaps him and hurls objects at him. She ridicules his masculinity and pushes him out the door, ordering him to find a job. He is upset by her curses; even though he is a "free thinker," he does not think God's name should be mentioned in vain.

By means of humiliation, physical violence, and threats to commit suicide, Mrs. Domínguez has achieved control over her husband, thereby reversing the usual pattern of dominancy which is characteristic of families in the control group.

HUSBAND-SCHIZOPHRENIC FAMILIES

The schizophrenic husband experiences aches and pains which come and go, a feeling of overwhelming fatigue, and excruciating anxiety. His anxieties revolve around his feeling of inability to fulfill the basic social roles of an adult male. He finds it difficult to hold a job and to fulfill his conceptions of male sexuality. The fear of unexpected events and of unknown dangers is problematical to him, since the creed of the *macho* stipulates that a man should be fearless even in the face of danger. For a man to show fear in the absence of objective danger is to exhibit an effeminate weakness. When Mr. Espinosa is unable to avoid friends, he puts his hands deep into his pockets so that no one will observe his trembling hands which are *cosas de mujer* (attributes of a woman), unbecoming in a man. Symptoms of illness are interpreted by the sick person, as well as by others, in terms of the behavior appropriate to the sex role.

The central role of the husband is that of provider for his family. The sick man suffers many impairments, and at work he embroils himself in interpersonal conflicts in which he becomes the object of hostility and punishment. Consequently, the schizophrenic man is less likely to be employed full time than is the man not afflicted with this illness. Two of the seven schizophrenic men married to well women are employed full time: one is a janitor, the other a clerk in a small grocery store. The remaining five in the husband-schizophrenic families are either unemployed or have irregular part-time employment consisting of ambulatory barbering or odd jobs.

The economic crisis that results from the inability of the sick man to provide adequately for his family is of considerable importance because the manner in which the wife confronts and copes with the problem of family subsistence is woven into the patterns of authority and control that emerge in her relations to her husband. Neither the control families nor the families in which only the wife is sick experience the problem of economic survival as acutely and as dramatically as do the families with sick men. The families with schizophrenic husbands, therefore, provide an opportunity to examine the impact that a disabled breadwinner, with a galaxy of disturbing symptoms of personality, has upon his marital relations.

The typical sick man receives from his well wife full dispensation as a provider. The wife views her husband's illness as a case of nerves that is genuinely incapacitating and, in most cases, she accepts the fact that he is unable to be an effective provider. She does not pressure him to keep working nor does she urge him to work if he is unemployed. Conflicts that center on a disabled and recalcitrant person unable and unwilling to fulfill the obligations imposed by his spouse do not emerge in six of the seven families with only husbands sick. The one exception to this pattern, the Herrero family, is discussed later.

The norm to be *conforme*, which so strongly influences the life and outlook of the women in the control group, leads the wife of a sick husband to accept his disablement. Moreover, these wives have considerable insight into both the inner turmoil from which their husbands suffer and the interpersonal conditions which aggravate their illness. The typical wife perceives with remarkable clarity her husband's imperfect motor skills, his low tolerance for annoyances, and the many dysfunctions of a "disorganized mind." She does not see these symptoms as defects in his "character"; she does not moralize about them, nor describe them in pejorative terms. Much of her behavior as a therapeutic partner to her husband is premised upon her insights into his illness.

In addition, such a wife moves to fill the economic vacuum created in the family by her husband's unemployment or part-time employment. Whereas only one of the twenty wives in the control group earns an income and none of the schizophrenic women married to well men works, four of the seven well women married to sick men are employed full time away from home. The women in this group were prohibited from working at the time of marriage by their husbands, as were the women in all groups. The general desire to work, so evident in the control group, is fulfilled by the women in this diagnostic group since it is clear to them and to their sick husbands that the family must have a stable provider.

Thus the sequence of adjustment initiated by the withdrawal of the sick man from work terminates in the employment of his wife. For example, Mr. Cardona earned $33 a week as a movie projectionist, but his symptoms were causing a disturbing absentee record. He had chills and uncontrollable trembling and weeping spells. "His blood froze in his body," according to his wife, "and his legs were paralyzed." He had chronic diarrhea. He had an intense fear of the dark room in which he worked, and this fear was aggravated when the film broke and the audience whistled, stamped their feet, clapped their hands, and shouted vulgar insults at him. "I had to quit," he says. "That was too much."

After Mr. Cardona left his job as a movie projectionist, he did minor electrical repairs for his neighbors which did not produce a sufficient and stable source of income. Mrs. Cardona then attempted to earn money by selling codfish and crabmeat fritters that she made at home, but proceeds of the sales did not cover the expenses. The family was heavily in debt; they owed money to the grocer; they could not meet the payments on the refrigerator; they were under threat of having their furniture repossessed; the water and electricity bills were overdue; and the rent for the lot on which they live was long unpaid.

Mr. Cardona's father-in-law, who lives next door, supported them by bringing groceries to them. Mrs. Cardona states, "It is one thing to eat, and quite another to eat adequately. During this period we just needed to eat." Mrs. Cardona secured her husband's approval to find work. For 2 months she went from one factory to another, and finally she found work sewing dresses at a doll factory where she earns $30 per week. The *desperate* financial problems of subsistence have been solved by the Cardonas. Now they confront the *ordinary* ones.

The Cardonas illustrate a sequence of coping with economic problems. This sequence starts with the husband's withdrawal from full-time employment, continues to the erratic and unsuccessful efforts that are made to subsist, and finally concludes with the wife seeking stable employment away from home. Financial problems are focused progressively on the wife who has a deep commitment to the preservation of the family.

Some sick men remain unemployed but most work part time on those days when they experience relief from the symptoms. Part-time work consists of barbering and odd jobs that involve nothing more than cutting lawns, washing cars, and miscellaneous work around higher-class houses; some men remain in their homes doing light repair work and minor carpentry. Some men become ambulatory barbers who work in the vicinity of their homes; the capital investment required to establish such a business is small—nothing more than the price of clippers, scissors, a comb, hair oil, perhaps a straight-edge razor, and a small wooden box for customers to sit on—but a successful day's work brings only $2.00. One mentally ill barber makes his rounds muttering to himself in a barely audible voice, "Anybody want the barber." When a customer hails him to have his hair cut, the sick man is surprised and confused. Another sick man, who quit his job as a waiter in a tourist hotel in San Juan because his hands trembled, is now an ambulatory barber in his neighborhood; although his hands still tremble, mistakes in barbering resulting from unsteady hands can always be rectified by cutting more hair.

As the wife gravitates toward, and the husband away from, the role of breadwinner, the rhythm of daily activity in the family changes. The husband centers his life at home; no longer does he arrive home after work demanding service and imposing obligations on his wife. Gradually, he abandons the enforcement of the conventional expectations so apparent in the life of the control families—that the wife diligently do the housework, that children be kept clean, that his meals be served on time, that a woman's place is at home.

The vacuum created in the household when the wife becomes the breadwinner is filled by the sick husband who, unlike the well man married to a sick or a well woman, is not aloof from the mundane affairs of the family; he is deeply involved in the details of family life. When his wife leaves the home to work, the sick husband cooks, takes care of the children, washes and irons the clothes, and scrubs floors. He becomes adept at doing housework. Mrs. Ramos and Mrs. Cardona repeatedly comment on how useful and cooperative their husbands are at home. These two husbands do *all* of the housework, and these wives are permitted to rest when they return home from work.

Reversal of economic roles takes place in most husband-schizophrenic families, even though neither spouse exerts pressure upon the other to assume the new role. In contrast to the activities of the husband in the control group and to those of the well husbands of schizophrenic wives, the activities of a sick man can be observed or inferred by his wife. Since he has retreated from full-time employment and no longer spends many hours in the communal street-corner groups composed of friends, a major source of marital tension is relieved. This source of tension, as we have seen, appears and reappears in the control families, but the wife of a schizophrenic man has no reason to quarrel about the infidelity of her husband or about his going from one bar to another.

By working outside the home the wife attains a freedom desired by the other women who are not ill. This has a double effect on the sick man. First, he feels humiliated; in the words of Mr. Berríos, "I am supposed to be head of the household. It is humiliating for a man to depend on his wife." Second, although he knows where she works, her hours of work, what she does at work, and how much she earns, he feels uneasy and uncomfortable that his wife is away from home for many hours of the day, involved in social relations with persons he does not know. He is concerned with the possibility that men at work are making sexual approaches to her. When he was employed he knew that his wife was restricted to the home and bound by a network of social relations composed of relatives and friends who were nearby. Under those circumstances, only an unusual wife, perhaps only one afflicted with sexual *furor*, would risk the consequences of an unfaithful act. The sick man is suspicious of his wife, more so than the husband in the control group.

As the social relations between the spouses are reshaped, the wife protects her sick husband from upsetting incidents. She believes her behavior, as well as the behavior of her children and other persons, toward her husband has an effect on his illness. For instance, when Mrs. Cardona found out about the sexual misbehavior of a stepdaughter (the product of her husband's former marriage) through gossip and by reading the girl's diary, she endeavored to keep this information from her husband because it would upset him seriously.

The wife of a schizophrenic husband returns home immediately after work. Often her husband meets her either at her place of work, at the bus stop, or at the place where the *carros publicos* (jitneys) commonly stop to discharge passengers. Mr. Berríos always goes to the bus stop to meet his wife and escort her home. He wants to find out as soon as possible what she has been doing, whom she saw, and how her employers have treated her. What is more important, the Berríoses' neighborhood is congested with whores, dope addicts, and *atomicos* (indiscriminate drunkards and addicts who inject themselves with, eat, or drink any substance known to produce a "charge," including sandwiches of menthol). According to Mr. Berríos, the police never patrol the neighborhood and are afraid to come into it even after a crime has been committed. Although Mrs. Berríos once prevented a man from attacking her husband by denying him admission while Mr. Berríos hid cowering in the house, Mr. Berríos attempts to protect his wife by escorting her home. Mrs. Berríos appreciates her husband's efforts to protect her; she thinks not many husbands are as attentive to and as concerned about their wives as is her husband.

A woman married to a schizophrenic maintains strict control over the children so that they will not make noise or be too unruly. Commotion upsets the sick husband, and if the children are responsible he beats them severely. The wife then intervenes to protect her children and to pacify her husband.

In addition to protecting their husbands, the wives guide them toward therapeutic outlets. Druggists, spiritualistic mediums, doctors, and psychiatrists are consulted, and their advice and prescriptions are followed to the letter; wives administer everything from tranquilizers to boiled medicinal herbs. The wife assumes an active role in therapy by satisfying her husband's needs. If he cannot sleep, she gives him a massage with rubbing alcohol; if he experiences hallucinations, she interprets the world in a reassuring manner. His anxieties and fears are discussed sympathetically. She gives him advice as to how he should behave. One husband states: "My wife has become a mother to me."

As the role of the mother is linked to that of the dependent child, the husband, in the process of being nurtured, becomes subservient. In the vernacular, "the husband sits on the trunk," a saying which conjures up an image of a ventriloquist's dummy being manipulated. Correlatively, during the process of becoming breadwinner, protector, guide, and therapist, the wife gains increments of control over her husband. The acquisition of power by the wife is, however, an unplanned result of the efforts both spouses make to cope with the illness. Although the husband adapts himself to a subservient role, the process is not always smooth. He feels a loss of authority and masculinity, even though the power he once enjoyed has not been dramatically challenged or forcefully wrested from him by his wife. A schizophrenic man may suddenly and unpredictably hurl bitter accusations at his wife for wanting to take over, or immediately after a nightmare he may pummel her or choke her as Mr. Cardona has done. When Mr. Berríos is sober, his wife maintains control over his behavior; whenever he gets drunk, he rebels violently against his wife's control. On one occasion, he threw her on a bed and stood over her for several hours with a wooden plank, threatening to beat her if she moved. On another occasion, he brought a male friend and two prostitutes to his home and insisted that Mrs. Berríos prepare dinner for his guests.

The manner in which the wife exercises control helps the husband to adapt to the subservient role. Wives do not shout commands and impose restrictions upon the behavior of their sick husbands. Rather, they give soft advice to receptive and anxious ears. For the husband to reject the advice is to reject therapy since his wife is acting in his behalf to help him get well. To strike back, to defy her requests, is to impugn her motives and to be *malagradecido* (ungrateful). Since the wife has been extremely self-sacrificing in her efforts to solve the problems created by the illness, she views herself, and her husband views her, as a symbol of martyrdom. The legitimacy of her power in the family stems from this.

The *modus operandi* of the wife is *a la buena* (by gentle persuasion). At no time is the husband's authority openly challenged and at no time does an issue of power become the object of controversy or of discussion. On the contrary, the wife often makes an effort to maintain an image of her husband's dominance. Employed wives give their earnings to their husbands who then disburse the funds. This money has special meaning. First, it represents the wife's total earnings. Second, the amount she hands her husband is a known quantity. This contrasts sharply with the practice of an employed husband who does not tell his wife how much money he earns, a form of institutionalized ignorance that sustains, and is sustained by, the pattern of masculine freedom outside of the home. Schizophrenic husbands do not fit into this pattern; they enjoy it symbolically.

The sick husband considers his wife the most important person in his life; he is dependent upon her. It is to her that he turns for support, not only when he suffers acute spells of anxiety but also on days when he experiences only a mild uneasiness. Although at times the schizophrenic man erupts in anger, he is soon calm again, reassured by the warm support of his wife. Psychotic breaks from reality which involve aggressive and uncoordinated outbursts against other persons are seldom experienced by the sick men who also rarely exhibit the trance-like episodes of going berserk, as do sick women.

The tone of marital relations in families with sick husbands differs from that of the control families. Husband-schizophrenic families are characterized by a great deal of harmony and communication and a sense of conjugal unity and solidarity which focuses upon the illness and upon efforts of the pair to solve the problems thus created; familial relations are not as strongly premised upon the pattern of *respeto*, extreme deference, to the male head of the household and of behaving properly according to the cultural norms that define husband-wife relations, as is the case in the control families.

When asked to describe the proper roles of the husband and wife, the schizophrenic husband gives the same reply as men in the other diagnostic groups, but the actual arrangement of family activities which he experiences is a gross departure from his stated expectations. The wife's deviation from the proper role of the woman is legitimate since it represents an effort to cope with problems that stem from the husband's illness.

Of the seven families in the diagnostic group of husband-schizophrenic families, *the Herreros represent the one and only clear-cut exception to the foregoing pattern of control and authority.* Mr. Herrero is 35 years old, his wife is 25, and their children are 5, 4, and 3. The Herreros live in a *caserío* apartment for which they pay $13 a month in rent. Mr. Herrero works as a grocery clerk in a small store and earns $25 a week. The usual difficulties experienced by schizophrenic men at work also afflict Mr. Herrero. His earnings are decreasing as his absenteeism increases. Undoubtedly, he will soon be unemployed. At present, his wife does not work.

If the Herreros could live their lives anew neither would choose to marry the other. Both find that marriage has been an extremely disillusioning experience and that few, if any, of their expectations have been fulfilled. According to Mr. Herrero, his wife does not understand him; she is not affectionate; she denies him sexually; she neither cares for nor caters to him; she disobeys him by visiting girl friends who have returned from New York City with bad moral reputations; she goes to parties without his permission. "She won't even bring me a glass of water when I ask her," complains Mr. Herrero.

Mrs. Herrero's frustrated desire for upward mobility is an important reason for this family's departure from the usual pattern of a nurtural, dominant wife married to a dependent and impaired husband so characteristic of the families in which only the husband is schizophrenic. Mrs. Herrero aspired to marry a professional man with a salary of at least $500 a month. She would like to live in a four-bedroom house with two bathrooms, a patio, a modern kitchen with built-in features, a dining room, a porch, a large yard enclosed by a fence, and a two-car garage. The house would be located in a quiet residential area with neighbors of "good class." If she were married to a professional man she could afford to go to the university to learn English; she would then become a professor and teach English. She finds the area in which she lives, her apartment, and her husband have all fallen woefully short of her aspirations.

Mrs. Herrero believes her apartment is too small, the neighbors do not mind their own business, and the furnishings with which she has to live are dilapidated and worn. The Herreros are deeply in debt; they are behind in payments on the refrigerator, the electric bill, and the rent. Symbolic of the wide margin between her desires and her possessions is a life-size doll in a pink dress trailing down the chipped chest of drawers on which it rests. Mrs. Herrero blames her husband for not being able to achieve her social and economic aspirations. She sees him as a man without energy, without spirit, without imagination; he has trouble earning even a miserable wage doing work that any man of the street could do better. He does not bathe or change his clothing; he is subject to wild fits in which he runs around the apartment or out into the darkness of the night, screaming that he is being attacked and that he must defend himself. This is hardly the kind of man that Mrs. Herrero dreams about—one who would be gay and *simpatico* in interpersonal relations, who would take her to movies, parties, and nightclubs.

Several months ago when Mrs. Herrero noticed that her husband was becoming sullen, taciturn, and withdrawn from her, she decided to make special efforts to entice him sexually. She groomed herself, dressed provocatively, and assumed an inviting attitude in his presence. To Mr. Herrero, these special efforts demonstrated that she was bent on being or was already unfaithful. Confronted by accusations of infidelity, Mrs. Herrero retreated sexually and emotionally from her husband. They sleep in separate rooms and, for a period of 4 months, have hardly spoken to each other.

Mrs. Herrero's attitude toward her husband differs sharply from that of the other wives married to schizophrenic men. She does not believe that he cannot work; on the contrary, she urges him to continue to work and to try to get better-paying jobs. When he falls short of her desires, she condemns him for the impoverished life she is forced to live. Also unlike the other women married to schizophrenics, Mrs. Herrero does not work to solve the financial problems of her family which have emerged from the growing inability of her husband to provide for the family's needs. Nor has Mrs. Herrero become a therapeutic marital partner. The idiosyncratic behavior of her husband, the bewildering symptoms from which he suffers, the accusations of infidelity, all repel her.

Underlying Mrs. Herrero's failure to become a breadwinner, a protector, a guide, and a therapist is her strong emotional identification with the style of life of the middle and upper classes in Puerto Rico. She wants the material advantages which she has observed in the modern residential areas. She sees women of her age driving in shiny new cars, taking their children to private schools, shopping at supermarkets with attendants to carry to their cars heavy bags loaded with canned goods or attractively wrapped products. She sees these women spending money freely at beauty parlors and clothing stores. To her, the women of the affluent classes look gay and carefree, unencumbered by the restrictions and prohibitions that husbands of the *caserío* and slum group impose on their wives.

Physically, Mrs. Herrero is an alluring, seductive, and prepossessing woman. The reports of the female fieldworker who interviewed her and the male fieldworker who interviewed her husband are dotted with frequent descriptions of Mrs. Herrero's attractiveness. She recalls that her relatives, friends, and casual acquaintances have complimented her from early childhood on her beauty. When she walks to and from the apartment, men on the sidewalk turn their heads to catch her eye and to compliment her with *piropos* and *flores*. Drivers of cars stop and with elegant gestures of masculine cordiality allow her to cross the busy thoroughfare. Mrs. Herrero is aware of the premium the Puerto Rican culture, at all class levels, places upon physical beauty. She knows also that she is at least as attractive as most women in the upper classes. She cannot understand, then, the irony of a life that condemns her to live with a disheveled and incapacitated husband who is devoid of all charm, with increasing debts, and in a *caserío* apartment with furniture that is rapidly deteriorating.

In brief, although Mr. Herrero's schizophrenic behavior is not significantly different from that of the other sick men in this diagnostic group, his wife's response to his behavior is atypical. Mrs. Herrero's commitment to a higher-class level makes it difficult, if not impossible, for her to cope with the problems which stem from her husband's mental illness. (After our interviews with this family were completed, Mr. and Mrs. Herrero separated and were planning to be divorced.)

SUMMARY

Most of the 20 families in which neither spouse is schizophrenic are dominated by the husband. The wife is a homemaker who stays at home or in the neighborhood while the husband earns a living away from home and often roams widely after work to participate in the entertainments associated with the male role. Thus, the wife's activities can be observed by her husband, but those of the husband are most often unobserved by the wife. A husband can also freely demand from his wife an account of her day's activities, whereas she is not free to make similar demands of him. The typical wife would like to work outside the home to earn money, but her husband does not permit this. Although he gives his wife a portion of his earnings for family expenses, she does not know how much he earns or keeps for himself. He sometimes purchases groceries and clothing, but this is usually done by the wife; the typical husband reserves the right to veto his wife's decision to purchase more expensive items which they have not selected together. With the exception of emergencies and occasional trips to the stores or to nearby relatives, the wife must have her husband's permission to leave the home. No doubt exists in the mind of either spouse that the husband has the right to forbid his wife heterosexual social contacts.

The typical wife waits on her husband by keeping his home running smoothly, catering to his needs, and granting his desires. By means of such gestures which have meaning in the culture, she recognizes him as the head of the household.

If a woman's behavior does not suit her husband, he orders her to behave, he becomes sullen, or he reduces the amount of money he gives her. If she repeatedly defies or insults him, he beats her, and he also makes use of his avoidance of the home as a punishment; as a final measure, he threatens to abandon her. On the other hand, if a woman disapproves of her husband's behavior she argues with him, denies him sexual relations, brings up the memory of former boy friends or husbands to arouse his jealousy, or becomes negligent in attending to his comforts.

The typical wife is deferential toward her husband and accepting of his efforts, however irregular, to provide for the family. The real or alleged infidelity of her husband is the one issue most likely to provoke her into anger. Although subordinate to her spouse, she gives him socioemotional support by consoling him if he is unemployed, sympathizing with his problems at work, and, if he is sick, nursing him to health. The husband does not reciprocate by performing therapeutic services for his wife. If she needs emotional support, a female relative is more likely than her husband to provide it. From day to day, however, the tone of marriage in the control families is harmonious, and neither spouse has to make repeated or extreme efforts to regulate the actions of the other.

Overt evidence of a struggle for power is barely apparent in families with a schizophrenic husband and a well wife. As a result of the illness, the definition of the illness, and the mutual efforts made by both spouses to cope with the problems produced by the illness, family roles are reversed. The woman becomes the primary breadwinner and her sick husband gravitates toward the homemaker role. However, the role of the emotionally supportive partner, which she learned in the culture to assume as a woman, becomes an even more important facet of her new authority. The wife in the control group has the potential to give comprehensive emotional support, but it is the wife with a mentally sick husband who has both the need and the opportunity to apply herself as a therapist.

The schizophrenic man is mild, meek, and defenseless, just the opposite of the dominating and powerful *macho*. He is home-centered, and even though he occasionally strikes out against the power and stability represented by his wife he is thoroughly dependent on her. The union in husband-schizophrenic families resembles a type of relationship between an emotionally supportive, martyrlike but controlling mother and a tyrannical but dependent son. The mother assumes two general attitudes toward her son: she relegates him to a superior role by viewing him as a *machito*, a diminutive *macho*, and she views him as subordinate and defenseless, needing care, protection, and sympathy. As a dependent person, the son is the object of the *Ay bendito!* attitude of the mother. (*Ay bendito!* is an exclamation of grief or sympathy directed at a person who has experienced some misfortune.) This attitude is usually accompanied by a welter of advice designed to make the son feel better, to correct the misfortune, and to alleviate his pain or discomfort. Whether or not this type of mother-son relationship is widespread in Puerto Rican society or at which points of the social structure it may be concentrated is not within the bounds of this study. This relationship is frequently discussed, however, by articulate Puerto Ricans who have a specific interest in family patterns on the Island and a general interest in *nuestra manera de ser* (our way of being, our identity), and this relationship we found to be typical of the marriages of sick husbands and well women.

Husband-schizophrenic families depart from the modal control family in several different ways. The sick husband's illness gives rise to a marital relationship in which the self-sacrificing wife dominates her husband by soft words and therapeutic guidance. The new relationship has the stamp of legitimacy, for both are anxious to cope with the problems created by the illness. The pattern of *respeto* is no longer a salient feature of their lives, and the style of life derived from cultural prescriptions of husband-dominance is not operative. The solidarity of the marriage rests firmly upon the mutual endeavor to cope with the mental illness.

16

Social Control in Marriage. II

WIFE-SCHIZOPHRENIC FAMILIES

The schizophrenic wife has had many unpleasant symptoms since she first experienced her "nervousness." Aches and pains invade her body on some days, only to disappear inexplicably on other days. Anxiety brings fear that tragic events are going to occur; she believes that danger lurks nearby. A deep fatigue overwhelms her as she braces herself to meet imaginary attacks.

Her many symptoms make it difficult for the sick woman to focus on the work required by her roles of wife and mother. Although her capacity to do housework is impaired, she desires to do the work she is not able to do. Daily life then becomes a hodgepodge of distasteful, frustrating, and often incomplete tasks. She thinks that because of her nervous condition she is entitled to partial but not full respite from work. She believes her husband could help, particularly on those days when most of the housework remains undone. The typical husband does not give his wife the help she desires unless she suffers a severe psychotic episode. Mrs. Feliciano's comment about her husband serves to describe the uncooperative attitude of the men married to sick women. "When I have to go on an errand, my husband will not even put a pot of beans on the stove."

Even though the well husband considers his sick wife to be afflicted with a nervous condition, unlike the well wife married to a sick man he demands that his spouse fulfill her familial role. Clothes must be washed and ironed; food must be served to him on time. From the husband's point of view, because there is no obvious physical injury his wife is not incapacitated. He reprimands her for not keeping an orderly home. At first, the wife pleads that she has not felt well, but a full recital of symptoms does not diminish the husband's anger as he has heard the same complaints many times before. Despite frequent admonitions, his wife refuses to comply with his orders that "things in the house should be done properly."

Mrs. Janer feels that her husband is unjust. He does not sympathize with her distressing symptoms. Moreover, he expects her to cook all the meals for his senile father and for his mentally deranged mother who has been feared in the neighborhood as a dangerous *loca* ever since she buried a neighbor's infant in a ditch. Mrs. Janer does not question her obligations to her in-laws, but, because she fears that her *loca* mother-in-law will injure or kill her children, she spends a good part of the day with one eye on her children and the other on her meandering mother-in-law. As a result of this and of the incapacities that stem from her illness, Mrs. Janer is frequently unable to complete the housework. "My husband always finds something wrong. He thinks I can be responsible for *everything* that happens in this house," she says. When she explains why the house is in disorder, he thinks she is unjustly attacking his mother; when she complains about the ailments from which she suffers, he considers her a whining wife. Out of resentment, Mrs. Janer slams his food on the table, sometimes spilling it on his clothing.

The well husband whose sick wife is often remiss places special emphasis on the importance of a well-kept orderly house. On his return home from work he inspects the household and demands a full accounting from his wife. Mr. Urrutia is angered when he sees that his wife has not combed their daughters' hair. "The children's heads look like sea-urchins," he tells her and then demands, "What have you been doing all day?"

Compounding the sin of careless housekeeping is the sick woman's tendency to meander. She walks here and there in the house, in the neighborhood, and in the shopping and residential areas; although to her there is a purpose in her movements, it is not apparent to others. She wants to do so many things that she embarks on a second task before she finishes the first. To her husband, this is senseless, gadabout, and irresponsible behavior. Moreover, the sick woman is taking the privilege of leaving the home without his permission, which could easily lead people to think of her as a "woman of the street." The efforts a husband makes to confine his wife to the home can be inferred from Mrs. Nieves' complaint: "If I leave home and my husband does not know where I have gone, he should not beat me until he learns where I have been."

Arguments between husband and wife give way to physical violence.

The sick woman shows little reluctance to engage her husband in a physical brawl, although she may end up badly bruised and with a black eye or a bloody nose. Mrs. Lebrón relates:

> When he makes me angry I tell my husband that he is without shame, that he is the son of the grandest whore. Then he beats me until I cry like a dog. This is what has made me sick like a dog. He will make a *loca* of me.

Physical force is used habitually by a number of husbands to coerce their wives to follow orders. A husband who does this has found it fruitless to control his wife *a la buena*. The belligerence of the sick woman disposes her to start an endless round of arguments whenever her husband makes a request. Mr. Feliciano insists that his wife take the tranquilizers prescribed by the psychiatrist; she is just as insistent that she will not take them. Then Mr. Feliciano slaps his wife until she takes the tranquilizers. Mr. Nieves has therapeutic reasons for using physical force on his wife. Every day when he returns home, his wife is agitated and upset because she quarrels with neighbors or believes that a clerk at the store took advantage of her inability to read by overcharging her. She attributes bad motives to everyone including the interviewer whom she accused of taking money from her pocketbook. At the end of the day, after feeling herself assailed, stolen from, and ridiculed, Mrs. Nieves fulminates, hurling insults at her children and at her husband. Mr. Nieves then slugs his wife, because, in his words, "she needs it to get better."

Husbands also use force to control wives who experience episodes of aggressive acting-out behavior. Such behavior poses a danger to the neighbors, and the husband is then called on to restrain his wife; he accomplishes this by holding her, sitting on her, and lying on top of her. Strong-arm methods are used by the men both to coerce their sick wives into following orders and to subdue them.

All the well husbands married to sick women are employed; none of their wives have jobs. The husbands work as janitors, assistant bakers, utility men, kitchen helpers, service workers, and unskilled construction laborers. Although the typical husband has relatively stable employment and receives regular wages, he feels that his job is threatened by his wife's illness which interferes with his work. Sometimes he has to stay home from work to care for his wife; other times he is called from work to subdue his wife who is creating a commotion in the neighborhood. Insecure in his work and unhappy in his home life, the husband attempts to understand, in his own terms, his sick wife's behavior in order to cope with it. If his wife fails to keep an orderly house it is because she is lazy and disorganized; if she is vociferous, argumentative, and explosive it is because she is *malcriada* (spoiled); if she meanders it is because she is a gadabout. These explanations are often nothing more than pejorative descriptions of his wife's unacceptable behavior; in contrast to the well wives of sick husbands, these men have little or no insights into the mental illness.

The husband believes that his wife's conduct is attributable to events and situations which *he* does not like. Mr. Feliciano believes that his wife's illness is aggravated by the care she gives their 12-year old daughter who was severely crippled by polio. Mrs. Feliciano is devoted to this daughter, nicknamed "the Eel" by the neighbors because she cannot walk and must drag herself along the floor to get from one place to another. Mrs. Feliciano carries her up and down stairs and lifts her into bed and into her chair. Her husband, however, is disdainful of his daughter, who, he tells us, is the exact opposite of their oldest son, killed by a truck. The dead son was an athlete, according to the father, destined to become a baseball player in the major leagues. The crippled daughter is a living reminder to him of the loss of the son. He complains when his wife carries the paralyzed girl back and forth to school about a half-mile away. Mrs. Feliciano wants her daughter to learn how to read and write, to have friends, and to live as normal a life as circumstances will permit. Consequently, she defies her husband's commands that she not carry the girl to school. Mr. Feliciano notes that when he argues with his wife about this problem she becomes upset, which convinces him that the physical burden of carrying the girl is, in fact, worsening his wife's illness. Much like the other men married to sick women, he seldom, if ever, entertains the possibility that his own behavior seriously harms his wife. The husband is unwilling to consider this explanation even though his wife often tells him that his excessive rectitude, his authoritarian comportment, and the severe beatings he inflicts are making her illness worse.

In addition to verbal and physical punishment, the husband responds to his sick wife by avoiding her. After work, he spends long hours away from home drinking, talking, and gambling with his friends. Often, he engages in extramarital affairs. Finally, the husband responds to his sick wife with indifference. The wife, however, is absorbed and preoccupied with the discomforts of her symptoms, their meaning, thoughts of becoming a *loca*, and the possibilities of getting well. Beside the usual aches and pains, she has many strange experiences about which she wants to talk. Mrs. Urrutia periodically feels a drop of water rolling around inside her head; when she moves her head to one side, the drop of water rolls downward to the lower part of her head; if she shakes her head, the drop of water whirls inside her brain. At his wife's urging, Mr. Urrutia placed his ear against her head and shook her head like a *maraca* in an effort to hear the drop of water, but he hears nothing. Now when his wife complains about the drop of water, Mr. Urrutia disregards her; when she describes her symptoms and troubles, he looks out of the window, turns a deaf ear, tells her to shut up, or leaves the room. The schizophrenic wife feels that she is neglected because her husband will not listen to her troubles.

The sick wife responds to the treatment she receives from her husband primarily by rebelling in anger against his authority. Although the husband informs her that "the only loud voice to be heard at home is my own," the wife's "loud voice" also is heard. An accusation is met by a counteraccusation, as are commands and even physical beatings. Mrs. Iglesias puts the point simply: "When he hits me I hit him back." The cultural ideal that a wife should bestow respect upon her husband is contradicted sharply by the sick woman. She is not *conforme*; she blatantly reminds her husband that he does not provide enough for the family. "When I come home from work," says Mr. Nieves, "my wife and children search my pockets to see what I have brought them." The husband hesitates to give his wife too much of his earnings because he believes that she is an irresponsible spendthrift. When the sick wife goes shopping, she acts as if she could compensate for her overwhelming poverty by buying quickly. Her level of living falls far short of her aspirations, and she blames her husband for the disgraceful and wretched poverty in which she is forced to live.

The sick woman resents the freedom her husband enjoys as a man. She asks herself why a man should come and go as he pleases, whereas a woman is so restricted and burdened. In her inner life, in her thoughts, and in her hopes, she tries to escape from the subordinate position society has imposed on her. The sick woman acts as if she were on a par with her husband. To her, how well she performs as a wife depends on how well her husband performs his own role. Her husband then makes the reverse assumption, awaiting an improvement in his wife's behavior before he does what she wants. Mrs. Lebrón does not do housework because her husband does not provide her with the proper equipment with which to work; her husband, on the other hand, does not provide her with these things because she is a slovenly housekeeper. Reciprocity becomes retaliation, and in the words of Mrs. Lebrón, "Two equals join together." The husband's authority is challenged by his wife even though she is physically weaker and dependent on his earnings for subsistence. Should he abandon her, she would be left with the burden of providing for the children; other men would be reluctant to marry her because sexually she is "damaged goods." As the marriage deteriorates further, the husband wields the more telling sanctions. Nevertheless, day in and day out, the sick wife engages her husband in a struggle for power, each employing coercion, threats, indifference, and insults to control the other.

The schizophrenic wife is an angry woman who is easily provoked. If she tries to restrain her hostility, the strain she is undergoing is apparent to persons who are with her. Mr. Feliciano at times tells his wife, "Woman, speak out! If not, your tongue will be eaten by cancer." Few sick women need the encouragement to "speak out." In Mrs. Feliciano's psychotic episodes she acts like a dangerous *loca* who has gone berserk.

In contrast to the sick man who is dependent on his spouse, the predominant orientation of the sick woman is one of hostility and attack. One day, Mrs. Urrutia lost her temper with a troublesome hen, one in her husband's flock of chickens, that repeatedly flew into the house to eat leftover scraps of food on the table, on the floor, and in the kitchen sink. The hen also ate rice and beans from the pots cooking on the stove or flew to the table where food was set for dinner and glutted itself on the Urrutias' meager servings, then defecated on the floors, the chairs, and the table. Mr. Urrutia attaches great value to his chickens, particularly to the hens, because the eggs they lay feed his sick and destitute mother. He has instructed his wife to feed and care for the chickens and to guard them from theft and injury. On that day, while the hen was inside the house, Mrs. Urrutia locked the doors and windows, caught the hen, and pummeled it with her fists. By the time the attack had ended, the hen's legs were broken and it was almost featherless. "I hit that hen as if it were a grown man," she says, describing the incident; she draws an analogy between the torment she suffered because of the hen and the torment she suffers at the hands of her mother, of her husband, of her children, and of her hymn-singing neighbors who keep her awake at night. In her eyes, the world has scorned her, maltreated her, and punished her.

Unlike the control families, the spouses in a schizophrenic-wife family do not share disillusionments, hopes, or aspirations. There is little cooperation between them in the pursuit of common goals. They speak to each other in a harsh and belligerent manner. Topics that are of interest to the wife are of little interest to the husband. Differences of opinion are aired, but agreement is seldom reached.

Of the nine families with sick wives and well husbands, *only the Oliveras family does not fit the main outline of the foregoing description.* Mrs. Oliveras differs from the other sick women in that she is a meticulous housekeeper and an attentive wife. She makes special meals and desserts for her husband. Mr. Oliveras has no complaints about his wife's management of household affairs; on the contrary, he is proud of and satisfied with the efficient and diligent manner in which his wife takes care of their home. Mr. Oliveras is a good provider. As a meter-reader for a utility company he earns $120 a month, and in addition to this he receives $160 a month from the Veterans Administration because he is studying in high school at night under the Korean Bill. Mr. Oliveras wants to be an IBM technician. Through his efforts he has lifted himself and his wife from the depths of a muddy slum which borders the black waters of the Martin Peña Channel in San Juan. The prospect of plunging back into the slum frightens him. Consequently, he works hard to stabilize his level of achievement and to make greater gains.

Since their marriage, Mr. Oliveras has suffered through several of his wife's psychotic episodes. He is terrified that she may have to be hospitalized permanently. If this were to happen, his home life would be shattered and his children would be raised by his mother-in-law in the slum atmosphere he despises. Mr. Oliveras sees a clear connection between the manner in which he behaves and the state of his wife's nerves. Unlike the other husbands in this group of families, he believes that his wife's health depends on how pleasing he is to her. He has observed that her tantrums always lead to long-lasting flights from reality in which she behaves as if she were "completely out of this world."

Mrs. Oliveras is an astute, natively intelligent woman. She understands both her husband's concern over her illness and his willingness to defer to her so that she will not be upset. This knowledge enables her to wield a degree of control over her husband that is unknown in the other families. Mrs. Oliveras confides to the interviewer that whenever her husband is reluctant to follow her requests or when he does something she does not like, she feigns being upset. He obeys her requests out of fear that she will have a temper tantrum. Thus, Mrs. Oliveras dominates her husband. She made him resign from the

Army, which he thought of as a career, because she was lonely in Germany where he was stationed; she prefers slum life in San Juan to Germany any day. She made him stop drinking; she prohibits him from seeing his friends who used to join him in escapades with women of the "happy life." After work and after his evening classes, he returns home immediately. He has become a home-centered husband. Mr. Oliveras' change in career plans, as well as the changes in his personal comportment, has been heavily influenced by the manner in which his wife *employs* her mental illness. Recently, after a slight difference of opinion, Mrs. Oliveras commanded her husband to kneel before her and to beg for her forgiveness. He complied with her request, lest she "erupt like a volcano."

Thus, the Oliveras family deviates from the pattern of a domineering husband confronted by a rebellious wife which is characteristic of the families with schizophrenic wives.

DOUBLE SCHIZOPHRENIC FAMILIES

Both husband and wife are suffering from schizophrenia in the Aponte, the Gallardo, the Quiromo, and the Santano families. The husbands and the wives in these families view themselves as ill; reciprocally, they think their spouses are ill. The following is a translated and punctated paragraph taken from Mr. Quiromo's handwritten report of the problems he experiences in his family.[1]

> I sometimes see myself as sick and other times as better. Now what worries me most is my wife. I get sick so that on some days I don't have the energy to go out to work. I get weak and I get dizzy spells, and I can hardly sleep thinking of so many things. Some days I don't eat at noon and return to eat late. Sometimes my wife does not even take care of herself because she complains about many pains, and she has always been slow and unconcerned in doing things. I suffer seeing her sick and incapacitated. . . . Since she had our son, she has been ill in her organism [sic—i.e., sexual organ] and, moreover, by her carelessness she hits her head. It is as if her sight were poor. Objects fall from her hands because she is nervous. She suffers because of her false teeth.

When a schizophrenic is married to another schizophrenic, his behavior is even more disorganized than if he were married to a well

---
[1] For a reproduction of part of the original, see Appendix 4.

person. The experiences of the fieldworkers attest to this fact. Often, the sick person is excessively verbal in his reply to the questions addressed to him, rambling from one topic to another, or he is noticeably withdrawn so that on each visit the interviewer has to reestablish rapport almost as if prior interviews had not been held. Episodic flights from reality are more common among schizophrenics married to schizophrenics than among those who have well partners. The evaluations of the psychiatrists contain frequent references to the persons being diagnosed as "burned out," "vegetable-like in behavior," and "extremely weak ego structure."

Mr. Gallardo, who worked as a stevedore on the docks of San Juan, is the only husband employed full time when the families were first visited. During the time we studied the Gallardo family, he left work and by the time of our last visit he had been out of work for almost 3 months. Two of the sick men in this group work part time on their own. Early in the morning Mr. Aponte walks through some of the higher-class residential areas of San Juan and stops at each house offering to mow lawns, wash windows, trim hedges, or wash and polish the family car. As a roving handyman, Mr. Aponte does not know from day to day whether or not he will work or for whom. Mr. Quiromo is a part-time ambulatory barber in the semirural areas on the outskirts of San Juan. The remaining sick man in the double schizophrenic group, Mr. Santano, is unemployed. Thus, when the field work was completed, none of the sick men married to sick women was employed full time.

Mrs. Aponte is the only one of the four wives who is employed. She works as a domestic servant and earns $8 a week scrubbing floors, washing clothes by hand, and ironing; she does not cook or take care of her employer's children. Mrs. Aponte's complaints about her work resemble those of the sick men. Small annoyances upset her; it is difficult for her to do the work because she is always tired, and the instructions her employer gives confuse her. Although Mrs. Gallardo is unemployed, she speaks vaguely about getting a job as a beautician; she observes, however, that her movements now are slower and that she no longer has the required manual dexterity. At work or in anticipation of work the sick woman recognizes the problems that employment brings.

Neither the schizophrenic husband nor his sick wife is a full-time provider for his family. In this respect the four families with both spouses sick differ from each of the other three diagnostic family groups. The vigorous efforts of the well wife to cope with the economic problems produced by her sick husband's disablement are not repeated in the double schizophrenic families. Rather, subsistence comes from feeble and sporadic attempts to work and also from the help the wife's relatives provide. Although they do not approve of the husband's economic dependence on them, he benefits from their assistance as a *de facto* member of the family.

Correlatively, the schizophrenic woman with a sick husband is as unable to be a good homemaker as the sick woman with a well husband. She is incapable of organizing her household in an orderly manner which, we have seen, is an important part of the solidarity of the families that are free of schizophrenia. Irrespective of the sex of the person who is afflicted, schizophrenia incapacitates him to perform his social roles. Mr. Quiromo summarizes this point concisely: "I do, but I don't have a wife."

Each person understands and believes in the common expectations associated with the roles in the family even though he cannot fulfill them. Each spouse observes the discrepancy between expectancy and behavior in the other spouse. Both have ample opportunities to make such observations since the husband is not employed full time and spends more time at home than does the man who is not afflicted with schizophrenia. Does the husband or the wife influence his mate in any way to behave more appropriately? Does he compensate in any way for his partner's inability to perform his role adequately?

Before we present case material on the four families to bear on these questions, one point should be made. With the exception of Mrs. Gallardo, each sick person insists that his spouse fulfill his familial obligations; these obligations are not eliminated or relaxed despite the fact that the person imposing the obligations upon his mate views him as "sick of the nerves." Thus the attitude of each person toward his spouse resembles the attitude of the well man toward his sick wife rather than that of the well woman toward her sick husband.

Mr. Aponte's neighbors consider him to be an aloof and belligerent person, easily provoked into explosive outbursts of anger. When they see him coming from work they quickly disperse from the passageway that leads to the door of his apartment in the *caserío*. Mr. Aponte's attitude toward his neighbors is equally unfavorable: "If you live in this neighborhood you don't have to go to the movies—around here you can see anything." The neighbors have often heard screeches and wails coming from the Aponte apartment. They know on these occasions that Mr. and Mrs. Aponte are embroiled in bitter strife.

Mr. Aponte demands that dinner be served immediately upon his return home, but Mrs. Aponte finds it degrading to serve him. She remembers the many beatings he has given her: "How can I serve my husband when he has been so cruel and inconsiderate?" She thinks of the time several years before when her husband fell in love with a young girl. When Mrs. Aponte discovered this, she went to her rival's house pretending to be her husband's sister. The girl's mother told her that he had proposed matrimony and that the marriage would soon take place. This incident started a round of vicious wrangling between the Apontes which continues to the present. She also cites as evidence of his lack of interest in the family the fact that, although he occasionally brings food or clothing to the family, he never discusses the purchases with her so that often what he buys is unneeded. Many grievances have become so deeply imbedded in Mrs. Aponte's memory that to do anything at all for her husband involves a loss of pride.

Under the impact of economic problems some persons develop new expectations inconsistent with the prevailing ones to which they still adhere. Although Mr. Aponte holds the conventional idea that a woman's place is at home, he would still like to have a wife who earns a salary. If he could live his life again, he indicates that he would marry a different person. He is worried because he knows that the $13 a week he provides for his family and the $8 a week his wife earns as a servant are not enough to support his 6 children who range in age from 4 to 15 years. If he could live his life anew, he "would look for a woman who knows something, who is not ignorant. Someone who could help me. Someone with training who could earn a good salary to help me take care of the home."

The interpersonal relations between the Apontes are of two kinds: they either fight or do not speak. The marital situation is seldom if ever emotionally neutral. They avoid contact with each other, except to reprimand, accuse, or punish. They go to bed at night and arise in the morning at different times. The husband tells the eldest daughter when he will return home; the neighbors warn Mrs. Aponte of his approach at which point she usually goes to the bedroom and locks herself in. The 15-year old daughter serves him dinner. This state of silent war punctuated by aggressive outbursts prevails in the Aponte household. Neither spouse can make the other behave in a more acceptable manner.

The marital relations of the Santanos resemble those of the Apontes, except that the Santanos air their grievances openly without ever retreating into a grudging silence. Mr. Santano spends his days at a neighborhood bar, at his mother's home, or at his mother-in-law's apartment where he lives with his wife and children. At present he does not work but receives $37 a month in unemployment compensation. Ideally, he would like

> . . . to have a job, to return home and find an affectionate wife waiting for me with a smile. Then I would go to bed and drink a cold beer without having to leave the house for anything. I would stay home with my wife and children in a tranquil atmosphere. I would have a peaceful, cooperative wife.

Mr. Santano's ideas do not match his experiences at home. Conflict between the couple started about a year and a half after their marriage. At first he was convinced that with "strength of character" he would soon subdue his recalcitrant wife, but, as he says, "Once I beat her she was no longer afraid of being beaten. She threw herself at me, slugged me with her fists, and scratched me with her fingernails. Now she rides me like a pony."

Mrs. Santano's tongue-lashings, her disdain of threatened beatings, and her pungent ridicule cause Mr. Santano to flee from his home and go back to his mother. According to him, his mother is the only one who understands his illness. She cares for him, feels sorry for him, and encourages him to stay at her home and rest, relax, or do anything he pleases. However, Mr. Santano pays daily for his moments of rest and relaxation, for when he returns to the apartment, his wife greets him with caustic reminders of the many ways he has defaulted in his promises and obligations. "Why don't you work like a man?" "When are we going to have a home of our own?" "You promised to take me and the children for a walk; why weren't you home to do so?" "Were you sitting on your mother's lap all day?" "If you return home drunk once more my mother will throw you out of the apartment." Mr. Santano is confused by the rapid-fire questions and threats, for he does not know whether his wife wants him to leave or to stay. His wife, in his words, "has driven me to desperation, to the point of madness or of committing some barbarity. She has completely shattered me. She does not even want me to visit my mother."

To brace himself against his wife's diatribes, Mr. Santano often stops at a bar on his way home from visiting his mother. His confidence returns after a drink or two, and then he is ready to confront his wife, to exchange acrimonious insults, and to take part in the dispute to the point of physical violence; sometimes, he becomes *macho*-like in his comportment and coerces her into having sexual intercourse. Early the next morning while Mr. Santano is sober, suffering from a hangover, and only partly awake, she shakes him out of bed, hurls fierce invectives at him, and evicts him from the household demanding that he not return unless he find a job. This initiates another round of arguments which continue from one day to the next. Neither one is successful in forcing his mate to behave in a more acceptable manner.

The Santanos are too deeply involved in strife to solve their problems, even those that can be clearly foreseen. The afternoon after the first visit by the interviewer, Mrs. Santano began to feel the birth pangs of her fourth pregnancy. She decided to go to the doctor at the health unit of the *caserío* where she lives. Neither of the Santanos had consulted a physician about the pregnancy, nor had they made arrangements for the delivery of the child. When the pains began Mrs. Santano went to the bathroom to shower. As she showered, the intensity and frequency of the pains forced her to squat on the floor of the bathroom. Soon the head of the fetus appeared, and after what seemed an interminable ordeal the rest of the fetus emerged. Mrs. Santano, bleeding profusely, managed to drag herself to the door of the bathroom, open it, and scream for help. The neighbors who came were unable to get a doctor since the only one nearby was out for lunch. They summoned a midwife who cut the umbilical cord, made the mother comfortable, and called for an ambulance. Mrs. Santano was given blood transfusions for 16 days at the hospital until she was finally permitted to go home. Upon her return home, although she was exhausted from her experience, she immediately engaged her husband in a row. Relations between the Santanos are so fiercely antagonistic that neither thinks of scarcely anything but his hatred of the other.

Marital relations between the Quiromos are not as tumultuous as between the Santanos, but considerable discord is apparent in the family. The Quiromos argue over her reluctance to cooperate sexually, over his infidelity, and over his punishment of their son, which according to her is excessive and severe. The Quiromos argue a great deal about their religious differences. She complains about his inability to provide adequately for the family and about their economic dependence upon her parents. Neither spouse has any appreciable influence on the other's behavior.

Mrs. Quiromo is an extremely withdrawn schizophrenic. She does not cook, clean house, or wash and iron clothing. She sleeps in the clothes she wears during the day; her hair is tangled and uncombed, hanging far below her shoulders. According to the psychiatrist, she has retreated into a vegetable-like existence. She is encapsulated in a world of fantasy in which she plays the role of a nun in a convent, aloof from mundane affairs; most of her energies are inwardly directed. This attitude upsets Mr. Quiromo who yearns for her to respond to him, to recognize his presence. He has learned, however, that she does respond to events which she believes are dangerous and threatening to her, and he employs a variety of attention-getting devices to stir her out of the psychotic lethargy which makes her oblivious of his presence. Mrs. Quiromo is fearful of everything from the sharp crowing of a rooster to the ominous rustling of the leaves outside the house. Mr. Quiromo hides behind the house and makes deep guttural noises until she comes to investigate; then he jumps out to scare her. At other times he throws small pebbles at her and watches, in hiding, her disconcerted efforts to discover where the pebbles come from. Another scheme is to feed the hungry chickens in the yard a handful of rice, then imbed a grain of rice into the head of his son's uncircumcised penis. The chickens chase the naked 4-year old around the yard in an effort to get at the grain of rice. Mrs. Quiromo yells at her husband because she does not find his efforts to scare or confuse her funny.

Above all, Mr. Quiromo wants his wife's sympathy and respect since, he believes, he has had a series of revelations in which the word of God was communicated to him by a voice that also commanded him to become a prophet and spread the gospel. The indignity of a wife who does not appreciate the gift of splendid charisma upsets Mr. Quiromo and makes him feel lonely and isolated. No amount of argument, cajoling, or persuasion, has convinced Mrs. Quiromo that Catholicism is wrong and that he is chosen and right. On Sunday mornings when Mrs. Quiromo listens to religious services on the radio, her husband stands nearby trying to drown out the program by singing hymns that he himself composed. As she turns up the volume, he intensifies his voice until finally the noise of the blaring radio competing with the shouting hymn singer becomes unbearable to both the Quiromos and to her parents who live next door.

Mr. Quiromo strives for recognition, understanding, and sympathy from his wife. It angers him that she suffers from frequent sore throats and chronic diarrhea, which makes her pity herself and robs Mr. Quiromo of the sympathy he feels he should receive from his wife. Mrs. Quiromo sympathizes with their son who is often afflicted with severe attacks of asthma. When the mother or the son is sick, Mr. Quiromo gets down on his hands and knees and acts like a bull or horse, or he squats and becomes a chicken; he has also feigned nervous attacks to gain sympathy. These measures have not influenced his wife.

In contrast to the Apontes, the Santanos, and the Quiromos, the Gallardos seldom, if ever, clash overtly. The furious exchanges, the dogfights, the hostile wrangling so characteristic of the relations between the three couples just described are absent in the Gallardos' marriage, as Mr. Gallardo is an explosive man given to violent and savage outbursts of aggressive behavior and Mrs. Gallardo is terrified by him. He keeps a knife handy which he often sharpens and claims he will use on the neighbors who disturb his sleep and who have several times urinated and defecated on the stairway leading to the Gallardos' *caserío* apartment. "When I get done with the neighbors," he threatens, "twenty coffins will be needed." Mrs. Gallardo fears that her husband will carry out his threats.

Almost daily, Mr. Gallardo slaps, kicks, and slugs his two daughters and son who are 3, 4, and 7 years old. Once as he was lashing his son with a razor strop, the strop wound around the boy's head and the buckle hit his ear. According to Mrs. Gallardo, if the strop had been longer it would have put the boy's eye out. The mother and the children are afraid of the sick man; they cower in a corner of the living room or hide in the bedroom when he becomes violent. Every night, Mrs. Gallardo gets up from bed two or three times to check on the safety of her children. She is panic stricken by her husband's violence and is deeply concerned about the children's safety. Consequently, when her husband commands her to do something, she leaps to obey. She runs to the grocery store and back, skipping through dangerously heavy traffic, fearful that her husband will accuse her of lingering or consorting with another man. She keeps the front door of the apartment closed, no matter how hot it may be, lest her husband charge her with eyeing the men in the neighborhood. She keeps the children away from him so that he will not be provoked into wrath. When he orders her to tell the neighbors to be quiet she goes out to the front porch, reads the Bible for a brief moment, and returns to tell her husband that they will soon be quiet.

Although Mrs. Gallardo is terrified by her husband, she feels obligated to him. For 7 of the 8 years of their marriage, he was an exemplary husband. She is the only sick person married to a sick partner who would choose the same mate were she to live her life anew: "I would marry him thirty times if I had to do it over." From her point of view, his violence is due to his illness which she believes will not last forever. She listens to his many complaints, consoles him, calms him, rubs him with alcohol, strokes his head affectionately, takes him to the psychiatrist, and encourages him to participate in church activities.

The leader of the church group to which they belong frequently visits them, listens to Mrs. Gallardo, and advises her husband. Moreover, Mrs. Gallardo's father is the political boss of the *barrio*. Mr. Gallardo is impressed with, and respectful toward, his influential father-in-law. Mrs. Gallardo often summons her father, particularly when her husband is acting dangerously. The father wields significant control over his son-in-law and is usually able to pacify him.

Even though Mrs. Gallardo is attached to her husband, gives him therapy, and makes use of the religious leader and her father to control his behavior, the marital situation has begun to have an effect on her illness. Voices have told her to poison herself. Other voices have told her to take her children and abandon her husband. Several times she has left home in a semiconscious trance, walked to a local park with her children, and stayed the entire afternoon, relatively oblivious of her surroundings. She is awakened from the trance by one of the children who cries, wanting to go home. Since then, she has discovered in herself a conscious desire to leave her husband.

Perhaps as Mrs. Gallardo orients herself toward her husband according to her desire to leave him, her family will begin to resemble the other three families in this diagnostic group. The Apontes have abandoned each other seven or eight times. The Santanos are only a partially formed family since the sick husband repeatedly gravitates toward his mother and away from his wife and children. Mr. Quiromo once abandoned his wife to live with Juana the Cripple, a local prostitute.

In brief, the marital bonds of the double schizophrenic families are fragile and unstable. A sick person with a sick mate is not exempted from normal responsibilities by his partner; rather, each partner uses extraordinary effort to make the other's behavior more acceptable. Although each spouse makes innumerable efforts to modify the unacceptable behavior of his sick partner, these efforts are relatively futile. Moreover, no spouse with the exception of Mrs. Gallardo makes any effort to modify his own behavior so as to avoid aggravating his partner's symptoms, nor does he make any effort to control situations in the family for the benefit of the sick mate.

SUMMARY

In contrast to the wife in the control group, the sick wife married to a well man is unable to perform according to the expectations associated with her sex and family roles. The order, the serenity, and the routine in family life characteristic of the control families are absent in such a marriage. The schizophrenic wife believes she should be relieved of normal responsibilities, but her husband does not. She neglects to do things she ought to do and does things she should not do. She is vituperative toward her husband; she is rebellious instead of *conforme*. The husband views her actions as misbehavior. He strikes back verbally and physically, or he becomes indifferent toward her, escaping into "street-corner" activities which are a part of the masculine world. He makes little or no effort to compensate for his wife's impairment. A power struggle embroils the spouses into a mutually unsatisfactory relationship; as the husband employs all the influence of his masculine role, he is countered by a frenzied, rebellious wife.

A sick wife is incapable of being either a servant to a well husband or a therapeutic mother to a sick one. To fulfill either mandate is difficult because of her weakened ego structure. Her theme is rebellion against obligations and demands and, in particular, against persons who try to impose them on her.

The double schizophrenic families differ from the wife-schizophrenic families in that the spouses spend more time together and thus have more opportunities to search, probe, and attack each other's sensitivities. In contrast to the well man with a sick wife, the sick man with a wife also afflicted cannot use threats to withdraw from his role as provider. His wife does not recognize him as the legitimate head of the household, and, moreover, he does not have the institutional support that stems from full membership in male peer groups. In these marriages, each sick spouse tries to change the other's unacceptable behavior by physical violence, verbal tirades, rude frightening jokes, ridicule, and sullen reluctance to speak. Neither mate is dominant in this inconclusive struggle.

Among the double schizophrenic families, Mrs. Gallardo is an exception in her efforts to preserve the little solidarity that remains in her marriage. The atypical response to a sick husband in this one family is probably attributable to the recent origin of the schizophrenic process. We were able to observe Mrs. Gallardo's illness as it developed and we noticed, even at that time, that she began to show traces of alienation from her husband.

The exceptions to the modal family pattern in the three remaining diagnostic family groups—the dominant wife in the Domínguez family of the control group, the dominant wife of the Oliveras of the wife-schizophrenic group, and the breakdown of social controls in the Herrero family of the husband-schizophrenic group—all show one important characteristic in common: at least one spouse is deeply immersed in his own personal world of fantasy or aspiration which significantly affects his relations to his spouse. Mrs. Domínguez (control group) is intolerant of her husband because of her erroneous self-conception. She has convinced her husband that he is not worthy of her, which enables her to wield considerable influence over him, much more so than the typical wife in the control group. The aspirations of Mr. Oliveras (wife-schizophrenic group) and Mrs. Herrero (husband-schizophrenic group) are not as unrealistic as Mrs. Domínguez' fantasy. Their understanding of life on a higher-class level, with style, comfort, and power, is a significant part of the slum- and *caserío*-dweller's image of the affluent groups. There is a consensual basis to their aspirations. Both Mr. Oliveras and Mrs. Herrero are more deeply committed to the achievement of their hopes than is the usual person who is not afflicted with schizophrenia. Mr. Oliveras can see that the modest social gains he has made have freed his family from the worst slum, and he realizes that the goal toward which he is working will open new opportunities for employment and further gains for him. His desire to consolidate these gains, and to achieve more, leads him to accept his sick wife and to adapt to her efforts to dominate him. Mrs. Herrero considers the fact that she is unusually attractive as sufficient credentials for entry to a higher class. She views her sick husband as a heavy burden that anchors her to an acceptable status in the lower class. Since the pressures she put on him to be successful were fruitless, her solution is to withdraw from the marriage.

In sum, the husband habitually and pervasively dominates his spouse in the control families; in the husband-schizophrenic families it is the wife who does this; in families with schizophrenic women married to either sick or well husbands neither spouse is clearly dominant. Thus we find that the structure of authority relations *is* related to the mental status of the husband and the wife.

17
Sexual Conflicts

Cultural values and practices regarding sexual behavior by males and females structure the sexual relations of husbands and wives. The cardinal cultural prescription pertinent to this discussion is the double standard of morality prevailing in Puerto Rican society. The sexual behavior of husbands stems from the widely held beliefs that sex is necessary to a man. A woman can live without sexual intercourse; a man cannot. In accordance with this belief, a man is sexually aggressive, in the vernacular *mujeriego* (a woman chaser). He is expected to create and capitalize upon sexual opportunities.

We mentioned in Chapter 8 that the mother is an important agent in the socialization of her son. She helps transmit to him the cultural image of the sexually aggressive male. She interprets the size of her son's genitals as evidence of his masculine equipment, his masculine "documentation," and the armament he can use to "defend" himself in a life of sexual conquest and sexual adventure. Even a wife who suffers the infidelities of her husband refers to her father with subdued pride as a man who has "women on the left." The process of socialization is influenced and supported by the father and by peer group members with whom the boy associates.

A woman who is as sexually aggressive as a man is expected to be is viewed with opprobrium because she departs sharply from the cultural norm of feminine modesty. If she also is sexually promiscuous, she will be thought to have *furor*, a vaguely conceived affliction with symptoms that are likened to those of a "bitch in heat." This behavior is incongruous with the norms and values that define the role of the ideal woman. To a man, an encounter with a woman afflicted with *furor* is a happy experience, but he is frightened by the prospect of a wife with *furor* because in his absence she would have affairs with other men; she would make a cuckold of him. Moreover, a wife with *furor* would impose excessive sexual demands from him. "What if I were too tired from work?" "What if I had been with another woman and could not 'lift pressure' for my wife?" These troubled questions are asked by the husbands. A woman with *furor* would upset marital relations and undercut his masculinity.

The different sex norms for husbands in comparison with wives are highlighted by a person's belief of what a spouse *should* do when confronted with infidelity. To investigate this point, we asked each person two questions: "What should a husband do if his wife is unfaithful?" and, "What should a wife do if her husband is unfaithful?" Each person selected a reply of: "divorce"; "separate"; or "give him (or her) another chance." In our report of the findings, we have combined the replies of "separate" and "divorce" because they involve the rupturing of the family, in contrast to "give him (or her) another chance." The findings indicate that (1) 85 per cent of the wives and 95 per cent of the husbands think a husband should divorce or separate from an unfaithful wife, and (2) 35 per cent of the wives and 18 per cent of the husbands think a wife should divorce or separate from an unfaithful husband. To test the stability of these findings, the sex of the person replying, his mental status, and the mental status of his spouse were controlled at the same time. The imposition of these controls does not affect the pattern of findings. Husbands and wives agree on this point: an unfaithful wife should be accorded more severe punishment than an unfaithful husband.

In brief, the different sex norms that apply to men and women are imbedded in the culture. A man is given wide latitude in his sexual conduct and is, indeed, encouraged and expected to seek sexual outlets, but a woman who departs from sex standards transgresses against the mores of society. These norms outline the major sex conflict in marriage.

Two points of tension pervade the marital relations of almost every spouse pair: the sexual demands one spouse makes on the other, and the real or alleged infidelity resulting from the denial of sexual intercourse to one member of the spouse pair by the other. The issue of infidelity focuses chiefly on the husband's behavior. Seventy per cent of the wives in the 40 families have accused their husbands of infidelity; 70 per cent of these husbands accused by their wives voluntarily admit to the interviewers that their wives' accusations are correct. In contrast, only 25 per cent of the wives have been accused by their husbands of infidelity. No wife admits the correctness of the charge. It is interesting to point out, however, that the percentage of husbands in the present generation who have been involved in adulterous behavior is almost the same as it was in the parental generation. In Chapter 4 we reported that 68 per cent of the husbands and 65 per cent of the wives claimed their fathers had been unfaithful to their mothers. Adulterous behavior by married men appears to have been relatively constant in the two generations under study.

In a schizophrenia-free family the wife has had relatively restricted, controlled, and supervised heterosexual contacts through childhood and adolescence. Her parents have admonished her that men will try to "feel her up" and to damage her by doing strange and evil things. On entering marriage, she may have a relatively vague idea about the mechanics of sexual intercourse. Her role as a wife obligates her to submit to the sexual requests of her husband, and her husband insists that she fulfill her sexual obligation to him. They both believe that this obligation is an expression of God's will, a way of fulfilling a sacred duty, of perpetuating humanity. Although such appeals legitimatize coitus in marriage, they do not induce a wife to be a cooperative sex partner. To cooperate sexually is incongruous with the modest behavior she has been taught since childhood. Her interest in sexual relations is less lively than that of her husband. Mrs. Cortés says:

> I could live very well without sex relations, but I give in to him because it is a man's life. A man enjoys it very much. If it were up to me, I would sleep all night, every night.

As Mrs. Julía puts it: "If it were up to me to start the sex act, we wouldn't have it as often as when he starts it."

The husband does not confront such a discontinuity in his sexual behavior. He approaches his wife by stroking her, by fondling her genitals, and by verbally requesting her cooperation. The wife seldom cooperates immediately. Rather, she rejects him diplomatically by introducing other topics of conversation or by withdrawing from his reach. Often, she pleads that she is too tired from housework, or she waits until he is asleep before she goes to bed; she may remind him that the children or the neighbors are within earshot. The husband knows that as a man he is sexually stronger than his wife and that women are reticent. Nonetheless, if his wife continues to be uncooperative, he gets angry. He addresses biting comments to her, reminding her of the many other times she has turned him down. Soon, in the words of one wife, the husband "becomes sulky, irritable, and sharp with the children." To avoid bitter conflict, she submits or even initiates the sex act. By rewarding her husband she believes that she is discouraging his infidelity. The wives say:

> A woman should not always reject her husband when he wants sexual contact because if she does she is inviting him to go out to women in the streets.
> My husband gets mad if I don't give it to him. I am afraid he will go out in the street and get another woman. He goes for walks, but I think it is to forget about sex.
> My husband is sexually satisfied. This is why he hasn't given me any problems. If a man does not have sexual satisfaction in the house, he will go outside for it.

In brief, the wife does not allow her reticence to become a serious marital problem. If the conflict promises to become recurrent and bitter, she submits. Sexual intercourse is one of the few rewards a wife can offer her husband to keep him happy, to control his behavior, and, in particular, to discourage him from having extramarital affairs.

Correlatively, the husband feels a measure of justification in philandering because his wife is reticent, but this is a rationalization for doing what he may do in any case. In all probability, he is aware that his father, brother, uncle, and other male relatives have had extramarital affairs, and the male peer groups that abound in his locale encourage him to behave like a real he-man. He is loath to be looked upon as a "pubic hair," a term of ridicule that points to a socially ineffective person, in particular a man who is dormant in the face of sexual opportunities. From the point of view of his peers, a man should be alert to sexual opportunities. Through his friends he hears of a house servant, a widow, a divorced or separated woman, or a girl who has returned from New York City with liberal sex ideas. By approaching one of these women he confirms his masculinity to himself and to his peers. A man who overlooks an opportunity for sexual intercourse is either a fool or a homosexual. Mr. Rosado tells us:

> My wife worries about my affairs because she knows I am a man, and a woman that gives it to me is a woman that I will take. This is the way I am, but she should not be concerned about it for I bring her what she needs around the house and I give her affection.

A suspicious wife makes dire threats to leave with her children, but she is not likely to do so, as then she, alone, would be saddled with the responsibility of supporting the children; she would encounter many difficulties in finding a place to live since her brothers, sisters, parents, and other relatives are equally impoverished and cramped for living space. Although these considerations do not prevent her from pushing the marriage to the point of dissolution by hurling acrimonious insults at her husband, by rebelling against his control, and often by refusing to prepare his food and clothing, she fears the loss of her husband. In Mrs. Hidalgo's words:

> I worry very much because some day my husband could find a *señorita*, a virgin, and he could damage her and then have to marry her. Then I would be left with the rope and no goat. Some other girl is going to tie him up and take him away from me.

A husband does not discuss with his wife many of his activities away from home, since he assumes these activities should not be of concern to her. As long as he provides some modicum of financial support for his family, he believes he is discharging his chief obligation as a husband and father. The wife feels she has a right to know more about her husband's activities away from home.

The wife discovers the real or alleged infidelity of her husband primarily through neighborhood gossip she hears from a friend or relative, usually another woman. Neighborhood gossip, which is a communicative network operating in part to keep track of husbands, is by no means her only source of information. A husband may tell his wife of his affairs when he is angry at her, or she may surreptitiously spy on him and, in some cases, even find him in bars with other women. Lipstick stains, the odor of perfume, and sucker-bites are telltale signs that give the husband away. Occasionally a wife inspects her husband's undergarments after he has returned home and gone to bed. One wife, after her husband has gone out for the evening, counts the contraceptives which he keeps in a bureau drawer. A wife also infers that her husband has fallen in love with another woman because suddenly he is generous, effusive, euphoric, expansive, and splendid, or suddenly he is taciturn, surly, and indifferent toward sex. A husband who is frequently absent from home and whose behavior has changed abruptly arouses the suspicions of his wife.

The discovery that her husband is spending money to entertain or support another woman is bitterly resented by a wife. She recites the unsatisfied needs of the family, emphasizing that an immoral woman of the street is taking food from her children; it enrages her to know that the clothing she washes and irons for him is worn for other women. To be robbed of the support she feels is hers and to be used as a servant is humiliating. Some wives attack their sexual rivals and, as one wife put it, "We hit each other like grown men." Other wives who know the whereabouts of their rivals avoid them out of fear that their faces might be slashed. A scarred face carries the stigma of a woman of the "happy life."

The extramarital affairs of the husbands range from the transient *pica flor* (flower nibbler) relationship to the more or less enduring relationship with a mistress or concubine. The transient affairs are usually with a woman of the "happy life" who is unmarried and is not living with parents; thus, widows, divorced or separated women, and house servants are vulnerable to these affairs. To initiate an affair, the husband may introduce himself as a single man and perhaps make vague and indefinite promises of matrimony, or he and the woman may agree verbally or tacitly that their relationship is for "fun" and make no plans to establish a more enduring bond. In either case, the essential feature of the transient affair is that the man does not feel obligated to support the woman and has not institutionalized his commitment to her. Transient affairs result in the mistress arrangement when the man fathers a child he recognizes as his own or when he withdraws from his marriage. A man incurs some obligation to support his mistress and any offspring that are produced. Two husbands in our study group support two families. Another husband abandoned his wife to live with a mistress but returned to his wife. To a husband, the transient affair is more desirable than the mistress arrangement; usually his income is too small to allow him to discharge his economic obligations to two women, and, moreover, both his wife and his mistress bring extraordinary pressure to bear on him because they find it disturbing and repugnant to share the same man.

Mrs. Julía is haunted by the idea of her husband's mistress, *la Pinta*, the freckled one, who has a daughter the same age as Mrs. Julía's son. Both children were fathered by Mr. Julía. Mrs. Julía found out about *la Pinta* when her husband, in anger, told her that few men could brag, as he could, of having two women pregnant at the same time; he then told her about his affair with *la Pinta*. When Mr. Julía first found out that his mistress was pregnant, he threatened to beat her but he finally accepted the obligation of his illegitimate daughter. Although he provides $33 a month for her support, he tells his wife that it is only $12 a month. Mrs. Julía says:

> The biggest problem I have is *la Pinta*, the freckled turkey egg. My husband got tied up with her when he got drunk and took her to the

beach. He ate her pork chop that night. Now I always suspect him. I think he takes condoms out of our chest of drawers to use with *la Pinta*. Our fights are because of *la Pinta*. I mention her name to him and he gets mad. It makes me mad to know that I am a servant to him so he can show off in front of her.

Mr. Julía boasts:

Sometimes I tell my wife to hurry and iron my shirt because I have to see *la Pinta*. We argue about her all the time. My wife takes this seriously. I don't like to argue. Lower-class people argue. I am a man. I am not going to let a pubic hair of a woman tell me what to do. If a thousand women give it to me, I will take a thousand. I will stick it into them. I am not a duck [homosexual].

The endless round of arguments between the Julías occurs also in families in which the wives know that their husbands continuously engage in affairs. Wives feel humiliated, insecure, and disgusted by this knowledge. However, Mr. Julía's bravado in bragging about his mistress to his wife is not typical; husbands are usually circumspect, discreet, and tight-lipped.

To summarize, families in which neither spouse is afflicted with schizophrenia have two prevailing sexual problems. The first involves the reticence of the wife to submit to her husband's requests for intercourse. She submits before conflict erupts, however, because she feels obligated as a wife, who wants to avoid conflict, and she fears her husband will seek another woman. The second problem is the real or alleged infidelity of the husband. The wife does not willingly accept the husband's adulterous behavior. Conflict disappears when the wife believes that her husband no longer sees the other woman. Her hostility is not cumulative, nor is it long lasting; she is, however, more prone to suspect him after such an affair. At the moment, she may deny him sexual access but, soon, the former pattern of submitting after grudging delays to his requests for intercourse is reestablished.

In families in which the husband is afflicted with schizophrenia and the wife is mentally healthy, marital relations are generally harmonious, partly because the wife is prone to comply with the requests of her sick husband since he is not as demanding as he formerly was. Of greater importance is the power of the wife over her sick husband and the husband's withdrawal from friends and associates.

The wife of a sick husband is vigorous, active, and resourceful. New responsibilities have given her a considerable measure of control over her husband. She copes with the economic plight of the family. She ministers to his aches and pains by massaging him, giving him medication, and being a sympathetic listener. She is philosophical and accepting, inured to his grating idiosyncrasies. She may respond to her husband's requests for intercourse by trying to convince him that something unfavorable will result. Mrs. Cardona says:

> I feel that since my husband is sick, he should stop having sex, but he cannot restrain himself. I have asked him to restrain from having sex relations because I am afraid I will become pregnant and if I had a child it would turn out to be nervous the way he is.

Similarly, Mrs. Ramos reports:

> When my husband felt better we had sex every night and during the day at siesta. Now that he is sick we only have sex about four times a week and I feel that more sex would harm him. He is sexually active and I have to control him.

The advice offered by the wife is not designed merely to circumvent her husband's sexual desires. Rather, it expresses her fear that intercourse will bring harm to her husband or to possible offspring. Since the husband depends on her for economic and emotional support, he accepts her advice. The wife uses sex also to influence the behavior of her husband. Though she often indicates the undesirable consequences of coitus,-she just as often entices him to have sexual relations when he is depressed or in a bad mood. Sex is part of the therapeutic treatment she administers to her husband. Mrs. Cardona reports:

> I wait until my husband comes to me, and, no matter how tired I am, I never say no. He is always affectionate and after he finishes he always asks me whether or not I have been satisfied. I actually don't care, but I say that I am satisfied.

Mrs. Espinosa says: "I never turn my husband down. Never! I would really have to be feeling very bad."

The sick husband centers his activities in his home, away from the usual focus of masculine life. His behavior is more visible to his wife and is, therefore, within the bounds of her control. He is no longer exposed to the stimulus of the peer groups to participate in extramarital affairs, nor are the usual channels to sexual adventure available to him. The sexual satisfaction he enjoys with his wife probably makes him less inclined to be unfaithful. Should he have an opportunity to have an affair, his wife intervenes forcibly. Mr. Ramos spends his time doing housework while his wife works in a factory. During the hours his wife is away from home, a young girl who lives in an adjoining apartment visits him, teasing him into an affair. She tempts him by not wearing undergarments. "So far," according to Mr. Ramos, "all I have done is to kiss and squeeze her. I would like to take her to a hotel." Recently, Mrs. Ramos came home from work and found the girl in the apartment. She chased her out and threatened to thrash her if she ever returned; she also spoke to the parents of the girl. Mrs. Ramos does not inveigh against her husband. She removes temptation from him. Her attitude is one of protection for her husband against the philandering girl.

The usual sexual conflicts disappear in families with sick husbands. Other points of tension emerge, however. The sick husband experiences many doubts about himself because his masculine autonomy has vanished. Repeatedly, he dwells on his sexual powers, recounting past experiences when he was more sexually adequate. Memories of his bravado with women of the "happy life" are brought up unsolicited, recited, and presented as his credentials to the listener. He fantasizes plans of future sexual conquests. Although he admits that his wife gives him beneficial advice about sexual relations, he insists that he is active, she is passive; he rules, she follows. Purporting to speak about himself, he talks of the ideals of masculine dominance and feminine subservience. These ideals are not fulfilled in his family life.

The sick husband more often than the well husband has a fear that his wife is being unfaithful to him. Mr. Cardona says,

> After three years of marriage, I began dreaming my wife was unfaithful, and I began to be jealous of her. If she gets up to give the children a drink of water I want to know if she has been with another man. We have bad arguments.

Similarly, Mr. Herrero tells us:

> My wife visits on the third floor, and I don't like this as there are women there who have returned from the United States. These girls are always talking to their boy friends in parked cars and coming home late at night. I have even heard these girls say bad words. I have reminded my wife about these things and told her not to associate with these girls because people will gossip about her and confuse her with the others. They will speak bad of her. I am jealous of her. One day I let her go to a movie and I followed her all the way to avoid the possibility that others would talk about her.

In an ironic reversal of roles, the sick husband spies on his wife. Mr. Cardona shuts the bedroom door on bits of paper after his wife has gone to bed. If the pieces of paper have fallen on the floor in the morning, his wife has to explain why she left the bedroom during the night. Mr. Herrero keeps his eye on his wife even when they sit on the front porch of their apartment. In an attempt to alleviate suspicion, the wife assures her husband of her fidelity and attributes his accusations to his nervousness.

The schizophrenic woman ascribes less importance to sex than does the well woman. Sexual intercourse causes her to feel physically ill. The following comments from the interviews in wife-schizophrenic families illustrate this point:

> When I have sexual contact, it makes me feel very bad. I feel a heaviness in my brain, a nausea, and a desire to vomit without being able to.
> When I have sexual contact, it makes me feel nervous, headachey, and restless. It upsets my stomach. When I have sexual contact it makes me feel bad.
> Sex is a bother. I'd just as soon not have sexual contact. I don't feel like having it. I feel weak and a man is bothersome. I don't enjoy it. Ever since I had my first child, I began to feel weak and sickly. I feel tired. After so many years, one gets tired and one's batteries wear out. Once in a while I give it to him to keep him from pestering me all the time. When I do, I feel a pain in my stomach. I am physically hurt and upset all the next day.
> His needs are repugnant to me. I want to vomit when I have this animal on top of me. To a man it is necessary, but when he is hooked into me I get violently ill.

Sexual intercourse exacerbates the sick wife's anxieties: she fears pregnancy; she recalls the pain of childbirth; she fears that her children or the neighbors will hear or observe her during the act; her overwhelming fatigue makes intercourse an exhausting experience. Consequently, the sick wife repeatedly and obstinately rejects her husband. The husband is insulted and angered. When she gives in, she is likely to vomit. To the husband, this is an intolerable personal affront. A cycle that alternates between rejection and explosive outbursts is established in marital relations. Mrs. Feliciano describes this process:

> My husband curses and damns around the house a lot. He is angry because I don't give in to him. He gets up the following morning in a bad mood and says bad words. This bothers me as it makes me uncomfortable to hear him damning things. I am quiet when he acts

this way, but he tells me I am going to get a cancer in my tongue if I don't speak out. When I reply he goes out to the street. When he returns he is even worse.

The indignity of an uncooperative wife often leads the husband to be contemptuous of her and, finally, to reject her. Mrs. Padilla relates:

Sometimes I feel I don't have enough in me for him. He would like it every night, and I can't give it to him that often. Sometimes I tell him no because I am tired, and he replies that someday he will leave me for another woman. We have fought over this and most of our problems are because of this. We get along well when I let him do what he wants. He has bad teeth and bad breath, and for this reason I don't want him to kiss me so I turn him down. Then he says I don't love him. We fight in bed. He tells me that he doesn't sleep with a *macho* and pushes me out of bed. One time he got up and put on his clothes as if to leave. I cried and begged him not to go. He goes to bed early and I go to bed late. When I go to bed, he is asleep. Then he awakens at 4:00 in the morning and begins to caress me. I think it is a dream and finally wake up. I am in a bad mood. I tell him to stop and he stops but he is mad. When I see that he is mad, I give in to him, but then he says no.

The scene of love-making becomes an arena of conflict. The husband vents his anger against his wife by insults and physical beatings. He leaves the house to seek another woman or threatens to do so. To mask her injured pride, the irate wife screams that he should go ahead. Soon, the anxieties concerning the unfaithfulness of her husband begin to haunt the confused fantasies of the schizophrenic wife. She knows that her husband is sexually dissatisfied, but since she has withdrawn from the neighbors she is relatively isolated from gossip and it is difficult for her to test her suspicions. From her viewpoint, the moment he steps out of the house he is exposed to a world of sexual opportunities; and she knows a *macho* transforms such opportunities into actualities. The pangs of suspicion lead the sick wife to spy on her husband with more persistence and anger than the well wife. Surreptitiously, she trails him to work, to bars, to the race track, or to his usual meeting place with his friends. One wife found her husband in a bar drinking with a woman and attacked her rival with her fists. Another woman chased her husband out of a neighbor's house before he could put on his pants. During the chase she lost the scissors she was going to use to castrate him; when she couldn't catch him she returned to the house to pummel her rival.

The schizophrenic wife is accusatory and insulting to her husband, as she is convinced that he is unfaithful. The husband, already dissatisfied with his wife's recalcitrance, reacts with pronounced hostility. Bitter words are exchanged. As a result, the husband withdraws from the family, spends more time in activities outside the house, and feels all the more justified in his sex adventures. This generates another self-perpetuating cycle of frustration, accusation, and aggression. "One of these days," says one of the exasperated husbands, "I am going on a long trip to New York."

In the double schizophrenic families the repugnance of the sick wife toward sex is typical of the other sick women. The sick husband's sexual demands exceed his sick wife's willingness to submit. To protect herself against her husband's approaches, the wife goes to bed after her husband is asleep or rejects him outright before they go to bed. Mrs. Santano states, "I go to bed at midnight and when I go to bed I am tired. I don't like to be bothered." The wife's rebelliousness provokes her husband to physical attacks, to accusations of infidelity, and to coercion. Mr. Aponte says, "I initiate the sexual act. When she rejects me or fights me, I tell her she must have another man, and then she gives in to me." Mrs. Aponte tells us: "I have always been forced to have sex. He never caresses or pets me. He is brutal and I am forced to do it. It isn't because I want to."

The violence associated with sexual relations in the double schizophrenic families is greater than in the families with sick wives and well husbands. Sexual intercourse is often a means of striking back to humiliate the spouse. Mr. Santano describes the way he and his wife make love. It starts when Mrs. Santano goes to bed late at night, tired and wanting to sleep. Her husband approaches her. She rejects him. He subdues her and coerces her into having sexual intercourse. He achieves sexual orgasm; she does not. She accuses him of being less than a man, a duck (homosexual), and a pubic hair because he cannot satisfy her. To defend himself, he replies, "I am not an animal." Following advice given to him by a friend, Mr. Santano subdues his wife again and places his penis in her anus. The friend told him that this would make her fall deeply in love with him. Mrs. Santano has not developed a deep love for her husband, however; she screams insults at him and ridicules his efforts to prove his masculinity.

Sexual tensions in these families are cumulative. The wife harbors many grievances against her husband because she is coerced into sexual relations, and the husband is angry at his wife for not cooperating.

Moreover, he is incapable or ineffectual when he attempts to pursue adventurous romances with other women. Although he has retreated from masculine social groups, he periodically strikes out in search of a woman with whom he can have an affair.

Mr. Quiromo is married to a deeply religious woman who does not fulfill her sexual obligation to him. (She always wanted to be a nun.) She obstinately denies her husband sexual access. Mr. Quiromo was the leader of a small congregation of his own private faith who revered him as a prophet. During services he brought the word of God to them and also read and sang hymns he himself had composed. Recently, Mr. Quiromo became infuriated with his wife's rebelliousness and abandoned her to live with Juana the Cripple, known throughout the locale as a prostitute. When his followers discovered that he had abandoned his wife to live with Juana the Cripple, they left him. In committing sins of the flesh and forsaking his wife for a disreputable woman, he lost his charismatic appeal. Because Juana the Cripple told him he was worthless and lazy, he returned to his wife. Mrs. Quiromo has not forgiven him, nor have her parents who live next door; they remind him every day that he is guilty of the worst sin.

Mr. Quiromo is now making efforts to regain his following. He does this by visiting the former members of the congregation, spreading the gospel, and singing his original hymns. Recently, as he was singing a hymn to a young girl and her mother, a man living nearby leaned out the window and called: "Hey, you with the voice! You, singer of hymns! Aren't you the one that Juana the Cripple threw out of her house because you could not even support her?" Mr. Quiromo was deeply humiliated; he sought consolation from his wife, but she replied that he was being punished for abandoning her.

The efforts of a sick husband to have affairs are relatively unsuccessful even if he gravitates toward a woman who is marginal in the community, as is Juana the Cripple. Irrespective of her status in the community, the woman has a set of expectations the sick man is unable to fulfill. Thus, Mr. Quiromo was unable to provide for Juana the Cripple as she expected. Moreover, since his friends, associates, and neighbors have begun to view him as a *loco*, his attempt at adventurous romance exposed him to taunts, ridicule, and punishment.

Charges of infidelity are exchanged by the sick husband and his sick wife. Neither one accepts the accusations with equanimity. Mrs. Aponte relates,

We have sexual contact about once a year. When he makes advances I reject him. Then he accuses me of having another man. I reply with accusations of my own. We end up in an argument, in a struggle.

SUMMARY

The sex problem in the four groups of families have been described. Families free of schizophrenia are not continually confronted with sex problems. Although the wife does not submit at once to her husband's requests for intercourse, she does so later before it disrupts her marital relationship. The issue of infidelity emerges now and then; it becomes persistent when the wife realizes that her husband philanders routinely, or when she knows he has a mistress, which occurs in a minority of families. Sexual problems are not experienced on a day-in-day-out basis. They emerge, disappear, and return, separated enough so that they do not have a deleterious cumulative effect on the relationship of the husband and the wife. This general description provides a base from which to examine the sick families.

Schizophrenic-husband families experience an opposite pattern. The usual problems associated with sex are resolved by the cooperative and powerful wife who ministers to her husband's aches and pains. She orients her husband in spheres of conduct not ordinarily accessible to wives. The husband spends his time at home away from the temptations and avenues that lead to the wife's sexual rivals. Although the usual problems of sex disappear, others that are not as disruptive emerge: the husband fears the loss of his masculinity and fantasizes himself in the role of the conquering he-man; he also suspects his wife of unfaithfulness.

The schizophrenic-wife families have chronic sexual problems. In contrast to the well families, latent sexual tensions erupt under the impact of the illness of the wife. A crisis over sex is met almost every day. To the sick wife, intercourse is repugnant and traumatic. Her husband, viewing this as a personal affront and an act of rebellion, soon withdraws from her and stays away from home. This confirms his wife's suspicions that he has another woman. Vitriolic exchanges between the husband and wife are commonplace.

Sexual conflicts in families in which both the husband and the wife are afflicted with schizophrenia are similar to those in families in which only the wife is sick. Grievances associated with the hostile rejection of the husband by the wife and charges of infidelity are repetitive and cumulative. Sexual intercourse is employed by each spouse to humiliate and degrade the other. These problems engender bad feelings that are unequaled in the other families.

We conclude, therefore, that the effect that schizophrenia has on sexual problems in marriage depends on the sex of the afflicted person. If families that are free of schizophrenia are used as a basis of comparison, conflicts over sex are alleviated when the husband is schizophrenic, but intensified when either the wife or both spouses are sick.

18
Nuclear and Extended Families. I

Interrelations between the nuclear families in an extended family group may be explained clearly by tracing the pattern of mutual help that prevails among the different components in the kin group. When a man and a woman marry, they wittingly or unwittingly share an extensive set of rights and obligations in relation to one another, to their parents-in-law, siblings-in-law, and other more extended kin. The marriage multiplies the familial connections of each person who is enmeshed in the network of family ties. The newly acquired relationships with in-laws entangle each spouse in a new family network. Bonds of obligation and rights are maintained with one's consanguinal relatives; simultaneously, a new set are acquired with the marital tie.

Mutual help within the kin groups is the focus of this and the following chapter. In this chapter we discuss the pattern of mutual help between the husbands and the wives, on the one hand, and their affinal and blood relatives, on the other hand. In the first part of the chapter mutual help is defined; then we show how the pattern of mutual help operates in a well family, the Escuderos, in which neither husband nor wife is afflicted with schizophrenia. In the third part of the chapter, the data on the Escudero family are analyzed to show that they are representative of the control families. The next chapter focuses on the sick families.

Mutual help applies through time and space: through time because of an ascribed norm that binds a person permanently to his family of origin, and through space because even relatives who are separated by wide distances behave in accordance with this norm. Thus, persons living in San Juan exchange help with relatives who have migrated to the United States. A person is expected to help his parents, grandparents, siblings and half-siblings, uncles, aunts, nieces, nephews, and cousins. A married person is obligated to render help to the spouse's relatives to the same degree of kinship. Other relatives also may be helped, but the compulsion to do so is not strong. The bonds of obligation are most solid between parent and child. In the hierarchy of disparaging labels, one of the most insulting is to be described as a "bad son" or a "bad parent." These terms usually signify that the accused has defaulted in his responsibilities to the designated person.

Of the forty husbands and forty wives, 89 per cent either support parents who cannot support themselves or expect to do so if the necessity arises. The remaining 11 per cent are orphans or have parents whom they believe will be able to support themselves through social security or other means. Persons of both sexes, and in all diagnostic groups, feel obligated toward their parents. Finally, 99 per cent of the persons state that sons and daughters *should* support their parents when the parents are unable to do so themselves.

The web of mutual help does not include the ritual kin of the godparent relationship. Traditionally, a child acquires a godparent through baptism; however, the relationship between godparent and godchild is not as socially important as that between godparent and parent of a child—the coparent relationship. Among urban dwellers this relationship lacks a religious significance. Many persons enter into a coparent relationship and address each other properly as *comadre* or *compadre* without having undergone a religious ceremony; frequently, this form of address indicates nothing more than an intimate friendship. There are periodic exchanges of favors between coparents, but the norm of mutual help does not apply in full measure.

The husbands and wives often have parents, grandparents, siblings, half-siblings, uncles, aunts, nieces, nephews, and cousins living with or near them. Eighteen per cent of the families have at least one relative living with them permanently; these relatives perform stable roles in the families. Another 18 per cent of the families have relatives who are living with them temporarily. An additional 15 per cent of the families live next door to relatives or in dwellings that are physically contiguous. In brief, one-half of the families need not leave their homes to visit with affinal or consanguinal relations. Persons who move into the San Juan area stay with relatives until they can establish a household of their own. Others who are on their way to the mainland use the home of a relative in San Juan as a point of departure. Some relatives live with the families because they are unable to support themselves.

The effective kin horizon includes more families; 93 per cent of the families have relatives living in the San Juan area. The geographical clustering of relatives reflects and facilitates mutual help, with obvious practical results. During the course of our interviews, 88 per cent of the nuclear families received material help from or exchanged material help with relatives. Nevertheless, many persons express feelings of guilt for not being able to give more help; similarly, a common topic of family gossip is the deviant relative who has not helped in time of need. The double edge of guilt and criticism sustains the pattern of reciprocal help.

Help varies from total to token support. Total support usually, but not always, depends on the donor's command of resources. Even families experiencing desperate economic problems provide for relatives. Money is given for food, clothing, transportation, water and electricity bills, rent, schooling, medicine, and so on. Material items given also include: lumber, clothing, dishes, furniture, and personal items. Groceries are given; some families save part of the food they have cooked for their relatives. In brief, there is hardly an item of consumption that does not pass between relatives.

We have selected the Escudero family as representative of the mutual help norm in the control group. Because of family assistance, the Escuderos who live in an established slum, *Buenos Aires,* enjoy a level of affluence unusual among families in the slum. Their house has 2 bedrooms, a combination dining room-living room, a kitchen, an outside latrine, and a shower stall. They have wrought-iron living-room furniture covered with brightly colored plastic cushions. Their dining table seats six persons; near it is a china cabinet in which half a dozen wine glasses are displayed. They have two beds made of mahogany, a radio, and a television set.

While we interviewed the Escuderos, several laborers were repairing the house: decaying walls were being replaced with new lumber; old corrugated-iron sheets were torn off the roof and new ones hammered on; the house was jacked several feet off the ground while new posts, which serve as stilts to keep the house above mud and water, were put under its corners; crushed stone was spread on the mud underneath the house. Before these repairs, rains combined with the high tides of an adjoining lagoon inundated the floor of the house which began to rot as a result of the constant soaking. According to the Escuderos, these improvements raised the estimated value of the house to $1,200.

The laborers who worked on the house were employees of the city government. The Escuderos were enjoying one of the benefits of their integral association in the monolithic local political organization. Arrangements for this help were made by Mr. Escudero's eldest brother, who is the Popular Party's political "president" in that neighborhood. This brother is an articulate spokesman for the Popular Party. As "president," he makes use of many of the resources and services of the city government. Ostensibly, his primary job is to improve living conditions and solve problems for families in the local community. If he cannot cope with the problems of a neighbor, he makes an appointment to have the person see the Mayoress of San Juan who usually helps.

Mr. Escudero left school after the third grade. He is 27 years old, works in a garment factory cutting patterns and earns about $50 a week. According to the psychiatrist, Mr. Escudero is free of mental illness. Mrs. Escudero, who is a 25-year old housewife, completed the fifth grade. She is diagnosed as a cyclothymic personality: she experiences "mood" changes from irritation to dejection, fantasizes being attacked, has morbid dreams, and has a compulsion to look under beds and check locked doors. They have three boys whose ages are 4, 3, and 1. Mr. Escudero's parents are separated. His father lives on the southern coast of the Island, working as a cutter of sugar cane during harvest and as a planter of fruit trees during the dead season. Mr. Escudero supports his mother who lives next door in a smaller house, also built with the help of municipal workers; because of her propinquity, her needs are visible, and her wants are heard. Mrs. Escudero approves wholeheartedly of helping her mother-in-law because she is fond of her. She is also grateful to her mother-in-law for taking care of the two girls who were fathered by Mr. Escudero in his former marriage.

Mrs. Escudero does not object to taking care of her stepdaughters. Early in her marriage she did so because her husband's former wife married a man who would not accept them. However, Mrs. Escudero fiercely opposed the weekly visits the real mother made to see the girls. She says, "I become furious when I see that woman come to my mother-in-law's house. It is like seeing the devil. Imagine how I felt when she used to come here." To avoid conflict, arrangements were made for the girls to live with their grandmother who has assumed full responsibility for their care. Mr. Escudero's mother also looked after the three children of his present marriage while the fieldworkers interviewed his wife.

Gambling is the most persistent point of conflict between husband and wife. Mr. Escudero is an addicted gambler; he places bets at the race track, at cockfights, and at boxing matches. He buys lottery tickets regularly. He plays cards and rolls dice almost daily. When he goes to a *cafetin* to drink beer, he inevitably gravitates toward the domino players to bet on a player. After payday, he sometimes stops here and there to wager a few dollars, and arrives home penniless. He believes that some day he is going to win big, but that day has not arrived. Mrs. Escudero has made innumerable attempts to convince her husband to stop gambling. She has threatened to take the children and abandon him. She asked him to work overtime and spend only the additional income on gambling, but her efforts to cope with this problem have been frustrated by the influence her brothers-in-law have over her husband. These men, particularly the *politico*, also love to gamble.

On a typical evening, Mr. Escudero was watching television with his wife. Soon, his eldest brother came to invite him to a card game with high stakes. His wife was outraged by this, but Mr. Escudero left with his brother. A few minutes later he returned home to pick up money he had forgotten. His enraged wife assailed him, ripped off his shirt, and scratched him with her fingernails. He punched her in the face and left. She says,

> I called him a son of a grand whore. I called him a queer. I told him to go sleep with his brothers if he missed them so much. His brothers are always telling him that I manipulate him like a puppet. They say that I sit him on my lap and make him do and say things a real he-man would not tolerate. My husband tries to show his brothers that he is a real he-man by gambling to defy me. I tell him, "Does it look better for a man to sit on the lap of a man or on the lap of a woman?" His brothers have him sitting on their laps. His brothers are ruining him.

Mr. Escudero identifies with his eldest brother more than with any other relative. He is proud of his brother's political influence and political ideals. Both like to dress well. According to Mr. Escudero, the bond of unity he has with this brother stems primarily from "our sharing the same vices; we like to play cards, bet at races, and drink rum." Mr. Escudero appreciates the help and good advice his brother gives him. (The four other Escudero brothers also receive these benefits.)

In retrospective and serene moments, Mrs. Escudero thinks it is better to have a husband who gambles than one who chases women. She says, "No man is perfect. Every man has at least one vice; many men have them all." In addition, Mrs. Escudero is deeply grateful to her husband for the help he has given her relatives.

Two years ago, two of Mrs. Escudero's brothers migrated to San Juan from the mountainous interior and lived with the Escuderos until they were established. Mr. Escudero was helpful and hospitable. Through his eldest brother, he found a house they could rent; in addition, he obtained jobs for them as assistant pattern-cutters in the garment factory where he works. Immediately after the brothers rented the house and found employment, they brought their mother and five younger siblings of school age to live with them. These persons subsist from the wages the brothers earn. All were anxious to move into San Juan in search of a better living, away from the hand-to-mouth existence of picking coffee beans.

The brothers also wanted to bring their mother and younger siblings to San Juan to protect them from their father, a violent alcoholic. The life history of this family, and of Mrs. Escudero before she left home, is the chronicle of a drunken, wrathful man terrorizing his wife and children. Before they left the mountains, the father vowed to kill them all. He began to sleep with two knives and swore to use one on his wife and the other on his children. Recently, the father migrated to San Juan in search of his family. He found the Escuderos and was allowed to live with them on the condition that he not drink. He soon started to drink, however, which led to hostile disputes between him and his daughter and son-in-law. These incidents were usually provoked by the drunken father's recommendations to his son-in-law that his daughter, Mrs. Escudero, needed to be subdued. From the father's point of view, she was too critical, too bossy, too belligerent. In the face of such accusations, Mrs. Escudero retorted to her father: "Those are the parts of my personality that I inherited from you." In a drunken rage the father grabbed a knife and chased everyone out of the house. He screamed at his daughter to buy herself a dress of mourning because he was going to kill her mother. The Escuderos called the police and had him arrested and jailed.

Despite their fears, the Escuderos soon felt sorry for the disheveled, incarcerated father. Three days later, Mr. Escudero convinced his politician brother to post bond, and the prisoner was released. The father is now living with his wife and children; his sons support him. Mrs. Escudero is happy to have her mother living nearby. During her last pregnancy, the mother cared for her through labor and the post-partum period. She also took care of the newborn infant. In turn, Mrs. Escudero occasionally gives her mother food and clothing.

At the age of 14, Mrs. Escudero migrated to San Juan to live with an aunt, where she stayed until she was married. About every other week Mrs. Escudero visits this aunt, a short bus ride away. According to Mrs. Escudero, her aunt's teen-age son is in love with her, and Mr. Escudero is very suspicious of his wife's cousin. Whenever she returns from a visit, he quizzes her thoroughly. Mr. Escudero feels uncomfortable when his wife's cousin comes to visit. If the cousin visits when he is not present, Mrs. Escudero has to explain his reason for coming.

Mrs. Escudero has been helping a number of other relatives during the past year. She takes small gifts to an aunt who is paralyzed from a cerebral hemorrhage. This woman reclines in a hammock day and night, speaking words no one can understand. Mrs. Escudero also took care of two of her husband's nephews. These children who are 2 years old are unable to walk; they suffer from chronic diarrhea, have bloated stomachs, and, according to Mrs. Escudero, they have "legs that look like toothpicks." To help them, she fed them starchy root vegetables mashed in milk. Another nephew of her husband was hospitalized for "having water in the stomach." Mrs. Escudero spent evenings with this child and consoled the mother who was afraid he was going to die.

Mrs. Escudero worries about relatives she seldom sees and hardly knows. She has a cousin who has been in and out of psychiatric hospitals several times since World War II. This man became a widower a short while after his release from the Army. He then began to drink, eventually became an alcoholic, and suffered a nervous breakdown. Mrs. Escudero would like to know more about her cousin. Although the Veterans Administration pays for his psychiatric treatment, she wonders if there is anything she and her husband can do to help him.

The Escudero family has many characteristics common to families in which neither the husband nor the wife is schizophrenic. The nuclear family, the wife's relatives, and the husband's relatives are bound together into a broader family group that functions to cope with problems. The norm of mutual help operates within the context of the broader family, as it did in the problematic behavior of Mrs. Escudero's father. His conduct forced his sons to leave home and come to San Juan. When they arrived the Escuderos provided them with room and board. Mrs. Escudero's politically powerful brother-in-law arranged for housing and jobs. The brothers then brought their mother and younger siblings to live with them. Now the mother helps Mrs. Escudero.

The Escudero family represents the rule, not the exception. Virtually all the control families have problems that are transmitted from one relative to another. As one problem is solved, new ones emerge, and new opportunities for solving problems are sought. The quest for solutions moves back and forth between blood relatives and across the nexus of conjugal bonds.

An economically marginal life creates a rash of problems which range from the malnourishment of a child to the drunken behavior of a father. Health problems are paramount: influenza, tuberculosis, kidney operations, hysterectomies, miscarriages, hernias, heart ailments, and so on enmesh the family. The initial symptoms of illness are perceived, interpreted, and treated by the family members. Folk remedies from boiled herbs to the therapeutic gestures of spiritualism are administered within the context of the broader family. Patent medicines are purchased and widely used. If the home remedies and cures are efficacious, the afflicted person is not taken to a medical or a paramedical person for help. Before a sick family member is taken to a clinic, a hospital, or a physician, virtually all the medical know-how in the kin group has been applied without success.

Conversations between relatives are focused on their problems. Information is exchanged and efforts are made to solve the problems. Thus the broader family represents a reservoir of both resources and problems. There is usually one person or one nuclear family that distributes more help to relatives than it receives. Problems gravitate toward these persons or families. The problems experienced by Mrs. Escudero's blood relatives flow toward her and her husband. To solve some problems—securing a house to rent for her brothers, posting bail for her drunken father, or repairing their own home—the Escuderos appeal to the politically powerful and prestigious eldest brother who is president of the *barrio* in which all of the relatives live.

Mutual help between families has an overall effect on the subsistence level of interconnected nuclear families. When one family begins to tumble into the depth of impoverishment, the adjoining nuclear families cooperate in an effort to solve its drastic economic problems. Correlatively, a family that begins to experience some affluence is immediately burdened by the convergence of needy relatives. The fortuities of a marginal life are such that, in the future, the flow of help may be reversed or arranged into a different pattern.

The arrangement of help depends on *who can help* and *who is perceived to be in need of help*. Mrs. Escudero's relatives consider her and her husband to be in a position to help. Mr. Escudero has a reliable and relatively well-paying job. The evidences of his affluence can be seen—his good home, his radio, his television set, his dining-room set and china cabinet, and his mahogany beds. These relatives view the Escuderos as "in the potatoes," an expression more accurately translated as "living high off the hog." Moreover, Mr. Escudero's name is linked to that of his *politico* brother, a man held in high esteem in the neighborhood. And, if his brother is in a position to help neighbors with whom he does not have blood or affinal ties, why should he not help his own relatives?

The Escuderos are also in a position to help because they live in San Juan. Six out of seven persons in the sick and well families moved to San Juan during the course of their lifetime. They migrated because of economic pressures that combine with an idealized image of the opportunities available in the capital. The migration has been accomplished in large part through the family. Earlier in their lives, Mr. and Mrs. Escudero came individually to San Juan and were aided by relatives who were in residence; the Escudero home was, in turn, a stopping point for her two brothers. Urban dwellers bed, feed, and help the new migrants settle. One beachhead leads to the establishment of another, thus facilitating future moves by other relatives. Beyond San Juan, there is New York.

The needs and problems of a person are usually known to his relatives; as Mrs. Escudero commented, her mother-in-law's needs are conspicuous since she lives next door. But relatives are *socially* visible even if they are out of sight and out of earshot. Their problems are disseminated widely through the give and take of opinions and information in the broader family.

Persons who receive help over a long period of time, or who receive a great deal of help at a particular time, may come under the influence of their benefactor. Mr. Escudero's inability to resist his eldest brother's invitation to gamble illustrates this point. Admittedly, Mr. Escudero likes to gamble and also admires his brother; nevertheless, the help he receives from his brother obligates him to accept invitations despite his wife's vehement objections. As displeased as Mrs. Escudero is over her husband's gambling, she does not inveigh personally against her eldest brother-in-law. This would be improper treatment of a person to whom she is indebted.

When a person lives with relatives and subsists entirely from their earnings, he must accept their control to a large extent. Sometimes the culturally prescribed, superior-subordinate relationship between parent and child clashes with the flow of influence that is associated with the flow of help. When Mrs. Escudero's father was head of the household, living with his family, he drank rum and did as he pleased with impunity. He was unwilling to accept the subordinate position his dependency entails. He endeavored to assert his power as a parent in a situation in which he was entirely dependent on the Escuderos by insisting to Mr. Escudero that his wife had to be "put in her place." Eventually, he was ejected from the Escudero household.

A person who receives help is expected to follow the advice that accompanies the help. Generally, the advice is directed at the problem, need, or condition that elicited the help. Mrs. Escudero advised the mothers of the sickly children to pay special attention to their nourishment. A gift of money is accompanied invariably by recommendations about how it should be spent. To accept help while rejecting advice is to be branded *malagradecido* (ungrateful). A person who does not reciprocate in help is also *malagradecido*. This is a degrading accusation, especially if the donor has made sacrifices to give help. Mutual help, influence, and the social value of gratitude are interrelated parts of family life.

A person who receives help is not defenseless in the face of his donor's influence. If the help is accompanied by excessive advice, the recipient can counter with charges that the help is "being thrown in his face," which questions the "pure" motives of the donor. Gratitude is a value; likewise, unconditional generosity is valued. Their joint effect is to define the amount of influence and the spheres of influence the donor has in relation to the person he has helped.

Very few nuclear families, free of schizophrenia, receive more help than they give. These families exchange help with relatives on more or less equal terms or give more than they receive. They have earnings they can use to help relatives; 85 per cent of the husbands in these families are employed full time and 5 per cent part time. No person in the control group suffers from an illness which incapacitates him so he cannot help his relatives. The Escuderos are typical in these respects.

The wife is a better informant about family affairs than the husband. In comparison to her husband, the wife is more conversant with the problems of relatives. She understands family problems in greater detail and, in general, she is more comprehensively informed about family affairs. Often, she knows more about her husband's blood relatives than he does. Since the wife is restricted to her home and the immediate neighborhood, she daily sees and speaks to relatives who live with her or in the immediate vicinity. When she visits beyond the immediate neighborhood, it is usually to see relatives. Although her husband expects her to stay near the home, he respects her right to make family visits. The family system comprises almost the entire life space of the wife. The social horizons of the husband, in contrast, are not as limited. He has social relations with many persons outside the family. He has friends at work and at places where he goes for entertainment.

Mrs. Escudero describes how she and her husband differ in their orientation toward family affairs. Her husband confronts some problems, tries to solve them, and forgets them entirely. Mrs. Escudero dwells on all family problems; she internalizes the suffering of her relatives, even those she sees infrequently. She identifies the needs of relatives, interprets these needs, proposes solutions, and she, more than her husband, mobilizes the resources of the family. At any given time, a number of family problems engage her attention. Family business is the pre-eminent specialty of the wife.

Men and women make different contributions to the solution of problems. Responsibilities for bringing up children who cannot be cared for by their parents are assumed by the women. Women prepare meals and sleeping quarters for relatives who are visiting or living with them. Women care for sick children and other ill relatives. They help through pregnancy, labor, and the postpartum period. They console relatives in grief. Men help relatives by earning money to support them, by finding them homes, by securing jobs for them, by commanding the services of the city laborers, and by posting bail. Women provide domestic and emotionally supportive help, whereas the help men give derives from their associations with organizations and social groups. Women give help *in* the family; men give help *for* the family.

In five of the twenty well families, a mother or an older sister is a matriarch. These matriarchs, without foregoing the help women give, offer the kind of help normally associated with the role the men play in the families. They earn incomes by owning and operating small *cafetines,* working as domestic servants or in a factory, or by doing piecework sewing at home. The husbands of all of these women are incapacitated by chronic illness, not involved in family affairs, or dead. Blood and affinal relatives live with or near these matriarchs. Help exchanged within the family flows through them; they coordinate resources in one part of the family with the needs in another part. These women incessantly supply help to their offspring, their siblings, and their parents.

Husbands and wives turn to such maternal figures for help, advice, or orientation. There is no matriarchal figure in the Escudero family. Therefore, we draw upon other families for the relevant information. The extent of this dependence is illustrated by Mrs. Hidalgo who cannot even have her coffee in the morning unless it is served by her mother; the mother also prepares her lunch and helps her clean the house. She gives her daughter advice on what should be done about Mr. Hidalgo's problematic behavior. At the time of the interviews, Mr. Hidalgo was having an affair with a domestic servant a short distance from his home. His mother-in-law was well informed and deeply involved in this problem.

Mr. Molína's mother allows him and his wife to live in a small shack located in her back yard. He eats half of his meals with his mother, half with his wife. The mother is omnipresent, bringing food, clothing, and pieces of worn furniture. She also lends them money. When Mr. Molína comes home drunk and accuses his wife of unfaithfulness, his mother intervenes to care for him. She also advises her daughter-in-law to disregard his accusations which she knows are not true since she watches her daughter-in-law all day long.

Mrs. Toro is bitter toward her sister-in-law whom she describes as a dictator. Every day the sister-in-law instructs Mrs. Toro on how she should keep house, but the primary source of Mrs. Toro's resentment stems from her inability to control the three stepchildren, products of Mr. Toro's former marriage. Mrs. Toro cannot correct the stepchildren in any way because her sister-in-law does not permit it. According to the sister-in-law, the children are not Mrs. Toro's; although she is responsible for their care, she has no rights over them.

The dominant maternal figures in the Hidalgo, Molína, and Toro families are extensively involved in relations with other relatives. In no family is there a man with as widespread influence as these women. Perhaps this is because men are not as centrally imbedded in the communicative network of the families as are the women. Moreover, men are reluctant to perform the domestic work associated with the role of the female, out of fear that they will be viewed as effeminate.

SUMMARY

The norm of mutual help is a part of daily family life, bringing the nuclear family, the wife's relatives, and the husband's relatives together into a system of exchange. Help varies from token to total support. The operation of this norm is facilitated by the fact that relatives congregate in the same dwelling, the same neighborhood, and the same city. Nonetheless, the needs and problems of relatives who are not seen become known because family members speak to and about each other a great deal. The women are more centrally involved in this process than the men. The women also are more deeply and consistently oriented toward family affairs than the men. Women give domestic and socioemotional help; the help that men give is premised on their relationship to persons and agencies outside the family.

The giving of help is associated with the exercise of influence. The value of gratitude directs the beneficiary to accept advice with the help he receives. It is a value for the donor to restrict his advice or he will be perceived as offensive and intrusive.

Extended families are not riddled by conflict. The husbands and the wives in the well families have, in general, harmonious relations with their in-laws and with their blood relatives. Although conflicts occur, they are overshadowed by the cooperation entailed by the norm of mutual help. The matriarchal figure is found in a minority of families and, where found, is not always a source of tension. Thus, conflict in these extended families is sporadic, discontinuous, and not clearly patterned in blood or in-law relations.

19
Nuclear and Extended Families. II

We described the pattern of mutual help between the well families and their relatives in the preceding chapter. Now we turn to the question: How does the schizophrenia of the husband, of the wife, or of both affect the pattern of mutual help in the extended family? Three case studies are presented to illustrate the way in which schizophrenia affects the pattern of mutual help among nuclear families and component units in the larger kin group; each family depicts one of the three groups of sick families. The seven families with sick husbands and well wives are represented by the Cardonas, the nine families with sick wives and well husbands by the Lebróns, and the four families with both spouses sick by the Santanos.

The Cardonas, the Lebróns, and the Santanos demonstrate many characteristics common to each group of sick families. To show the way in which the mental illness of either or both spouses influences the help the families receive from or give to their relatives, comparisons between the diagnostic family groups are made.

The Cardonas, a husband-schizophrenic family, live in a semirural area immediately outside the main commercial and residential areas of San Juan. The house is on the side of a steep hill, among a number of other houses of comparable size and quality. To reach the Cardonas' house, the visitor must descend from a road on top of the hill on steps that have been dug into the red clay of the hillside. Periodically, heavy downpours erode the steps; then the visitor has to step here and there, avoiding slippery patches of clay, always holding on to the shrubbery or the lower branches of trees to avoid falling.

Mr. Cardona estimates the value of his house to be $800. He does not own the lot on which the house stands, nor does he pay rent for it. The house has three small bedrooms, a combination living-dining room, a kitchen, and a small front porch. The walls and floor are made of wood; it has a roof of corrugated-iron sheets, and it is raised on posts so that rain water streaming down the hillside does not flood it. In back of the house, underneath the kitchen, is a small room that the Cardonas rent to a middle-aged woman and her elderly mother for $7.50 a month.

There are many evidences of diligent housework in the Cardona home: furniture is dusted; the linoleum on the floor of the combination living-dining room is mopped several times a day; bedspreads, although yellowed by age, stained, and frayed, are freshly laundered.

Mr. Cardona has schizophrenia of a paranoid type. He is 36 years old and has an eighth grade education. Up to less than a year ago, he worked as a motion-picture projector operator; he left this job voluntarily when the symptoms of his illness began. At present, he is unemployed. His wife has no symptoms of mental illness. She is 38 years old, has finished high school, and is employed in a toy factory sewing doll dresses where she earns $100 a month.

The Cardonas have a daughter, 8 years old, and a son, 2, from the present marriage. A girl, 13 years old, and a boy, 11, from Mr. Cardona's former marriage live with them, as does a 16-year old niece of Mrs. Cardona. In addition to the two tenants, there are seven persons living in the small house. Mr. Cardona's parents are dead. Two of his brothers live in San Juan; another lives in the southwestern part of the Island. The brothers have defaulted in their obligations to Mr. Cardona at a time when he is in financial and personal distress. He reports:

> My brothers seldom visit me, nor do they ask about my health. They should visit me at least every other week to raise my morale. If they would talk to me I would forget my problems. They should give me financial help. My brothers have moved away from me.

Although Mrs. Cardona agrees with her husband's description, neither Mr. nor Mrs. Cardona makes an effort to secure assistance from his relatives. Instead of receiving help, they have given help. Recently, one of Mr. Cardona's brothers decided he did not want to work—he wanted to have fun; he abandoned his family to come to live with the Cardonas. He talked Mr. Cardona into borrowing money to have a party. "In my time of need," says Mr. Cardona with irony, "my brother came to take, not to give."

As Mr. Cardona was experiencing his first psychotic episode a few months before the field work began, a letter came from a social worker.

It informed him that a 2-year old nephew, the son of his fun-seeking brother, was desperately ill. The mother of the child was unable to care for him because she was ill. The Cardonas borrowed money to travel to the other side of the Island and brought the sick nephew to live with them. Mrs. Cardona reports:

> The child was weak and undernourished. He could not walk. Although his arms and legs were skinny, his stomach was swollen. We could count his ribs. When I stood him up, he fell down. He had no strength. He would not eat or drink milk. He was always vomiting. I gave this child part of the food I had for my own son. His guts were hanging out of his butt. We nicknamed him "the Lump."

The Cardonas took the child to a doctor in a public health unit. They nursed him back to health by feeding him, massaging him with olive oil, and putting him in the sun every morning.

Mrs. Cardona's mother is dead. Her father and a sister live next door. Her father is dependent on social security and sharecropping; he gardens for the owner of a small farm nearby and, as payment, receives half of the fruits and vegetables he grows. Two other sisters and the only brother live in San Juan. A fourth sister has migrated to New York City. These relatives are a closely knit group. When one of the sisters is pregnant and after childbirth, the others spend long hours taking care of her and of the infant. Mrs. Cardona is particularly attached to her nearby sister and her father; she says, "I am very concerned with the problems of all of us."

Whereas Mr. Cardona's brothers have been indifferent to his problems or have sought help from him, Mrs. Cardona's family has helped in the fullest sense. When Mr. Cardona suffered his first psychotic episode, he left his job. Debts began to accumulate; the electricity and water were about to be cut off; the family was living on meager rations. By the time the economic problems began, Mrs. Cardona's relatives were aware that her husband was ill because of his "attacks." During one "attack," his body trembled, he was short of breath, and, finally, he collapsed, unable to walk. Mrs. Cardona's brother-in-law was summoned to bring his car. The ill man was carried to the car and taken to the municipal hospital. Her relatives accompanied him to the hospital. When he returned, Mrs. Cardona and her sister put him to bed and massaged him with rubbing alcohol. Every week now, Mrs. Cardona's father brings them fruit and vegetables from the farm where he works. Sometimes, he buys rice, beans, and salted codfish for them. He also helps by paying their water and electricity bills. Mrs. Cardona describes her father:

> My father is very poor. He shares the little bit of food he has with us. He does it in good form and with good will. My father was doing without food in order to help us out. I told him to eat with us. My husband feels ashamed when my father brings the groceries. When he sees him come in with the groceries, he looks at me and says, "Look at how good your father is." We have hope. As long as my father helps us, we are not badly off. My husband likes my father.

Mrs. Cardona's relatives affirm that they will help as long as they can. Recently, Mrs. Cardona secured the job sewing clothes in a doll factory, but she was worried about leaving her husband unattended. The prospect of his having an "attack" at a time when no one was home to help him frightened her. In addition, someone had to care for the children while she was at work. Arrangements were made for a niece to live with them. This niece, the daughter of the sister who lives next door, takes care of the children, does the housework, and keeps her eye on Mr. Cardona; when he is not feeling well, she summons an adult relative to help.

Mr. Cardona goes to his appointments at the psychiatric hospital secretly. By agreement with his wife, these visits are not discussed in the presence of other persons. Despite the frequent contacts and intimate relationship the Cardonas have with her relatives, she has not told them that her husband is going to the psychiatric hospital; she fears he will be identified as a *loco* and the relatives would then mistrust and avoid him. When they ask about his illness, she says that it is only a case of nerves.

The Lebróns represent the wife-schizophrenic families. Mr. Lebrón is a 24-year old veteran of the Korean War; he has had 10 years of formal education of which the last two were financed by the Veterans Administration. Mr. Lebrón earns $100 a month as a bill collector for a furniture store selling to persons in the low-income group. He does not have psychotic symptoms. Mrs. Lebrón is a 27-year old housewife with a seventh grade education. She has schizophrenia of an undifferentiated type.

The Lebróns have two daughters, aged 3 and 2. The older daughter lives with Mr. Lebrón's mother 6 days a week. Every Sunday, Mr. Lebrón brings the daughter home on the motorcycle he uses in his work. Before going to work on Monday, he returns his daughter to his mother. Mrs. Lebrón does not like her older daughter; the child makes her extremely nervous. During the interviews with the fieldworkers, both daughters cried incessantly and responded to friendly gestures with hostile outbursts.

The Lebróns live in a shed which Mr. Lebrón's mother purchased for $100 from a local factory where it had been used as a sentry guard box. She paid a trucker $10 to haul it to a clandestine slum located between a dirt road and a parcel of land owned by the government. As squatters are prohibited in this area, Mr. Lebrón fears the authorities will arrest or fine him. His mother disregards his fears, saying, "What if they fine you? I will pay the fine. Life is a gamble, and one must go ahead." Mr. Lebrón follows his mother's advice; he considers her to be alert, shrewd, and intelligent.

The shed which is a point of conflict between Mrs. Lebrón, on the one hand, and her husband and mother-in-law, on the other hand, is 10 by 12 feet; the wooden floor is black and gummy as if over the years it has been saturated with the used oil from an automobile crankcase. Food is cooked on a two-burner kerosene stove. By a broken china closet in one corner there are a bed and a crib, each covered with the remnants of ripped, soggy mattresses. The shed does not have electricity or running water. Illumination is supplied at night by a kerosene lamp. The toilet consists of a bucket which is emptied periodically out an unglazed window. Wet clothing is hung to dry on a barbed wire fence surrounding the government property.

To Mrs. Lebrón, the lack of electricity is bad enough, but the lack of running water is downright intolerable. Several times a day, she walks about one-third of a mile to a factory to draw water from an outside water faucet. Then she carries the water home in a 5-gallon lard drum. The drudgery of carrying water is not of as much concern to Mrs. Lebrón as are the factory workers who keep urging her to have sexual relations with them; she is afraid they will rape her. Her husband adamantly refuses to carry water; he considers it work for a woman or child and thinks it is degrading for a man to be seen in public with a can of water on his head. Mr. Lebrón and his mother believe his wife is seeking excuses to avoid the household chores that require water. He cites the fact that his wife also does not make the beds or sweep the floor—work that requires no water.

Mr. Lebrón eats most of his meals with his mother who gives him advice and money. He says:

If there is anything I am going to do or buy, I consult her. If she tells me not to buy it, I follow her advice. I don't talk things over with my wife.

To interview Mr. Lebrón, we went to his mother's home. He was often late or failed to keep his appointments. Meanwhile, we conducted informal interviews with his mother who spoke mostly about her daughter-in-law whom she has nicknamed "the Squirrel." According to her, Mrs. Lebrón is a *loca* who behaves in inexcusable ways. The children are always sick. She never bathes them, nor does she bathe herself. She puts on heavy make-up without first washing her face. She wears tight dungarees and wanders through the city, disregarding her obligations to her husband, her daughters, and her new home. She is an immoral woman because she had sexual intercourse with her husband prior to her marriage. The marriage is "a cat and dog fight." She is "a savage animal" who scratches with her fingernails. She even tried to slash her husband with a razor blade. She is a "filthy pig"; she keeps such a disheveled house that no sane person would drink her water out of fear of contamination. She is ungrateful; she does not appreciate having her own home. The worst thing that can happen to a man is "to have an old car and a wife who does not warm the house."

Mr. Lebrón says:

When my mother tries to give my wife good advice, my wife argues with her. My mother tells her that she should stay at home, but my wife does not pay attention. She complains to my mother about me and tells her that I come home late at night. My mother replies that no matter how late I come home, it is none of her business. Then they fight.

Even though Mrs. Lebrón disregards her mother-in-law's advice, she feels the effects of it. She knows when her husband has been at his mother's home because, when he returns, he barks at her. "Then," says Mrs. Lebrón, "I feel like going to my mother-in-law and knocking her out with one punch."

The admiration Mr. Lebrón feels toward his mother is unlike his attitude toward his father. He thinks his father is "illiterate," "stupid," and "a man without spirit or initiative." The father had a small business selling vegetables and fruits from a pushcart, but the mother insisted he could make a better living if he had a small store. When the change was made, his income was doubled to somewhat over $150 a month. To Mr. Lebrón, this is further evidence of his mother's wisdom.

Although Mrs. Lebrón's parents live 3 miles away, she goes every day to their home, usually carrying her younger daughter. She rarely has enough money to take the bus since her husband thinks she is an irresponsible spendthrift and does not give her money. As she meanders through the streets headed in the general direction of her parents' home, pedestrians occasionally give her pennies, nickels, and dimes, thinking that she is a beggar; on such "lucky" days, she uses the money for bus fare.

The most conspicuous feature of the house in which Mrs. Lebrón's parents live is that it is surrounded by a high fence of intermeshed barbed and chicken wire. The front porch of the house is barred from the street by a grid of rough wooden planks. Mrs. Lebrón's mother is mentally deranged. She was committed at one time to the insane asylum, but she escaped and now lives with her husband. To protect his wife from the taunts of neighbors and to protect the neighbors from physical attacks by his wife, Mrs. Lebrón's father constructed barriers around the house.

Several times, Mrs. Lebrón has left her husband to live with her parents, but her mother, who walks the floor all night, cursing imaginary enemies, interrupts her sleep. Mrs. Lebrón then returns home to her husband, saying, "Where can one go if one's mother is sick of the nerves?" Although she is fond of her mother, Mrs. Lebrón prefers her father, whom she describes as a "soul of God," and "an angel." In a normal week, her father earns $10 selling bananas and plantain from a small pushcart. He buys his granddaughters clothing and takes them to the municipal hospital when they are sick. The only fault Mrs. Lebrón sees in her father is that he uses a portion of his earnings to buy rum; then he gets drunk and fights with his wife. In Mrs. Lebrón's words, "Then, things get bad."

Mrs. Lebrón's two brothers and one sister who live in New York City were afraid the mother would be injured by the father when he was drunk. They decided to bring the mother to live with them, but she became homesick and returned to the Island. Mrs. Lebrón's oldest brother who lives in San Juan is considered to be the most successful member of the family; he is the chauffeur of a public car that takes passengers across the mountainous interior of the Island. Recently, with a loan of $4,000 he bought the car. Mrs. Lebrón is impressed both by her brother's ability to pay $50 a month rent and by the fact that he has American neighbors. Although she considers him to be conceited about his accomplishments, she is grateful for the vegetables and fruits he brings back to her from his trips across the Island.

All of Mrs. Lebrón's relatives see Mr. Lebrón as an irresponsible and cruel husband. Her family had taken her to New York City where she first met him. From the beginning, the family opposed her marriage; now they advise her to leave him. Conversely, Mr. Lebrón views his in-laws unfavorably, particularly his wife's parents. She describes her father as "a person who drinks"; he calls her father a drunkard. She describes her mother as "sick of the nerves"; he says her mother is a *loca*. "This is the reason," says Mr. Lebrón, "I no longer visit her relatives."

The Santanos (a double schizophrenic family) live in a two-room ground-floor apartment in a *caserío*. One room in the apartment has two beds shared by Mrs. Santano's 17-year old sister and her mother and Mrs. Santano's 4-year old daughter and two sons who are 3 and 1. The other room in the apartment is partitioned by a plywood wall. On one side of this wall there are a bed, in which the Santanos sleep, and a crib for the infant. The space on the other side of the partition serves as a kitchen-dining-living room for the family and bedroom for Mrs. Santano's 12-year old half brother. The mother pays $3.50 a month for rent and $2.00 for electricity for the apartment. Only the mother, the sister, and the half brother are authorized to live in the apartment; they fear a neighbor will report them to the officials of the *caserío* for allowing the others to live in the apartment with them.

Mr. Santano is 27 years old and has a seventh grade education. He recently left his job as a janitor, and he now receives unemployment compensation of $37 a month. His wife is a 24-year old housewife who left school after the tenth grade. Mr. Santano has schizophrenia of an undifferentiated type; she has schizophrenia of a paranoid type.

Mrs. Santano's mother works as a servant for several families, going to a different house each day. She earns from $10 to $12 a week; occasionally, she brings home left-over food given to her by one of her employers, but most of the food for the household she purchases. Meals are eaten in two shifts to avoid crowding the table. The mother arises at 5 o'clock each morning, warms the coffee, slices bread left from the day before, gives her son and daughter their breakfast, and departs for work. Then the Santanos eat breakfast. Mrs. Santano cooks the noon meal for herself, her children, and her husband if he is at home; her sister and half brother eat their noon meal at school. When the mother returns late in the afternoon, she cooks the evening meal for her son and youngest daughter. Then the Santanos eat the leftover food.

Mr. Santano dislikes these living arrangements. Not only is it too crowded, but also when he quarrels with his wife his mother-in-law intervenes in her daughter's behalf. He believes the way he is forced to live is making his sickness worse. He receives little sympathy from his wife or her relatives. They think he is healthy, and they criticize him for not working. They believe the money he receives from unemployment compensation should be used to feed the children; he squanders it on rum and beer. After a drinking spree, he gets into fights and sometimes spends a night in jail, or he returns drunk to the crowded apartment; then he curses his wife and in-laws, falls over the furniture, knocks freshly ironed clothing off the clotheslines which cross the inside of the apartment, tells his sister-in-law to get out of bed to cook for him, and orders his wife to prepare herself to submit to him sexually. His wife and in-laws counter by calling him a worthless, lazy, and inconsiderate drunkard. His enraged wife often chases him out of the apartment with a broom. Her violence is so uncontrollable that Mr. Santano admits, in his sober and reflective moments, to being afraid of her. Mrs. Santano says,

> Every day I tell him to get out of the house. He looks like a foolish bird. He walks aimlessly and talks to himself. I tell him to leave and not to return until he has established a household for me. He should stay with his mother.

Mr. Santano goes to his mother's home every day to talk to his brothers, to his father, and in the evening to his mother who also works as a servant for private families. Of her eight children the three youngest live with her. Her husband does not work because he is convalescing from a 2-year bout with tuberculosis. Before his illness was diagnosed, he and his wife had a lively business cooking and selling food. Now they subsist on her slim earnings as a servant and from the help their sons and daughters give them.

Mr. Santano's mother has been treating him better since he became psychotic than she did before the onset of his illness. The harsh treatment he receives in his wife's mother's home evokes sympathy from his mother. He says,

> She gives me money when I am broke. She gives me good advice. She tells me not to take my problems too seriously, to try to control myself. My father, my mother, and my brothers try to keep their problems away from me. . . . They have been better to me than I

could expect. My wife and my mother-in-law make me feel sad and restless. My mother gives me faith that someday I will feel better.

His wife thinks he is being spoiled by his mother who encourages him to be lazy. Several times Mrs. Santano has found him sleeping the afternoon siesta at his mother's home. It is unfair, she thinks, that her husband sleeps untroubled in the afternoon only to return late at night to awaken and disturb the many occupants of their apartment. If Mr. Santano fails to visit his parents, his mother sends for him. The younger Mrs. Santano is annoyed by this, and she frequently exchanges insults with her mother-in-law.

Beside paying rent and buying almost all of the food, Mrs. Santano's mother helps her daughter care for the four children. As they work, they talk about Mr. Santano's disgusting, lazy ways. Mrs. Santano wishes she had her own household. She does not like to clean the apartment that is not hers.

Mrs. Santano has a 22-year old brother who washes beer bottles in a brewery. He suffers from such severe stomach ulcers that he bleeds through the rectum. Mr. Santano, too, has suffered from stomach ulcers for 9 years. Although he was operated on 3 years ago for this condition, he still bleeds through the rectum. Both men spend many hours discussing the nature and treatment of their ulcers. Mr. Santano is sympathetic toward his brother-in-law because, "only a person who has had ulcers understands how painful they are."

Mrs. Santano does not have amicable relations with this brother. Recently, he came to visit his mother. Mrs. Santano told him to close the front door so her small daughter could not crawl out of the apartment. The brother who resented being ordered about by his sister threatened to slap her face. Before he could carry out his threat, she slapped him. Although he did not slap back, they have not spoken to each other since this incident. "He who hits first, hits twice," says Mrs. Santano.

Mrs. Santano dislikes an aunt who lives on the second floor of the same apartment building. The dispute started when Mr. Santano was at the aunt's apartment playing cards and drinking beer with her husband. To keep her husband from getting drunk, Mrs. Santano called him downstairs to go to bed. As he left the card game, the aunt ridiculed him for being dominated by his wife. Mr. Santano was insulted. Charges and countercharges were hurled and bad feelings ensued. The latest in a series of clashes occurred when the aunt's teen-age son was lighting firecrackers in the front yard as Mrs. Santano was putting her children to bed. She told her cousin to stop so her children could go to sleep. When the cousin refused, she threw an empty beer bottle at him. The bottle missed the boy but crashed against the side of the concrete building shattering into many pieces. The aunt came downstairs and was involved in an altercation with the Santanos which went on until the police finally came to disperse the crowd of neighbors that had formed.

Mr. Santano says,

> I don't like this place [his mother-in-law's apartment] or the persons living here. They call me a "bad mortgage," a lazy "piece of worthless furniture." I am not lazy. They don't understand how sick I feel. Only my mother really understands.

Correlatively, Mrs. Santano says,

> Some day, I would like to leave my children with my mother-in-law. I want to get away from everyone, from all the persons I know. I want to live a peaceful life.

Our general discussion of the extended families begins by focusing on financial help. Table 48 shows the percentage of families in each diagnostic family group that have sought financial help during the last year of the study and the sources from which they have sought it. No single comparison between percentages in Table 48 yields a statistically significant difference; but the overall pattern of difference is consistent.

During that year a larger percentage of families in each diagnostic family group sought financial help from relatives than from friends,

TABLE 48 Families Seeking Financial Help during the Last Year of the Study by Diagnostic Family Group

		AGENCY OF FINANCIAL HELP				
	N	RELA-TIVES, %	FRIENDS, %	NEIGH-BORS, %	GOV'T AGENCIES, %	COM-MERCIAL BANKS, %
Control families	20	45	35	20	20	40
Husband-schizo-phrenic families	7	86	14	29	14	29
Wife-schizophrenic families	9	67	56	22	44	33
Double schizo-phrenic families	4	75	25	50	25	0

neighbors, government agencies, or commercial banks. The importance of the extended family over other groups and agencies is clear when persons seek an impersonal item such as money. The amount of money sought is usually small. A wife may want two or three dollars to buy or make an item of clothing for herself or her children. She may need the price of a patent medicine advertised to cure a variety of ills and ailments, or an emergency may occur; the usual "emergency" is the illness or accident of a family member for which money must be found for transportation to a public health unit or hospital.

The well families either exchange material help, services, and advice with their relatives on a more or less equal basis, or they give more than they receive. Very few receive more than they give. The sick families are more dependent on their relatives than their relatives on them. Financial aid constitutes a small portion of the material help and benefits that sick families receive from their relatives. The Lebróns were given a house by his mother. Every week the Cardonas are given vegetables and fruit by her father. Services, such as transportation, child care, and therapeutic massages, are performed for sick family members, who also receive advice and orientation. To understand why the sick families are more often the beneficiaries of help, we must consider the impaired ability of a schizophrenic person to give help. The sick man is not a stable wage earner, and the loss of earnings represents a loss of money that could be given to needy relatives. In addition, the sick man loses membership in social groups of friends and fellow workers. The men in such groups talk about job openings, houses for sale or rent, where to secure cheap lumber, who performs this or that service. As friends, they refer each other to helpful persons and places. The benefits that accrue from this give-and-take are illustrated by the Escudero family. As Mr. Cardona and Mr. Santano gave up their jobs, they moved away from friends, as have the other sick men; in doing this, they have lost valuable social contacts that could be helpful to relatives.

The sick woman is equally incapable of fulfilling many obligations associated with her role. Mrs. Lebrón's inability to do housework and to care for her children, despite the pressures brought upon her by her husband and her in-laws, is typical of the sick women. A sick woman has serious difficulty in providing a supportive emotional response. The relative in search of a warm confidante finds the sick woman restless, preoccupied with herself, and prone to change the topic of conversation to her own tribulations; she is too troubled by her inner conflicts, her doubts, and her hostility to be a patient listener.

When only one spouse is sick, the family manages to give some help to relatives; the burden of giving help falls on the well person in the sick families. Mrs. Cardona nursed her husband's nephew back to health; unlike Mr. Lebrón, the six other well husbands married to sick wives give material help to relatives. It is Mrs. Cardona's relatives who provide food and money for them; they take Mr. Cardona to hospitals, minister to him during his "attacks," and, afterwards, join his wife in massaging him. They made arrangements for her niece to move into the house to attend to the children and the household chores and to alert the relatives in the event of another of Mr. Cardona's "attacks." The assistance her relatives provide is reliable and comprehensive, thus enabling Mr. Cardona, his wife, and their children to remain together as a family.

Of crucial importance in securing such help is the well wife who dramatizes her needs and problems to her own relatives. Then, as Mrs. Cardona has done, she mobilizes their efforts to cope with the husband's illness and with the economic plight of the family. The untold sacrifices of the wife's relatives are apparent to the sick husband and his wife. They are grateful for this help, as is illustrated by Mrs. Cardona's observation that her father does without food to help them. They are emotionally involved with her relatives and oriented toward them. Neither the husband nor the wife reminds his relatives that they are obligated to help. Gradually, the nuclear family develops stronger ties with the wife's relatives and, at the same time, becomes relatively isolated from the husband's relatives.

As the family exposes itself to the influence of the wife's relatives, it loses part of its autonomy and privacy. Because her relatives notice the husband's illness and address their help to the problems created by it, it is difficult to keep family secrets, particularly those pertaining to the psychiatric meaning of the illness. This is the most persistent source of tension between the wife's relatives and the families in which only the husband is sick. Thus the Cardonas agree not to tell her relatives about his visits to the psychiatric hospital. The bizarre and threatening behavior of the sick husband sometimes leads his in-laws to suspect that he is becoming a *loco*. The in-laws in another schizophrenic-husband family, the Espinosas, have been giving the husband and wife a considerable amount of support; yet, Mr. Espinosa observes that they avoid him in subtle ways, are hesitant and reserved toward him, and are unusually curious about the nature of his illness. Occasionally, they draw Mrs. Espinosa out of earshot to inquire about his behavior; they repeatedly give her advice to hide the knives, scissors, and razor blades, anything that her husband might use to harm her, the children, or neighbors. Mrs. Espinosa rejects this advice because to follow it would legitimize the idea that her husband is a dangerous *loco*. This idea is intolerable to her, and from her point of view it is detrimental to her husband.

The nine well husbands married to schizophrenic wives are employed full time. Consequently, their families have not experienced the economic plight that results when a husband is disabled. Nor have the extended families in which the nuclear families are enmeshed had to mobilize their resources to meet the problems that unemployment creates. Instead, a stable wage enables these families to aid some relatives. In this respect Mr. Lebrón is atypical, since not only does he not help his or his wife's relatives, but he also does not spend much of his earnings on his wife or children; his responsibilities as a husband and father are secondary to his drinking bouts and affairs with women of the "happy life." Even the money for his dwelling was supplied by his mother.

Unlike Mr. Lebrón, the usual husband in a schizophrenic-wife family is a help-giver, but primarily to his own relatives and only secondarily to his in-laws. His obligations to his in-laws are attenuated by the bitter conflict he experiences with his wife. As he dissociates himself from his wife, he moves away from his obligations to his in-laws. Seldom is help given because the husband *decides* to help. When his wife's family is helped, it is through no plan of the husband but because they attach themselves to the wife to "dip into" the available family resources, and in the culture it is a serious moral breach to withdraw help that is being given. The sick wife often turns to her relatives, even though her husband's earnings are equal to or more than theirs. She has little or no money to give her relatives because her husband views her as an irresponsible spendthrift. He buys the groceries for the family or gives his wife a small amount of money with orders to spend it for designated items.

Child care is the mother's responsibility, but the sick wife, as in the case of Mrs. Lebrón, has serious difficulties in filling the maternal role. Mrs. Lebrón is a careless and hostile mother. Relatives have to assume many of the responsibilities of child care, as Mrs. Lebrón's mother-in-law and father have done.

To get advice, consolation, or a sympathetic ear, the sick wife and the well husband to whom she is married each turn to their own relatives. In-laws are disregarded because the conjugal bonds are ruptured. Moreover, social support consists, in large part, of listening to grievances about the misbehavior of the husband or wife. In-laws are not good confidants because the primary allegiance is to blood relations. Mr. Lebrón's mother lashes back at her daughter-in-law when told that her son comes home late at night. Most well husbands married to sick women do not depend on their mothers as much as Mr. Lebrón. The husband married to a sick wife usually turns to his friends and companions to avoid marital conflict. Outside distractions keep him away from home for long hours, but he does not speak openly to his friends about his marital problems.

The sick woman is guarded and uncomfortable in her contacts with neighbors and friends because she fears they will view her as a *loca*. Thus her parental family is the only group to which she can turn for a supportive relationship. Although she must make considerable efforts to get there and often finds her mother agitated and unapproachable, Mrs. Lebrón still visits her parents every day.

Unlike the women in the husband-schizophrenic families who keep the truth about their husbands' illness from their relatives, the wives in the wife-schizophrenic families discuss their visits to the psychiatric hospital with their own relatives. These relatives do not foist the stigma of the *loca* upon her, as do her in-laws who use it as a means of condemning her. Mrs. Lebrón's mother-in-law voluntarily identified her as a *loca* to the interviewers.

The double schizophrenic families resemble the husband-schizophrenic families in one respect—economic support is provided by the wife's relatives, not his. The manner in which the economic support is given, however, differs in these two groups of families. In the double schizophrenic families, subsistence is provided for the husband because there is no reasonable way of excluding him from the help that is addressed primarily to his wife: if a bed is provided, he shares it; when rice and beans are cooked, he eats them. Although the help is given grudgingly, not in the spirit of preserving the unity of the family as is the case in the husband-schizophrenic families, the husband in the double schizophrenic family is a *de facto* beneficiary of the help extended to his wife and children. Concern and promises of greater generosity accompany the help received by Mr. Cardona, a schizophrenic whose wife is well, whereas imprecations accompany the help received by Mr. Santano, a schizophrenic whose wife is sick.

Double schizophrenic families and wife-schizophrenic families are very much alike. Each person turns to his own relatives, and away from his in-laws, for emotional support. Neither spouse dramatizes the illness of the other to his own relatives in order to receive help that benefits the entire family. Nor do the relatives of the sick persons mobilize their efforts to cope with the broader problems of disorganization in the family. Mr. Santano's mother is very concerned with the suffering of her son whom she loves but not with the problems created by his inability to do the things expected of a husband and father.

The husbands and wives who are both well have little conflict with their in-laws; relations are harmonious and cooperative. The pattern is very different in each of the three groups of sick families. Families in which only the husband is sick are closely tied to the kin network of the wife; they are isolated, in large measure, from the husband's relatives. The Cardonas not only are the recipients of a large amount of help from her relatives, they also are emotionally identified with them. Although they like them and get along with them, tension may stem from the possibility that the welcome, but intruding, in-laws may ascribe the role of the *loco* to the husband. The sick husbands and their well wives are disillusioned with his relatives because they fail to give the expected help. This does not create conflict as his relatives avoid becoming involved in his problems and are seldom seen.

In the wife-schizophrenic families, the relationship of the husband to his in-laws is characterized by strife or an effort to avoid each other. The families view the husband as cruel or irresponsible. They feel he is not fulfilling his obligations as a husband or father. This rule is also applicable to sick men married to sick women. Similarly, schizophrenic women married to sick or well men are engaged in an incessant war against their in-laws, particularly their mothers-in-law. To illustrate, 46 per cent of the sick women, in comparison with 7 per cent of the well women, were not on speaking terms with their mothers-in-law at the time of the interviews. (This difference is statistically significant beyond the .01 level.) Personal contacts with mothers-in-law are tense, strained, and often erupt into an exchange of insults.

As in the Lebrón and Santano families, conflict with in-laws is created when a person turns to his blood relatives, usually to his mother, to recount the misbehavior of his spouse. The parent listens and agrees because of the loyalty entailed by blood relations; a tacit coalition is formed against the spouse who is the focus of the grievances. The parent then acts on behalf of his offspring against his son- or daughter-in-law, or he is perceived by the son- or daughter-in-law to be acting this way. The in-law then is introduced as a third party in the conflict. Thus marital problems give rise to, and intermesh with, in-law troubles. The mother of a schizophrenic wife, Mrs. Urrutia, decided to put her son-in-law "in his place," despite the fact that she subsists entirely from his earnings. She felt degraded because her daughter was married to him. She told him he was nothing but a "fat, dirty Negro." Mr. Urrutia threw her out an open door and yelled, "You are not going to call me names and eat my food at the same time." Now, Mr. Urrutia rules the household with little overt opposition from his mother-in-law; his "suggestions" are followed by the reluctant woman.

SUMMARY

Schizophrenia impairs a person's capacity to help his in-laws and blood relatives, because the sick person's earnings, at best, are meager. His social contacts with persons outside his family are attenuated. He has few resources to draw on to give his wife and children the kind of help associated with the economic role of the male. Similarly, the sick wife cannot give to her husband and children the kind of help entailed by her role as wife and mother. The disablement of the sick person, male or female, prevents his giving help to relatives. Reciprocally, the sick person becomes the beneficiary of any help offered. For this reason, sick families, in contrast to well families, receive more help than they give.

The sources of help in the extended family depend on the sex of the person afflicted with schizophrenia. Families with sick husbands and well wives receive a great deal of help from the wives' relatives and very little from the husbands'. The wife draws help by dramatizing her husband's illness and the family problems created by it; the contributions of her relatives are diverse and reliable, thus enabling the family to continue to function. Tension between the husband and the wife, on the one hand, and her relatives, on the other, stems from the stigma associated with the role of the *loco*. The husband and wife try to protect themselves from those intrusions that might identify him as a *loco*.

The sick wife married to a well husband turns to and receives help from her relatives. The help is varied and addressed primarily to her welfare, not to the broader disruptive problems in her marriage. Each spouse communicates his marital problems to his relatives, but the husband can, in addition, seek the companionship of friends to forget and avoid the turmoil at home. The well husband can help his relatives, but his sick wife cannot help hers. Moreover, he is unconcerned with the needs of his in-laws because of the growing chasm that separates him from his wife.

In all relevant aspects but two, the double schizophrenic families resemble the wife-schizophrenic families. First, they experience a severe economic crisis because the husband is unable to continue to work. To cope with economic problems, the wife receives help from her relatives, and the husband benefits inadvertently. Second, the husband sees only his conjugal or blood family and does not have outside distractions as do well men.

Conflict with in-laws is not widespread in the well families or in the husband-schizophrenic families, but in families with sick wives, irrespective of the mental status of the husband, each person is entangled in disputes. As a person turns to blood relatives to confide the misbehavior of his spouse, the in-law relationship is contaminated with bad feeling.

In sum, organized patterns of cooperation between relatives observable in the well families break down in the sick families. Sick persons are not woven into closely knit family groups that include both sets of relatives. The problems experienced by a person's own relatives are not referred to his in-laws for solution. The husband-schizophrenic families are drawn into the wife's family group and away from the husband's. In families with sick wives, each person turns to his family of origin for emotional support. Thus, the conflict and isolation rupture the extended families of sick persons.

PART VI THE FUTURE

We have traced in preceding chapters the trajectory of the life arc of the sick and well persons from childhood, to the adult years, and on into the stormy period associated with the onset of schizophrenia. The web of interpersonal relations, the problems, and the conflicts as well as the patterns of mutual social and economic support which entangle the husbands and wives also enmesh their children.

Chapter 20 examines the behavior of the children in the context of the family and the neighborhood, with particular emphasis on parent-child roles, the punishment of the children, parental aspirations for the children, and evidences of mental disturbance in the children. Chapter 21 draws the study together and indicates points for further research.

20

The Next Generation

In Part V discussion has been confined to the grandparental and parental generations. This chapter focuses on the next generation—the children being reared in these families. Of the 40 families, 37 had children at the time we began to study them. Two of the three families without children were anticipating the arrival of a baby within a few months. Of the two pregnant women, one is in the sick group and one in the well group. The third family without children is likely to remain so, as the wife suffers from a venereal disease.

When we began the field work there were 134 children in the 37 families, ranging in age from a few days to 17 years. They are almost equally divided between the sick and the well families: 65 children in the sick group and 69 in the well group. The mean age of the children in the sick families is 7 years and in the well families 5.4 years. This difference is not significant. The ages and sexes of the children are proportionately divided between the four family diagnostic groups. The children in all the families are financially dependent on their parents.

In the phase of the family cycle we have studied, the children are undergoing the process of socialization for adult life. How does this process occur? What do the parents expect of their children? How do the parents view the neighborhoods in which the families live? What are the discernible effects of mental illness in one or both parents on (1) their own behavior in relation to their children and (2) the behavior of the children in the family, the neighborhood, and the school? The answers to these questions are the subject of our discussion in this chapter.

The data under examination are derived from direct questions to the parents and from observations in the family by the fieldworkers. The children were not interviewed, but the fieldworkers came to know them intimately. Many times, while one fieldworker took a mother to the psychiatrist for the mental health evaluation, another one cared for the children. Gifts of pencils, pads of paper, chewing gum, candy, and toys were taken to the children so they could entertain themselves during the interviews with the parents. After a number of visits to the family, the interviewers were referred to as "uncle" or "aunt" by many of the children because only relatives visit them so often. The parents were asked a series of questions, some of which sought to identify attitudes toward the children; others requested descriptions of the children's behavior. Both the interviews and the personal observations of the fieldworkers provide the data which are discussed here.

Puerto Rican culture is traditionally family centered. The ideal roles of mothers, fathers, and children are defined precisely. These mothers and fathers are almost of one voice in defining the ideal roles of a parent and a child. A good mother devotes herself to the physical and spiritual care of the children; she disciplines, teaches, and defends them; she sets a proper model by being morally impeccable and industrious; she shows an interest and imparts confidence to her children. Children who are clean and well groomed reflect credit on the mother. The values of the culture make motherhood a trust so elemental it may be said to be sacred. When her child is sick, a mother nurses him at all hours of the day and night, suffering through his illness. She displays her feelings for her children by embracing, kissing, and fondling them. She often makes poignant declarations of her love, vowing that she would die for her children.

The division of labor requires that the mother be more fully involved in the socialization of the children than the father. Usually, she is with the children many hours, the father few. Even when the father is at home, the main burden of child care falls on the mother. A father is not criticized if he is somewhat aloof from the children— one mark of a good father is the maintenance of respect in the family by not allowing excessive familiarity. Thus many fathers are not privy to the inner sentiments and deep affection which bind the children to the mother. Alternative ways of relating to the children are available to the father, but not to the mother; the role of the mother is subject to many more constraints. A mother who removes herself from the children in thought, action, or emotion to the extent that a father can deviates from the mores of good motherhood and is labeled *mala madre* (bad mother).

Much as the man who endeavors to validate his masculinity by posturing and behaving like a *macho*, the woman demonstrates her worth by fulfilling the sacred trust of motherhood. It is commonplace for a mother to deny herself food so her children can eat. Before she buys herself clothing she buys it for her children. She engages in ferocious brawls to defend her children from attacks by neighbors. She stays awake night after night to care for a sick child. Mrs. Feliciano, despite her own frailness, staggers a half-mile to school each morning with her crippled 12-year old daughter on her back; at noon she carries her back home again. Mrs. Ubarri's self-sacrifice centers upon her five starving children who eat only the occasional leftovers sent by relatives and neighbors. She says:

> Sometimes eight days will go by without our drinking coffee. We have gone three days without eating a mouthful of food. We have been hungry a long time. My stomach always aches.

Mrs. Ubarri is pale, scrawny, anemic, and tubercular, but to nourish her 3-year old daughter, who has eaten meat only twice in her lifetime, Mrs. Ubarri breast feeds her. Recently she weaned her 4-year old son because, "I was like a cow with two grown children suckling from me at the same time. My milk was not enough."

The responsibilities of a mother are incessant, compelling, and immediate. For the fatigued and anxious schizophrenic woman, the burden of motherhood is too much. Periodically, she withdraws from her role as mother into the fantasy of a life unencumbered by responsibilities. Her disgruntled husband demands that she respond to her obligations, however, as do her dependent children, by reminding her that morally she is "bound" to motherhood. The schizophrenic woman is torn between her desire to be able to do what society expects of her and her inability to do so. She screams at her children to leave her alone, only to kiss and hug them close to her at the next moment. Thus her children are trapped by a mother who alternates acceptance and rejection of them and by a father who exacerbates the family conflict in the brief time he spends at home.

The almost sacred sentiments of the good mother role are not an integral part of the role definition of the good father. The father is expected to provide sustenance, to discipline, and to teach his children respect. A good father is defined usually by proscription instead of prescriptions—he does not come home drunk to create discord and commotion; he does not maltreat his children by brutal, corporal punishment. A good father is ready to defend his children from attack by neighbors, police, or his enemies.

Some fathers express anxiety about the welfare of their children.

Mr. Domínguez is typical of the worried fathers in his concern for his undernourished 8-year old daughter. This child neither plays nor goes to school because she is feeble and pale, has lost weight, and is subject to dizzy spells. Mr. Domínguez fears that his inability to provide food will cause her to become tubercular. When he eats a meal he is guilt-ridden about the child's hunger, and sometimes he cannot sleep. A few fathers worry about the illnesses and the physical deformities of their children and the impact such deformities may have on the children. Mr. Porrata grieves about his 8-month old son who was born with a cleft palate and a harelip; the deformity exposes the infant's gums, the inside of his mouth, and his throat. Since he cannot be nourished normally, he is anemic and prone to respiratory infections. The doctors have refused to perform plastic surgery until he is older. The parents have struggled to keep him alive by feeding him with an eyedropper. Mr. Porrata worries that if the deformity is not corrected the child will develop "complexes" when he grows up.

> My child will be an unhappy person and think of himself as being ugly. He will rebel against those who scorn him and then he will become a delinquent. He will be afraid of going to school, of meeting other persons. He will be illiterate. He may even become a *loco*.

Beyond internalizing the problems of the children, as do Mr. Domínguez and Mr. Porrata, some fathers play with their offspring, listen to them, and discuss with their wives the aspirations they have for the children. If a son or daughter is graduated from elementary school, a father proudly celebrates the occasion. This type of involvement with the children is relatively frequent among the fathers in the control families. It occurs more often and is more intense among the sick men married to well women who, more than men in any other diagnostic group, spend many hours with the children because they have retreated from social contacts outside of the family. Even though the sick men are subject to erratic moments of explosive outbursts, they are, on the whole, benevolent, gentle, and emotionally committed fathers. On the other hand, rarely does a sick or well father married to a sick woman show such evidences of concern. To him, the children are part of a distasteful home life from which he tries to remove himself.

A good child is well mannered and deferential toward adults, loves and trusts his parents, and abides by the law. Most important, he is respectful. Respect is as important in the parent-child relationship as it is in the ordering of social relations between the husband and the wife. In the parent-child relationship, respect is considered to be more important than love: 90 per cent of the fathers and 73 per cent of the mothers volunteer the fact that a good child is respectful, and 78 per cent of the men and 83 per cent of the women choose respect over love from their children when asked to select between the two. One father says,

> When the children respect, things go well. Of what use would it be to me if they loved me but would not obey me? Respect brings order, discipline, and control.

Similarly, a mother says,

> When the children respect the parents, there is order in the house. If they do not respect, the house is disorderly; the children do what they want; they do not obey. They come home when they want and they govern themselves. Respect brings love.

It is believed that obedience results from respect. If a parent really commands respect he can correct the children by a stern look without having to raise a hand. Fifty-five per cent of the mothers and 68 per cent of the fathers evaluate their children as "very good"; 40 per cent of the mothers and 38 per cent of the fathers think of themselves as "very good" parents.

Schizophrenia is not related to a person's conception of the ideal roles of father, mother, and child; nor is it related to the premium a father or a mother places on respectful children and his or her self-evaluation as a parent.

Ninety per cent of the husbands and wives believe that discipline is a joint responsibility of the parents; in three-fourths of the families, both parents discipline the children. Three kinds of discipline are used. (1) Physical punishment which ranges from a light slap to a whipping with a leather strap or to a pummeling with fists; when a parent "goes blind with anger" because the child manages to evade blows, the child may be knocked down and kicked. (2) Physical restriction; a child is made to kneel for 15 minutes on the floor, but not "on the grate," a form of punishment the parent may have experienced during his own upbringing. Sometimes the child is made to stay at home for at least 1 day. (3) Reprimand or rebuke which is the most common form of discipline; a child may be reprimanded with mild admonitions or with bitter curses. After the initial outburst and the parent has "cooled off," the child is warned in more temperate language not to misbehave again. Seldom does a parent go into lengthy explanations about the reasons for the punishment.

A mother disciplines more often than a father because she is with the children more of the time. She uses all forms of discipline. The father tends to reinforce his warnings with physical force. Fathers are known to have a "loose hand," meaning that they are quick to slap or whip. Moreover, the child stands in awe of the father who is a symbol of respect and "strong character"; hence, the child is more afraid of him than of the mother. The mother is aware of this and often controls the child by threatening to report his misbehavior to the father.

A child is rebuked if he yells in the house, drops a glass or plate, or accidentally overturns a chair. Scuffling or wrestling, particularly among girls, is considered improper, but the greatest source of anger to a parent is disrespectful behavior. A disobedient child is disrespectful; every blow aimed at him is accentuated by *"para que cojas respeto"* (so that you will learn respect), an exclamation often heard over the screeches and wails of a child even during a short visit to a slum or *caserío*.

Discipline is a source of conflict in more than one-half of the families. The answers wives give to the question, "Do you argue with your husband over punishment of the children?" are summarized by diagnostic family group in the following tabulation:

DIAGNOSTIC GROUP	AFFIRMATIVE, %
Control families	50
Husband-schizophrenic families	14
Wife-schizophrenic families	78
Double schizophrenic families	100

The differences between these percentages are not statistically significant for the four categories. However, conflict over punishment is concentrated in the families with sick mothers who are married to sick or well husbands in comparison with the group composed of schizophrenic-husband families and control families ($p < .01$). These data are consistent with the findings reported in Part V which highlight the divisive effect of schizophrenic wives on family life.

In the control group, most arguments result from the mother challenging the father's use of physical force; neither restrictive nor verbal punishment is a point of contention. Few husbands contest their wives and still fewer couples have mutual recriminations over the discipline of the children. Occasionally, a husband tells his wife to beat the children when they do not follow orders. The dominant pattern of conflict over punishment in the control families is illustrated by the Badillo family. The Badillos have two daughters, aged 14 and 12, and a 17-year old son. The son is having an affair with an older girl of ill repute who lives in the same neighborhood. One night, the son came home late, took a bath, and washed his underwear. The parents inferred from this that he was washing away evidences of sexual intercourse. They fear that their son will be forced into a premature marriage if he makes the girl pregnant or he will be held responsible if another man impregnates her. The Badillos share this concern, but they have different solutions. The mother tries to gain the son's confidence with soft words and gentle questions about the girl; she advises him to be careful, that one intimacy leads to another, and that he is still too young to be burdened with a wife. She attempts to raise doubts in the boy's mind about the girl's morality; she discusses involvement with a girl who is "damaged," possibly afflicted with *furor*, and likely to be unfaithful after marriage. Mr. Badillo's reaction is in accord with his role of a strong father. Twice in one week he knocked his son to the floor, beat him, and ordered him not to see the girl again. The mother takes strong exception to such treatment but waits until her son is out of earshot to tell her husband so. Even though the husband and wife argue about it, she is convinced that slowly her husband is accepting her advice to solve the problem *a la buena*, with moral rather than physical persuasion. She reminds her husband with a touch of light humor that he has not always been pure sexually, either before or after marriage.

Few parents have children in the age of courtship, but the mothers in the control group resemble Mrs. Badillo in that they dislike their husbands to beat the children. An angry father's violence is uncontrollable so that, according to the mothers, even small children are beaten as if they were "grown men." The children are often left with long-lasting bruises, and the possibility of a serious injury is not discounted by the mother. Her strong emotional identification with the children usually causes her to suffer when they are slapped, whipped, or pummeled by the father. Rarely, however, does she intervene directly to thwart the father, as this would challenge his authority, an essential part of family solidarity. Arguments ensue when the mother discusses the subject with her husband away from the children, but she does not question his right to use corporal punishment; rather, as Mrs. Badillo does, she **expresses** doubts about its effectiveness in serving **the ends which they** both want. Disputes that do occur in the control group are short and appear to leave little residue of bad feeling between the parents.

In the husband-schizophrenic families, only one couple argues about the punishment of the children. The Herrero family is a clear exception to the unity and harmony found in the families of this diagnostic group. (This point is discussed in Chapter 15.) Almost every day the Herreros accuse each other of treating the children cruelly. The other parents in the husband-schizophrenic families do not argue over punishment and, in fact, seldom punish their offspring; this is surprising since sick men are subject to belligerent, impulsive, and aggressive outbursts easily provoked by noisy children. When the sick man erupts, however, the wife hastens to remove the children, and, apparently, the children learn not to irritate the father when the mother is away from home. Similarly, the wife's relatives, who often help care for the sick father while the wife is at work, learn to protect the children. At least as important are the bonds of affection, support, and mutual concern between the parents and the children. The mentally healthy wife and mother habitually defines the family situation for the sick husband. Should he be rough with the children, she speaks to him about it out of earshot of the children; when the Mrs. Berríos, Cardona, Davíla, Espinosa, Ramos, and Tirado speak, their dependent husbands listen.

Eleven of the parents in the thirteen families with sick mothers, married either to sick or well fathers, have bitter fights about punishment. Usually, the father openly accuses the mother of unjustified punishment for inconsequential annoyances. If the child trips, leaves the home without permission, stains his clothing, or makes a whining request, the mother is likely to beat him. A sick woman confesses that she often lacks self-control. She goes into a blind rage and beats the child; the father forcefully intervenes and soon the couple is embroiled in bitter conflict. The sick woman's anger toward her husband tends to be discharged on her children. (The fieldworkers observed this many times.) Mr. Santano says that when he quarrels with his wife she turns quickly to beat the children. Usually after a beating, the sick mother cuddles, kisses, and strokes the child and asks his forgiveness. Mrs. Janer expiates the guilt she feels after whipping the children by reassuring them of her love; this inconsistency confuses the father as well as the children.

Both parents in the Nieves family accuse each other of being cruel to the children, and each knows the other will intervene if a child is given a beating. To provoke his spouse, one parent slaps a child, and soon the conflict that embroils them excludes the children who stand aside to watch the fight between their parents. The Nieves children are accustomed to this sequence and have come to view their parents as idiosyncratic. They gossip about their parents and point to them with gestures meaning, "They're crazy."

In two double schizophrenic families the mothers have formed a united front with the children to protect themselves from the father. Mrs. Gallardo is terrified of her husband; the only time she defies him is when she rescues the children from his beatings. In the Aponte family, the mother and the children have identified the father as a common threat. For protection, they warn each other when the father is about to arrive home, and when he does they turn away from him. He is never told what has happened during his absence for fear that he will find fault and start a fight that will include the whole family.

Although the usual sick woman is punitive with her children, only one child in the thirteen families with sick mothers is the focus of abuse by all adult family members. The Lebróns' 3-year old child is a "flogging horse" for the mother, the father, and the grandmother. Mrs. Lebrón says, "She sickens me. I cannot stand her." The child spends weekdays with her paternal grandmother; on weekends she returns home. The grandmother sees a strong resemblance between the deranged mother and the child, and so she tries to whip the bad behavior out of the child. Her attitude stems from the bitter hatred between Mrs. Lebrón, on the one hand, and her husband and mother-in-law, on the other. To Mr. Lebrón and to his mother, the little girl is symbolic of the defiant, disheveled, sick mother. To Mrs. Lebrón, the daughter represents the distasteful responsibilities her domineering mother-in-law and punitive husband impose on her. Mrs. Lebrón slaps or lashes the girl with a belt on the slightest provocation; she immediately grabs away any object the child picks up, even a scrap of paper or a toy. If the little girl comes close to her mother, she is pushed away or hurled against a wall. When her presence becomes unbearable to Mrs. Lebrón, she carries the child to her mother-in-law's house, slams her down on the front porch, and leaves without telling her mother-in-law that the child is there. The fieldworker who interviewed Mr. Lebrón reports:

> I interviewed him at his mother's house because this is what he suggested. But sometimes it was necessary to interrupt the interview for periods of up to ten minutes because his daughter who stays with her grandmother would be screaming loudly, demanding the father's attention. He pushes her away in a brisk manner, saying, "Get away

from me; leave me alone. Don't you see I am busy?" When the child persists, he whips her with a belt. Other times the grandmother whips the child. They take turns. During the last two interviews the grandmother left a thick belt with me, instructing me to whip the child if she annoyed me. . . . I noticed that at all times the grandmother demanded adult conduct from the little girl.

The parents have rich and detailed perceptions of the class system of their society. To them, differences between social classes are based on education, occupation, the consumption of goods and services, membership in social groups, quality of friends, power, and morality. Nearly all view themselves as in the lowest social class and, regardless of mental status, would like to have their children achieve a higher-class position; 82 per cent of the fathers and 95 per cent of the mothers want their children to belong to a higher social class than they do. Specifically, they want their children to have occupations which will lift them to a much higher level of affluence, comfort, and social standing. In descending order of frequency the four occupations the parents desire most for their sons are medicine, engineering, law, and accounting; for their daughters it is teaching (elementary and high school), office work, nursing, and social work. If the wishes of these parents are fulfilled, only 10 per cent of the 134 children will be manual laborers—mechanics, carpenters, or plumbers.

No parent wishes his daughter to be a house servant, factory worker, waitress, or cook; nor does any parent desire to have his children do agricultural work as he himself may have done during earlier years. Agricultural work is manual work, and manual work, in the city or in the country, is stigmatized in the traditions of the culture. Parents know that manual work provides few opportunities for advancement. Mr. Urrutia left the cane fields at the age of 20 after 10 years of carrying water for the workers in the field, hoeing, fertilizing, and cutting cane; his best period of earnings brought him $12 per week during harvest, but during the dead season there was no money to be earned in the fields. By living in the city, he hopes to educate his daughters so that two of them will be teachers and the third will be a nurse; he says with this education they will be prepared ". . . to take care of themselves. I am an animal, but I want my daughters to be something."

The parents want the children to be in the professions, affluent business groups, or at least to join the ranks of white-collar workers. To wear a clean, starched, pressed suit of clothing to work, to have an inside job out of the blistering tropical sun, to sit behind a desk—these are symbolic of higher-class values.

Bound by their own economic position, the parents must take a telescopic view which virtually spans the entire hierarchy of occupations in the society. From this distance, the elementary tasks, the prestige, affluence, and power of a higher occupation are understood, but misconceptions about the required qualifications emerge. Although formal education is viewed as an important, perhaps the most important, avenue for ascending the occupational scale, most parents have unclear or erroneous ideas of the education necessary for many of the professions. It is not unusual for a parent to assert that after 2 years of college his child will become a physician.

The decision that a child should be a physician, teacher, lawyer, nurse, or mechanic is sometimes based on the parents' observation of the child. Two of the Urrutia daughters often play at being in school, alternating in the roles of teacher and student; the parents have decided they will both be teachers. The 4-year old Tirado boy argues frequently and proficiently, so he will be a lawyer. The 7-year old Quintero boy will be a mechanic because he likes to take apart and assemble toy cars; Mrs. Ubarri's 3-year old daughter will be a nurse as she is always doctoring her doll. Parents volunteer such observations and, according to them, with the will of God and the help of the government the children will receive the maximum benefits of an education. A common saying is: "Nowadays in Puerto Rico anybody can get an education. The government gives many scholarships to the poor."

Each parent was asked the amount of education he would like for each of his children. The amount of education varies according to a particular child and to the sex of the parent. Compared to their own educational levels, the parents have lofty aspirations for their children. The maximum and the minimum education desired by either parent, regardless of sex, for any or all of the children was used to classify each family into one of three groups with the following results: (1) 28 per cent want 1 to 4 years of high school for the children; (2) 40 per cent want 1 year of high school to 4 years of college for the children; and (3) 32 per cent want from 1 year of college to an advanced professional degree for the children. All parents would like each of their children to have at least 1 year of high school; 72 per cent would like at least 1 child to receive a year of college education.

Ironically, very few parents display an active interest in the education of their children. Seldom do they ask what the children are learning at school; there is no insistence that class assignments be completed, and it is an unusual parent who assists his child with homework. If a child is absent from school for a prolonged period of time or if he is held back in the same grade at the end of an academic year, the parent accepts this with passivity and resignation. Contact with a teacher, the principal, or a school nurse occurs primarily when a child is misbehaving and the parent is summoned to discuss the problem. Only two parents have ever attended a Parent-Teacher Association meeting. Although the parents aspire for upward mobility for their children, little is done to instill the motivation for such mobility in the child by giving him positive support for high achievement in school. Rewards and punishments in socialization are organized according to conformance with respect, obedience, deference, and morality rather than to educational gains. The parents place greater emphasis on the behavior of the child according to their rules for proper conduct than upon achievement.

Forty-five per cent of the children are 6 years of age or older; none is over 17 years of age. If we assume that all children between 6 and 17 should be in school and that a child of school age will complete one school grade for each chronological year of his age, we have a basis for making some assessment of the success or failure of a child's performance in the school system. Viewed in these terms, only one child in three is in the school grade corresponding to his age. Two children out of three are in grades below their chronological age. Not a single child was in a grade higher than we might expect for his age. The percentage of boys who are older than their placement in school is about the same as for girls. There is a difference, however, between the boys and the girls on the *amount* of incongruity between age and grade in school. The boys are 1.7 years older for a given grade than we would expect from our model of a grade a year; the girls are 2.7 years (mean) older than we would expect in terms of our model of a grade a year.

The incongruity between age and grade in school of the children is related to the diagnostic family group to which the children belong.[1] In descending order according to family diagnostic group, the incongruity is greatest in the double schizophrenic group, the mother-schizophrenic group, the control group, and, finally, the father-schizophrenic group. In brief, the effects of schizophrenia, as reflected in school performance, is most deleterious or retarding in families with both parents mentally ill, but where only the mother is mentally ill these effects are also strong. If the father is sick and the mother is well,

---

[1] $x^2 = 8.975$; 3 df; $p < .05$.

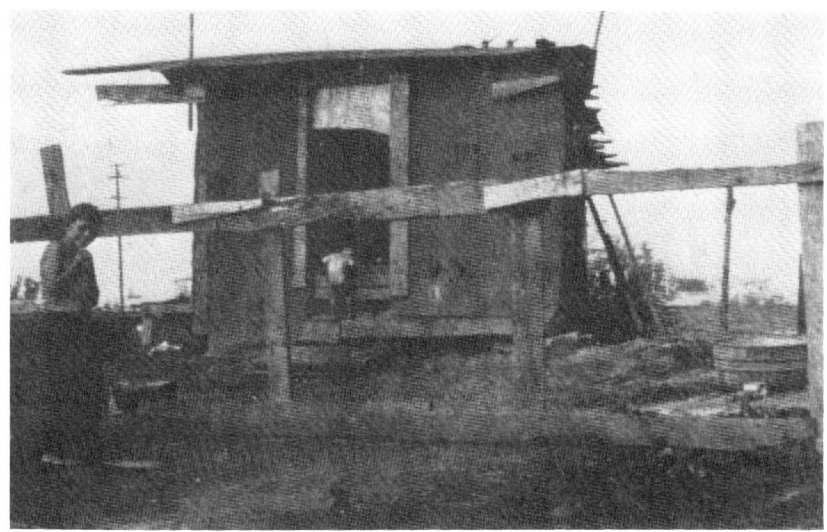

there is little effect on the grade level of the children. The effect that schizophrenia in the family may have in future years, as the children grow older, is subject to speculation.

The parents feel that the neighborhoods in which they live have an adverse effect upon their children. We asked: "Do you think this is a good neighborhood in which to raise your children?" In reply, 73 per cent of the fathers and 80 per cent of the mothers say that the neighborhood is not conducive to the proper raising of children. These percentages are not affected by mental status. Both sick and well parents voice innumerable complaints against the neighborhood: it is noisy, lacking in privacy, and has little or no police protection even though thieves abound; families are embroiled in malicious gossip, and physical violence is commonplace. Violation of the sexual mores is a frequent complaint:

> The woman next door is a prostitute.
> I care for a little boy whose mother has devoted herself to the bars and the happy life.
> The house across the road is a brothel.
> The family across the alley has two girls and one of them is pregnant. She does not know who the father is. Her mother and sister entertain men.

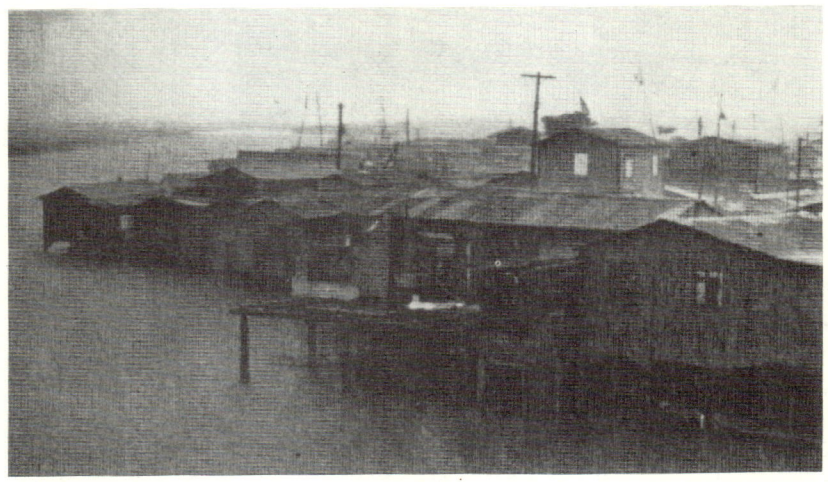

The woman upstairs is a whore.
The widow in the next apartment has three daughters. They entertain their boy friends in the apartment. They drink and dance and play loud music. The boy friends suck the girls' tits on the balcony.

One family was incensed by the proximity of a neighbor, a homosexual, who had been abandoned by his wife and left with several small children. The man hired a couple with a teen-age daughter to move in with him and care for his children. In a short time, the neighbor had seduced not only the teen-age girl but also her father. The wife was furious; she and her daughter left, but her husband stayed with the homosexual neighbor. This man is viewed as a menace in the neighborhood, but the family we studied believes it can do no more about the situation than to watch their children carefully.

Although practically all adults object to obscene words, they are heard daily. Curses, insults, vile names, and indecent phrases are uttered regularly by men, women, and children to express their feelings or degrade an opponent. One day a fieldworker was in the slum where the largest number of our families live. Children were coming home from school when suddenly two little girls, 6 or 7 years of age, began to fight. One girl hit the other, pushed her to the ground, and scattered her books in the odiferous muck which had oozed from the open sewers. The fieldworker asked her why she had hit her opponent. The little girl replied, "Because her mother told her to say bad words to me." Then, as a final justification, she added, "Anyway, she is nothing but the daughter of a grand whore. She doesn't matter." The fieldworker then questioned the other child. This one shouted, "That girl, may God shit on her mother, is the daughter of the grand whore, the whore!" As one mother says, "Here the children learn to say bad words before they can say Papa or Mama."

Children are often the focal point of conflict between neighbors, particularly when the mother is schizophrenic. Conflict between the children creates conflict between the embattled mothers who soon forget the precipitating incident. The angry mothers think they have been insulted, that there has been a breach of respect; the neighbor is henceforth an enemy. The sequence of the conflict is clear, repetitive, and straightforward. Mr. Padilla reports an incident in which his sick wife was involved while he was at work. A neighbor's child hit the Padillas' 5-year old son. Mrs. Padilla's angry complaint to the mother of the child brought out counteraccusations that on former occasions the Padilla boy had hit her children. Mrs. Padilla struck her opponent in the face with a hairbrush, and when the other neighbors intervened she used her hairbrush on them also. Before the fracas was over, she had soundly whipped the neighbor's child. According to Mr. Padilla, the incident left a lingering fear that ". . . the neighbors would have us arrested, that they would attack us without warning, or that they would injure one of our children."

The children were not diagnosed by a psychiatrist, but, as a result of the many visits to each family, the long interviews with both parents, and the close relations established by the fieldworkers with the children, information was collected about symptoms of possible relevance to mental illness in the children. In six of the forty families there is at least one child who suffers from conspicuous, dramatic, and problematical mental and behavioral symptoms. In five of the six families in which children evinced mental disturbances, the mother is schizophrenic. This clustering is significant ($p < .01$). The one exception is the Quintero family, in which the wife is mentally healthy but the husband suffers from nervous symptoms.

The oldest child in the Quintero family, a 16-year old girl who is in the fifth grade, hears an incessant rumbling in her head, feels a drop of water in her brain which rolls around when she moves, and meanders in the neighborhood with little idea of where she is going or where she has been. Once the police found her wandering many miles from home after she had been sent by her mother on an errand to a nearby relative. At night, the daughter dreams about cadavers and caskets; during the day, she hallucinates that a man accompanies her everywhere. When she is told that no man is present, she replies that he disappears when anyone else looks at him. Recently, she broke a double-edged razor blade into small pieces and stirred them into a pot of boiling rice. On another occasion she poured liquid bleach into the family food. Now the mother does not allow her to help cook the meals. The girl has not received medical care, nor has anyone in the family, the neighborhood, or at school suggested that she needs it.

The girl's bizarre and dangerous behavior may result, in part, from the discriminatory and pejorative label of *la Prieta* (the dark one) which the mother has attached to her (this girl is slightly darker than her seven siblings). The fieldworker reports:

> It upsets me to observe the attitude of the mother toward this girl. She calls her *la Prieta* and announces to everyone who listens that this girl is the coal stain of the family. When the girl went to pick up the 3-month old infant from the hammock, the mother screamed, "Leave her alone—if you touch her you will stain her with your color."

In none of the families with schizophrenic husbands and well wives is there a child with such conspicuous symptoms, although one family has problems with a 12-year old daughter who is being courted by a neighborhood boy. As Chapter 8 demonstrates, courtship is an inherently stressful experience because of the parents' desire to restrict the girl and the girl's desire to establish adult heterosexual relationships. Consequently, the girl's conflict with the parents cannot be taken as evidence that she has an inwardly ruptured psychic life. (Shortly after the field work was completed, this girl married the boy.)

In five of the six families in which the children displayed evidences of psychopathology, there is a schizophrenic mother married to either a sick or a well husband. The Lebrón child is seriously "ill of the nerves." According to the fieldworker:

> The little girl is whipped repeatedly. Sometimes the child takes the punishment with indifference. At other times, she strikes back in anger.

The efforts of the interviewers to establish rapport with her were fruitless, as she recoiled from them either in terror or anger. The child is isolated and has withdrawn into herself, away from the punitive adults who surround her.

The Gallardos' 7-year old son is "nervous." When he does not get his way he screams and vomits. He suffers from severe headaches, does not respond when spoken to, and is restless. At night, he falls out of bed and is frightened by dreams that someone has pried open the window and is creeping into the apartment. According to the mother, the son is being infected by the father's illness. Mr. Gallardo, however, attributes the abnormal behavior to the son's birth by Caesarean section.

The Aponte children share the hallucinations of their schizophrenic parents. They claim to have seen a spirit who invades their home, throws sheets from their beds on the living room floor, and rearranges the furniture in the house while the family is sleeping. The children explain that they crouch over their plates at mealtime, but the spirit somehow steals food from them, and they are always left hungry.

The Nieves' 13-year old son who is in the sixth grade is at war with his parents, his school teachers, and the school principal. He argues with his teachers and defies their orders and their efforts to correct him. He gets into trouble in the classroom, the cafeteria, and the hallways. Recently, his claim of ownership of a book which belonged to another student led to an argument, then to a fist fight, and finally to a fight with single-edged razor blades. This boy often hitchhikes to school. He carries a rock in his hand and if a car passes by without stopping for him he hurls the rock at the driver. Mrs. Nieves was advised by the school teacher to consult with the social worker about her son's behavior. She was told that both she and her son need psychiatric help.

There are other examples of children who act out against society, have rapid changes of mood, behave idiosyncratically like a "nervous person," are terrified by adults, become upset to the point where they vomit, and experience hallucinations. With but one exception, the Quintero girl, these children are all in the wife-schizophrenic and double schizophrenic families, but not all of the children in these two diagnostic family groups evidence symptoms of disturbance. Indeed, of all the children the interviewers saw, they were most impressed by the Quiromo boy whose parents are both schizophrenic. This boy is lively and spontaneous, expresses himself well, and is interested and curious about the world. The fieldworkers' accounts of this family contain frequent references to his healthy behavior. As the data were analyzed, the contrast between the healthy boy and the sick parents became clear. The parents are enmeshed in a deep and pervasive pattern of tension, hatred, antagonism, and conflict.

Four years after the field work was completed, Rogler returned to interview the Quiromo parents and the son. The parents still argue bitterly over religious differences. Violent conflicts still arise because Mrs. Quiromo is unwilling to meet her husband's sexual demands. Today, as four years ago, she accuses him of infidelity; now he is alleged to be having an affair with a neighbor woman. The husband makes determined efforts to draw his wife's sympathy, but, as before, she is encapsulated in a world of hallucinations. To interview the Quiromos is to enter an unreal world of revelations, apparitions, and spirits; simultaneously, one must cope with the bitter hatred, mutual recriminations, and almost hopeless disillusionment that envelop this couple.

The boy, however, now 8 years old, remains stable, alert, and likeable. Although he has lost one year of school because of recurring respiratory infections which confined him to bed, he has learned how to read and write Spanish. He reads "Jack and Jane" stories in English and writes a few words in English. He knows the basic essentials of arithmetic. The hard-cover assignment notebooks which represent his school work during the current year are marked with evaluations of "OK," "100%," and short complimentary statements written by his teachers.

Unlike most sick women, Mrs. Quiromo does not beat her son and then embrace him for forgiveness. Although she is withdrawn from and belligerent toward her husband and her own parents, she is convivial and outgoing toward her son. The inconsistency is apparent from one moment to the next as she addresses an insult to her husband, then turns to her son with warm and ingratiating gestures. Mr. Quiromo still unsuccessfully competes with his son for his wife's attention by assuming the role of a dependent child. Although at times he still plays cruel and painful tricks on his son, Mr. Quiromo is a loving father. In contrast to most fathers married to sick women, he is not aloof and reserved in relation to his son. He plays games with the boy, reviews his school work, and compliments him on his achievements with good-natured pats. Despite their own turbulent and unstable relationship, the Quiromos are joined together by affection for their son.

SUMMARY

When the field work began, 37 of the 40 families had children and, in addition, two wives were pregnant for the first time. The 134 children have a mean age of 6 years. All the children are being socialized into lower-class culture. The roles their fathers and mothers play are those defined for them by the culture in which they themselves had matured and those they learned by participation in their own families of orientation. The parents know what is expected of a father and a mother, and they attempt to fulfill the expectations. The children are cared for as the culture prescribes. The mothers are loving, nurtural, protective, and supportive of the children as long as they do what is expected of them. The fathers view themselves as providers, defenders of the home, and responsible men who teach their children respect. Mothers and fathers resort to punishment to ensure that the children respond to what is expected of them by their parents and the culture. The fathers are prone particularly to resort to corporal punishment.

The parents have high aspirations for the children. All the fathers and mothers hope their children will achieve more education than they themselves did; each parent hopes his children will move from menial, low-paid manual occupations into clerical, managerial, and professional pursuits. Most mothers and fathers have some definite ideas of how much education they desire for each child and the occupational pursuit they want the child to follow. Their stated levels of hoped-for education and desired occupational choices are incongruous with the conditions under which the children are being reared. The probability of realizing these aspirations is very small. The realities of the conditions under which the families live in relation to what would be necessary to achieve the stated aspirations are not understood; actually, they are hardly envisaged. The parents realize the neighborhoods where they live are undesirable; they do make an effort to insulate the children from the grossest instances of social pathology. However, two-thirds of the children in school are two grades below what might be expected for their age. The parents do not have the economic and intellectual resources to help their children realize the aspirations they claim to have for these lower-class representatives of the next generation. One boy has left school and gone to work full time; this boy never completed the seventh grade. He is employed by his father and, if he follows in his father's footsteps, he may eventually establish a back-yard garage under the shade of a tree and become a "businessman."

The effects of the mental illness on the development of the children are ignored by most parents. The mothers who are married to schizophrenic men are coping successfully with the family problems their husband's illness has forced on them. Their children are the least retarded in school, and none of these families has severe behavioral problems among the children. The families in which the mother is schizophrenic are severely disturbed. There is conflict between the parents and the children, and these are the families in which there is almost universal retardation in school. The sick mothers are unable to support their children emotionally and socially; the fathers do not concern themselves with their children. The significant association between a schizophrenic mother and severely disturbed behavior in the children indicates that the prospect for the children in future years is black.

21

Summary and Conclusions

We began this study with three basic questions to be answered: Do the life histories of persons who develop schizophrenia differ from those of persons who are not schizophrenic? When and under what circumstances do persons who become schizophrenic exhibit the symptoms characteristic of this affliction? What effect does schizophrenia in a husband or a wife have on the family?

The theoretical frame of reference we used to answer each of these questions postulates that a person's experiences in his effective social environment influence the development, onset, and consequences of schizophrenia. The effective environment is encompassed by the social groups, particularly the families of orientation and procreation, which enmesh the person throughout his lifetime. Other relevant social groups are composed of work associates, friends, and neighbors. Interpersonal relations in the effective environment are organized according to expectations of role performance, and the behavior of a person is analyzed according to the adequacy with which he performs or fulfills the expectations of his social roles.

To apply the frame of reference to the basic questions of the research, we made an exploratory study of families living in the urbanized area of San Juan, Puerto Rico. For our data we went to the sources: the men and women who lived through the experiences they related to us. Their responses, in repeated interviews stretching over several months, to our systematic, searching questions were supplemented by observations in the homes and neighborhoods in which they live. Repeated interviews of husbands and wives, combined with direct observations, enable us to study these families as they face the problems of everyday living in their natural setting.

To gather the data needed to answer our questions, we limited the study to families in which the husband and wife are between 20 and

39 years of age, are in the lowest socioeconomic class, and have never been treated for mental illness. To attain the objectives of the study, however, we had to be able to make comparisons between two groups of families; there had to be a schizophrenic husband or wife in each family of one group, whereas the other group had to be free of schizophrenia. The decision to divide the families into two such categories of equal size resulted in certain strengths and weaknesses pertinent to the conclusions we shall reach in this chapter.

Viewed from the perspective of strength, the families selected correspond to a previously defined population. We demonstrated in Chapter 2 that a Survey Sample of 1144 housholds interviewed in the first phase of this study is representative of the total population of the San Juan area. In addition, we proved that the forty families on which this study is based are representative of families in which the spouses are between 20 and 39 years of age, in the lowest socioeconomic stratum, and resident in the slums or *caseríos* of the urbanized area of San Juan. On the basis of the detailed comparisons between the forty families and the corresponding group of families drawn from the Survey Sample, we may proceed to the presentation of the summary and conclusions confident that the families in the Intensive Study are representative of a larger universe of families.

The small size of the group, however, presents us with limitations in the analysis of quantitative data. We were not able to pursue suggestive findings by dividing the sample into subgroups to check on the spuriousness of a relationship or to refine an inference. On the other hand, a large sample study would have limited the amount of information we could gather on each person and each family, and it would have made it impossible to collect intimate data which can be elicited only after repeated interviews. A control case study sacrifices for practical (not logical) reasons multivariate analysis, but it gains through the richness, depth, and scope of its data.

Throughout the analysis of the data, comparisons have been made between sick and well persons or between diagnostic family groups. The sick persons are all schizophrenic. None of the well persons is psychotic; they are either neurotic, have personality disorders, or are free of symptoms. Had we been able to select a symptom-free well group, more differences between the sick and well might have appeared. Statistical significance in a small sample study requires large differences between the groups being compared. A few exceptions to the hypothesis being tested require that the assumption of chance variations be accepted. The exceptional cases found through presentation of the data in our tables tend to concentrate among persons or families in the control group. Persons or families with neurotic symptoms often resemble the schizophrenic group more than the symptom-free group. Selecting a completely symptom-free group would have prolonged the lengthy field phase and added significantly to the cost of the study. On the other hand, refining the mental illness dimension during the analysis of the data so as to make comparisons between a symptom-free group, a group of nonpsychotic-symptom carriers, and a schizophrenic group would have led to further attrition in the size of the subgroups. Were we to do the study again, we would expend great effort to select a symptom-free control group.

The life history data are based on memories of past events and experiences. The use of retrospective data raises a number of questions: Were true differences in the life histories of the sick and well erased by distortions of memory? Were the few differences in the life histories of the sick and well artifactitious results of the retrospective process? Is the process of recalling past events distorted by the respondent's present psychiatric status? These questions can be stated but not answered. Our experiences indicate, however, that sick persons did not consistently falsify the events and experiences which we were able to observe as we gathered the data. The accounts of the sick persons were, with few exceptions, in accord with the accounts of their mates, although the opinions and evaluations of the event described often did differ. Generally, the sick persons were more spontaneous, revealing of themselves, and willing to describe their private and intimate experiences than were the well persons.

Our experiences demonstrate that detailed, intensive, control case studies, consisting of psychiatric examinations, repeated interviews, and direct observations of the family, the neighborhood, and the community, can be done. To secure the cooperation of the persons selected for the study without compromising the goals of the research, we explained the medical specialty of psychiatry in clear and unambiguous terms without resorting to falsehood or subterfuge, and we arranged for the psychiatric examinations to be carried out in the offices of the psychiatrists. This policy proved to be successful. The persons did not resist going to the private office of a psychiatrist. Our data demonstrate that persons will submit to psychiatric examinations in a field research study.

Field research must adapt to the rhythm of the daily activities of the persons who are studied. If the interviewee understands what is expected of him and is motivated to cooperate, he will respond to the repeated demands made on him by the researchers. The prestige associated with a visit from a higher-status interviewer and the psychological relief of speaking with a reliable confidant motivated the persons to cooperate with us. The norm of hospitality, the generosity, and the friendliness of the persons studied contributed to the successful completion of the field phase.

The effort expended in carefully recruiting and training a field staff was worthwhile. We believe that no amount of training compensates for the unwise choice of a fieldworker. The skills that a good fieldworker puts into play in the field result from personality characteristics which he or she brings to the research project. Prefield training, however, sharpens the required skills and gives them meaning according to the purpose of the study; it focuses the fieldworker's skills on the work which has to be done. This research demonstrates that field studies of the mentally ill can be carried out with little or no sacrifice of the "deep" data generally associated only with research done inside the walls of hospitals and clinics.

With these comments on the salient features of the research design and some of its strengths and weaknesses, we turn to our conclusions on each of the three basic questions that shaped the research. First, do the life histories of the schizophrenic men and women reveal meaningful differences in comparison with the life histories of those who are not schizophrenic?

The families of orientation into which the husbands and wives were born shared the culture of lower-status persons in Puerto Rico a generation ago. The parents were illiterate or semiliterate. The fathers were predominantly agricultural laborers employed in the sugar cane fields or on small hillside farms. Few mothers were employed outside of the home as they were occupied with the many chores of the housework, childbearing, and child care. The parental families were large; all were burdened with poverty. One-half of the families were broken by the death or desertion of one parent before our respondents were 15 years of age. Adulterous behavior by the father is reported to have occurred in some two homes out of three; excessive drinking of rum was often combined with adultery. Economic and interpersonal problems existed in approximately 95 per cent of the parental homes. Mental illness is ascribed to some member of one-half of the families of orientation. The basic conclusion we have reached is that the parental families of persons who are mentally healthy do not differ socially or culturally from the families of persons who suffer from schizophrenia.

The husbands or wives who are schizophrenic present no evidence that they were exposed to greater hardships, more economic deprivation, more physical illnesses, or personal dilemmas from birth until they entered their present marriage than do the mentally healthy men and women. Before the onset of their illness, the schizophrenic men and women took part in the same activities as the well men and women. They had as many friends as the well persons; they viewed their friends and think they were viewed by their friends in the same terms as the well persons think of their early peer relationships. The leisure time activities of the two groups were similar. There is no evidence that the sick persons were more prone to solitary activities than the well ones.

In sum, systematic comparisons between the mentally healthy and the sick persons indicate that they are remarkably similar in their assumption of the appropriate social roles for each sex at the customary age. The life histories demonstrate that in childhood, youth, and early adult life there are only a few significant differences between the behavior of those who are now mentally healthy and those who are suffering from schizophrenia. One notable difference is the more frequent occurrence of nightmares during childhood among the sick than among the well persons. The occupational histories are almost identical in the two groups, with the exception that the schizophrenic women were gainfully employed at an earlier age than the well women.

The effective social environment that enmeshed these young men and women during the years that have elapsed between the time they were under the control of the parental family and the present, confronted all of them with a series of social and personal problems. They have either solved these issues successfully, or they have become victims of them. The culture and their low socioeconomic status in the society present them with a series of tension points that are linked to the difficulties they have faced through the years. Incongruities between cultural values and role performance exacerbate the crises young people face. For example, marriage is an accepted goal in the culture; however, the parents of the girl strive to inculcate an attitude of modesty in her. To preserve her virginity, her contacts with boys are severely restricted. In contrast, the boy is given a great deal of freedom and, at the same time, encouraged to be sexually alert, aggressive, and promiscuous. This cultural difference is symbolized in the double standard of sexual behavior. The double standard clashes with the sovereign power of the girl's family. The family insists that the daughter subordinate her wishes and desires to those of the family. The solidarity of the family draws a clear distinction between the in- and out-group, between those persons who are its members and those who are not. The prospective groom challenges this distinction and poses a threat to the family's reputation.

Even those parents who grant the prospective son-in-law the *entrada* so that he courts the girl under supervision are suspicious and anxious until the courtship is brought to its fruition in what they hope will be a legal union. Quite often, however, the *entrada* is neither granted nor encouraged, thus forcing the girl into a clandestine romance. Such a romance is likely to culminate in a sudden, explosive, and bitter disengagement of the girl from her family. The girl then enters a consensual union, often with a reluctant groom who may have been seeking sexual opportunities rather than marriage. Although neolocal residence is the ideal, the young couple does not have the financial resources to establish a household. This problem is usually resolved by their living with the groom's relatives for a short period of time.

Upon marriage, a second set of crises emerges. The girl's first coital experience is charged with anxiety, repulsion, and, sometimes, panic. She has to unprotect herself and give her husband sexual access to her body. Her carefully inculcated sense of modesty is violated by sexual cooperation. Few wives are completely able to master the problems which stem from such a sharp discontinuity in social conditioning. The wife's reticence creates a problem for the husband, for he does not experience the same discontinuity.

With the exception of the obligation to submit sexually, the wife quickly assumes after marriage the responsibility of her new role, as she is no stranger to the work of a homemaker. If she lives with her in-laws, she is reluctant to work for them, but she serves her husband. Tensions emerge, however, as a result of the husband's reluctance to institutionalize fully his obligation to his wife. The freedom and prerogatives of a single man are not quickly surrendered upon marriage. The new husband, particularly if he is consensually married, continues to spend a considerable portion of his earnings on drink, gambling, and other women. Evenings after work are likely to find him in convivial exchange with his friends on the street corners and in *cafetines* or in continued pursuit of women. A wife's attitude of resignation, of acceptance, of being *conforme*, does not apply to her husband's infidelity. A wife who learns of her husband's unfaithfulness fights with him and even, at times, with her sexual rival. Thus, there is a strain for the male between the role of a good husband and that of the all-conquering *macho* which is not relieved as long as the husband continues to participate in the activities associated with the he-man role.

The disparity between the achieved and aspired level of living presents the husbands and wives with another major strain. The fact that five persons out of six migrated into San Juan from farms and rural villages is indicative of a desire to be socially mobile. The urban complex reinforces and increases their aspirations by exposing them to the most affluent characteristics of Puerto Rican society. In their minds, subsistence farming, cutting cane, picking coffee beans, and curing tobacco are things of the past. The new object is to secure stable employment and reliable wages. Within reach, but only to be grasped tentatively on credit, are pastel refrigerators, oriental lamps, mahogany beds, and all the items of consumption advertised on television and radio. The clearest symbol of emerging aspirations is to be seen in the description of the house in which they some day hope to live. The men and women are almost of one voice in describing their dream home:

The house is to be located on high ground on a paved street on a lot 50 by 100 feet. The lot is near schools, stores, a church, and a playground. There is easy access to public transportation, doctors, and a hospital. The lot is enclosed by a concrete wall high enough to provide privacy for the family and protection for the children. The house is built of concrete, with floors covered with glazed ceramic tile, and the roof and ceiling are made of reinforced concrete. The kitchen and bathroom have glazed ceramic tile on the walls. The interior is divided into a kitchen, living and dining area, a bathroom, ample closet space, and two or three bedrooms. It has a porch and a patio in back.

The families want electricity properly installed in the home. They want city water in their homes with sinks in the kitchen and bathroom. They want also underground, sanitary sewers. The desired neighborhood is a quiet one. They want to live in an atmosphere of mutual friendship and respect with their neighbors.

The discrepancy between what the husbands and wives have and what they would like to have is clear when they speak about their children. Nearly all parents want their children to be professionals, enterprising businessmen, or white-collar workers. They want to rid the children of the stigma of manual work. The progress of the children in school is not commensurate with their ages, however, a problem which the parents seldom consider. Nor are the children punished or rewarded according to achievement. Rather, socialization of the child is addressed primarily at inculcating *respeto*, a traditional value more consistent with older social structures and less adapted to the upwardly mobile urban social structure. *Respeto* demands that you stay in your place and behave according to your publicly recognized, traditional status. The intrinsic difficulties of emerging from the culture of poverty are reinforced and compounded by the socialization of the children into a value complex that is not conducive to upward mobility. (To what extent will the children internalize the aspirations which their parents have for them? To what extent will economic development in Puerto Rico provide opportunities commensurate with the growing aspirations of the persons in the slums and *caseríos*? If such development fails to fulfill their aspirations, how will the children cope with the frustrations and disillusionments that the future will inevitably bring?)

Migration into the San Juan area has forced lower-status families to live in slums and *caseríos*. Severe overcrowding is one consequence of the rapid increase in the population of the area. Consanguineal and affinal relatives tend to live with or near one another. The extended family functions to ease the transition of the new migrant into the urban condition. The ecological clustering of relatives reflects and facilitates the operation of the norm of mutual help in the extended family. Beyond the extended family, the neighborhood is not integrated on a cooperative basis; rather, relations with neighbors are conflict ridden. Almost all husbands and wives are quick to recite a history of accumulated grievances against the neighbors who are derogated as dirty, noisy, immoral, and inconsiderate.

In a crowded slum or *caserío* a person can be seen and heard by neighbors to a much greater extent than in the less congested and more affluent residential areas. In the absence of privacy, when a husband beats his wife, curses her, or returns home drunk, his behavior is known throughout the neighborhood. When a child cries at night, the neighbors are awakened. What and how much a person eats is a matter of public knowledge. The delivery of a new pink refrigerator is observed and discussed by the neighbors. When the refrigerator is repossessed because credit payments have not been met, this also becomes a matter of gossip throughout the neighborhood. In brief, physical crowding makes persons visible to each other. Few opportunities are provided for a person to deviate surreptitiously from the folkways and mores of his neighborhood. The culprit is quickly identified and punished through gossip, ridicule, or insult. Since there are few economic and social differences between families in slums and *caseríos*, persons are classified and evaluated according to their conformity with cultural norms. The desirability of privacy, so clearly reflected in the high concrete wall which surrounds the dream house, is as understandable as the schizophrenic person's yearning for peace and tranquility away from the oppressive density of the neighborhood.

The effective social environment creates a series of common and repetitive difficulties with which a person must cope. It often prevents a smooth transition from one stage of the life cycle to the next. It imposes competing and contradictory demands on a person at specifiable periods in the life arc. It creates aspirations without providing the means for their achievement. It generates social processes which lead to conflict, mutual withdrawal, and alienation between neighbors. All together, the problems and tension points confronted by the typical husband and wife form a maze which they have entered but from which they have not emerged.

Over and above such problems, the trajectory of the life arc of each person who now suffers from schizophrenia is broken at a discernible point in time. Our second question focuses on the circumstances under which the break occurs. The break in the life arc coincides with a complex of interrelated crises the schizophrenic person experienced during the 12 months preceding the perceived onset of his illness. He views these critical experiences as personal dilemmas with which he has to wrestle and, in some way, solve. His competence is called into question by the crises he faces. His adequacy in the performance of his basic social roles as a man and a husband, or a woman and a wife, is on trial. Coping with the difficulties that encompass him becomes the central issue in his life.

Systematic comparisons of the six types of perceived personal problems reported by the sick persons (and families) with those of the well persons (and families) demonstrate that each of the diagnostic family types in the sick group encountered many more problems than the well families during the problematic year. There are more economic difficulties and more severe physical deprivation in the sick than in the well families. There are far more interspouse conflicts among the sick families than the control families; difficulties with members of the extended family are more frequent and more severe. The sick families report more quarrels and fights with their neighbors. There are more physical illnesses in the schizophrenic families. Finally, more sick persons than well persons, male as well as female, note a disparity between their own perception of the difficulties they encountered and the ways they think their spouses viewed these same problems. Stated otherwise, the schizophrenic men and women think their spouses do not understand the personal difficulties they face, as well as the men and women in the control group do. In general, the person who is diagnosed as suffering from schizophrenia perceives himself as bombarded by a multiplicity of personal and family problems he is not able to handle. The behavioral evidence shows, however, that he struggles to solve them by every means available to him.

At the time the illness is perceived to have started, the schizophrenic men felt unable to do their accustomed work. They had difficulties with their associates on the job, and as they withdrew from employment their earnings went down and they lost their sense of the ability to provide for their families. The schizophrenic men have a history of employment before the beginning of the problematic year neither more nor less erratic than the well men. A similar pattern is observed among the sick women, with the difference that prior to the onset of their symptoms they played the roles of wife and mother in the home; they did their work and were congenial members of family groups; they did not have extraordinary interpersonal difficulties with their neighbors. Since the perceived onset of the illness, it has been extremely difficult for the sick women to establish meaningful relations with other persons.

The acceleration of problems in the life of the vulnerable persons and in the family, combined with the self-awareness of role failure, appears to be a factor in the development of the illness. A husband who inadequately fulfills the role demands required of him has this fact brought to his attention by his wife, relatives, or other persons outside the immediate family. As a consequence, his failure creates interpersonal difficulties in the home, on the job, and, often, in the neighborhood. The sense of inadequacy which results from a failure to fulfill normal role requirements becomes an intrinsic part of his very being. Relentless social pressures are converted internally into emotional stress. The besieged person, unable to cope with his external and internal crises, becomes physically and mentally distraught. He becomes the victim of his failure.

External stresses and internal strains in one area of role performance tend to give rise to role failure in other areas of a person's life space. A heightened sense of personal inadequacy on the job or in child care creates more difficulties in the family, as other persons react to the social and psychological conflicts engendered by the distraught person. He, in turn, reacts to others in ways that exacerbate the pressures and stresses he feels, giving rise to additional interpersonal difficulties. Failure to cope with the dilemmas which beset him becomes manifest in his behavior as a concomitant of the decompensation that is occurring in his personality structure. The way the anxiety-ridden and fearful person, as well as others in his life space, interprets his behavior is another aspect of the problem that engulfs him.

Every sick person realizes that he is unable to fulfill his primary obligations to his family. The husband's cardinal roles revolve around his position as head of the family and his maleness. He is expected to earn the family's living; he is expected to make the basic decisions regarding the family's welfare. A man who is unable to hold a job has failed as principal provider for his wife and children. A man without money cannot capitalize on sexual opportunities in the world of the *macho*. The men emphasize, time after time, their inability to work because they are afflicted with a variety of physical ailments; they lament that their associates at work do not treat them as they did before the onset of their symptoms.

The women complain about their inability to take care of the household and the children. We infer that every bereaved mother has a profound sense of guilt, but to the schizophrenic mother the child's death is a constant symbol, however irrational, of her failure in the performance of a cardinal role in the woman's life. Her guilt is an intolerable burden; in some way she has violated the sacred trust of motherhood, and she cannot hide her sense of failure from her husband, her self, and her family.

The sick men and the sick women change, as worry over their personal difficulties grips their thoughts both day and night. The afflicted person becomes tense; he prepares for attacks from persons and situations in his immediate environment and from within himself. He experiences an overwhelming fatigue that limits his capacity to fulfill everyday obligations. He begins to define himself as ill, but the unpredictability of his aches and pains is puzzling. During this phase of his developing illness, the sick man is punished for his symptoms by his boss, work associates, neighbors, and relatives. He reacts to insults by fighting back in some instances and by withdrawal in others. In his search for a way out of the social and psychological labyrinth that enmeshes him, he begins to exhibit the behavior that the society defines as *locura*. The ailing person is haunted by the dread of becoming a *loco*.

The idiosyncratic, erratic, and hallucinatory person begins to disengage himself from normal social intercourse, as he fears the stigma of identification as a *loco*. Simultaneously, the social groups in which he has previously participated move away from him. This process is mutual on the part of the sick person and on the part of his associates outside the nuclear family with only two exceptions. The first is that the schizophrenic man married to a well woman does not alienate himself from his wife; he integrates himself more into his family than he did before the onset of his illness. The second exception is the sick person's and his spouse's interest in spiritualism. Spiritualistic groups do not withdraw from the mentally ill person; on the contrary, they encourage him to become an active member. The ideology of spiritualism provides an acceptable meaning to symptoms which are otherwise stigmatized.

A series of secondary problems come into existence. The ailing person has to cope with the crises that have come upon him: the internalized strains associated with his failure to meet his social obligations, the symptoms he reveals to his associates, and, finally, the heavily charged social definition of his illness. The problems encountered by the sick person overlap. The failure to solve one dilemma appears to condition the development of an additional one; a snowballing effect occurs until the person, enmeshed in insoluble difficulties, is overwhelmed. This is illustrated by the culmination of a series of unsolved problems Mrs. Gallardo encountered in her family which resulted in the hallucinatory experience of a hammer that beat, and beat, and beat her until she was crushed by its pounding.

As the person unsuccessfully struggles to disengage himself from his manifold conflicts, a break with reality occurs, and he decompensates into schizophrenia. Some dramatic event, such as the pounding of Mrs. Gallardo's spectral hammer, marks the overt break with reality. When this occurs, the afflicted person experiences a life quake, and the trajectory of the life arc is radically altered. Gradually, he begins to see himself as inept, inadequate, and unable to fulfill the normal demands of the social roles he had managed to satisfy previously.

The person who decompensates into a schizophrenic solution to his personal difficulties, metaphorically speaking, is caught in a trap with two compartments: one is the intermeshed series of insoluble dilemmas he encounters in his failure to fulfill the role requirements of his society; the other is the culturally defined role of the *loco*. The sick man or woman fears, as he searches for a way out of his personal maze of problems, that he may spring the catch on the trap that will make him a *loco*. To be recognized and treated as a *loco* is to be truly an outcast in this society which places a mentally ill person outside the bounds of a normal social life. The men and women did not solve their problems by becoming a schizophrenic; each one drifted into this mental condition unwillingly and unknowingly. All of them are haunted by the fear that they will be branded as *locos*.

The mentally healthy men and women are a sharp contrast to the schizophrenic ones. The well persons are capable of meeting the demands of their sociocultural environment, and they perform their social roles in adequate ways. They have social problems to meet, but they manage to solve them in acceptable ways. They have adjusted successfully to the conditions congruent with their socioeconomic status in this culture. They do not exhibit the phenomenon of a cataclysm that has broken the trajectory of the life arc. Persons who have not developed schizophrenia continue to trace a relatively smooth course in their relations with other persons. However, as we have shown, in Parts IV and V, the spouses of schizophrenics show the effects of their spouses' illness in their behavior patterns.

The etiological processes culminating in the development of schizophrenia may be of relatively recent origin. Childhood and adolescent experiences provide meager clues for an understanding of the way the illness develops. In contrast, at a recent and discernible period in the life arc prior to the eruption of overt symptomatology, a rash of insoluble, mutually reinforcing problems emerges to trap the person. We suggest that further research focus on this critical period. To arrive at a more precise understanding of the experiences and events which transpire during this period, field studies must develop research techniques to identify and measure the complex interactional processes which bind the person into intolerable dilemmas. We suggest further that the analysis of role performance in sick and well persons and families is a promising approach to understanding the development of schizophrenia.

The third question of this research focuses on the effect of schizophrenia on the family. Affinal and consanguineal relatives in the extended families of the persons who are free of schizophrenia are bound together by a norm of mutual help. The economic help exchanged ranges from token to total support. Persons are advised by relatives on how to solve problems. A crisis such as illness or death brings relatives together with offers to serve and to help. The women more than the men keep the bonds of kinship active and intact by identifying problems and marshaling resources to solve problems. Through a process of collecting and disseminating information, the women preserve the social visibility of even those relatives who do not live nearby.

Whereas the well families give more help than they receive, the sick families receive more help than they give. By dramatizing the husband's illness and the financial problems of the family, the well wife married to a sick husband draws social, emotional, and economic help from her relatives. The help is continuing and pervasive, thus enabling her to maintain the stability of the family. As a result, the husband-schizophrenic families are more closely linked to the wife's relatives than to the husband's. In the wife-schizophrenic and double schizophrenic families, the relationship of the nuclear to the extended family is fragmented. Each spouse seeks help from his blood relatives but not from his in-laws. The help that each receives is designed for his or her own individual benefit and not for that of the entire family. Conflict with in-laws emerges as each spouse seeks solace and support from his relatives by complaining to them about his mate. The impact of schizophrenia on the extended family operates through the nuclear family, particularly the relationship between the husband and wife.

Role performance in the families free of schizophrenia are in accord with expectations common in the culture. The division of labor requires that the husband be the breadwinner, the wife the homemaker. At home the husband can be aloof from household details and problems, yet he maintains final control over the major decisions which affect the family. The wife accepts his authority, defers to him, and endeavors to serve him by keeping an orderly and tranquil home. With the perceived onset of the illness, a drastic change ensues in the husband-schizophrenic families. As the husband withdraws from social relations with colleagues, associates, and friends, the wife endeavors to cope with the economic problems created by his inability to work. Soon, the wife seeks full-time employment in a factory or as a servant. At home, she nurtures and protects the husband; she takes him to *curanderas*, spiritualistic mediums, and psychiatrists. An unplanned result of this process is that the wife gains increments of control over her husband who is relegated to a dependent role. The work roles are reversed as the family reorganizes itself to cope with the illness. By this method, many tensions in the family are alleviated.

The onset of the wife's illness has an opposite effect on the family, irrespective of the husband's mental status: tension points are exacerbated, and the family is disorganized. The sick wife repeatedly denies her husband sexual intercourse. She criticizes him for his meager earnings. She defies his authority, exchanges insults with him, and engages him in physical brawls. The well husband married to a sick woman often philanders, spending his free time away from home. If he also is sick, he withdraws into his home only to be confronted by a belligerent wife with whom he now has a greater opportunity to fight. The discord, confusion, and chaos of the families with a sick mother envelop the children who are more often psychiatrically disturbed and retarded in their educational development than are the children of well mothers. These findings clearly demonstrate that there is a relationship between the sex role of the afflicted person and the solidarity, harmony, and stability of the nuclear and extended family.

The most striking and pervasive characteristic of the sick man's relationship to his wife and to other members of the extended family is his dependence on them. This is incongruous with the cultural definition of the *macho*, which emphasizes strength of character, independence, and freedom. The theme of the sick woman is rebellion against both her husband and other figures of authority. Such a rebellious attitude is inconsistent with the ideals of feminine behavior; a woman is expected to be humble, deferential, and conforming. The disparity between behavior and the ideals embodied in social roles gives rise to problems for the sick wife which do not emerge when only the husband is sick. Irrespective of the mental status of the husband, a male is not attuned by attitude, temperament, or skill to cope with the problems created by a sick wife. He is indifferent to her complaints, strives to coerce her into behaving more appropriately, or escapes from the house to participate in street-corner activities with his peers. His behavior does not compensate for her lack of normal role performance as does that of the well wife married to a sick husband. In point of fact, the husband's responses are not only inflexible and unadaptive, given the requirements of the family situation, but also serve to provoke the sick wife into greater rebellion, irritation, and despair.

The complex coping sequence involving a reversal of roles in the husband-schizophrenic families is probably facilitated by conditions, facts, and events traceable to courtship and to the types of union formed. The men who are now schizophrenic, more often than the well men, married women their own age or older, courted according to the *entrada* pattern, and established legal unions at the beginning of the present marriage. Such findings suggest that the sick men paired themselves with women who would give them social support in a marriage to which they both had a strong commitment from the beginning. This hypothesis is probably more applicable to the sick men who married well women than to those who married sick women. The wife-schizophrenic families resemble the control families in the age differences between the spouses, the type of courtship pattern which led to the marriage, and the type of union, either legal or consensual, which was established at the beginning of the marriage.

To understand more fully the relationship between the sex role of the afflicted person and the dynamics of family life, it is extremely important to consider the successive pressures, problems, and constraints impinging on the husband and wife from the time of marriage. An examination of the husband-schizophrenic families demonstrates this point. At the beginning of the marriage, the sick men were working full time as breadwinners for the family. The occupational histories of the sick men show no evidence of erratic employment before marriage or during the first years of marriage. Correlatively, the well wives of the sick men did not work away from home during the early stages of the marriage. As in the other diagnostic family groups, the women who were employed left work when they got married because their husbands insisted they devote themselves to the tasks of a homemaker. The husband's performance of the several roles congruent with his position was no different than that of the husbands in the control group. The perceived onset of the illness occurred after marriage when the sick man encountered difficulties at work. He left work, withdrew from friends and associates, and entrenched himself in the nuclear family. In an effort to solve the economic problems resulting from a disabled breadwinner, the wife sought employment. Thus the reversal of work roles occurred after the perceived onset of the illness. Before the symptoms began the husband-schizophrenic families resembled the families who are free of schizophrenia. Similarly, the stormy relationship between the spouses in the wife-schizophrenic and double schizophrenic families can be traced to the decompensation of the ill persons into schizophrenia.

Here we have shown that schizophrenia is associated with inadequate role performance of the person who is afflicted. A disparity emerges between what the person does and what he ought to do according to the expectations embodied in his roles. As a result of this change, the role performance of his spouse is also changed. The sick or well husband married to a schizophrenic wife alters his behavior in such a way as to intensify and perpetuate the problems created by the wife's illness, but the well wife copes with the problems created by her husband's illness. Fundamentally, her ability to cope derives from the general role of women in the culture. Women more than men specialize in matters of illness, and it is the women who bear the burden of socioemotional support in time of illness and distress. Our data amply demonstrate the zest and vitality with which women pursue paramedical functions both in the nuclear and extended family. Beyond the family, the roles of women as midwives, spiritualistic mediums, and *curanderas* are deeply enmeshed in the culture.

Her role integrates the woman deeply into the extended family as a social system. Unlike the man who participates in a variety of activities which often compete with his obligations to the family, the woman's horizons, her social space, and the effective setting in which she enacts her role are encompassed by the family system of which she is a member. She is centrally located in the communicative structure of the family and is able to bring resources from one part of the system to bear on problems in another part. The sacred bonds of motherhood which unite her with her children reinforce her commitment to preserve order, consistency, and stability in family life.

Future research may show that when a wife confronts the problems resulting from a disabled husband afflicted with an illness other than schizophrenia she will proceed to cope with them, much as do the wives in the husband-schizophrenic families. An understanding of the functions which women perform in the family leads to this hypothesis. Further research should note, however, that schizophrenia impairs a person physically, mentally, and socially and that, consequently, the wife must face a peculiar combination of problems. In addition to the loss of the breadwinner, the well wife must cope with a husband who is fearful, nervous, fatigued, and withdrawn and who experiences pains and ailments that are as pervasive as they are fickle. Hallucinations and delusions afflict the sick man. Doubts about his masculinity emerge. Fears of becoming a *loco* haunt his thoughts. He behaves in odd and idiosyncratic ways, at times even revolting against the power of his self-sacrificing and benevolent wife. He is scorned, ridiculed, punished, and downgraded by his fellow men. Could it be that such problems provide an extraordinary test of the supportive, therapeutic, and family-centered dimension of the wife's role in the family?

Does such a test resulting from the husband's illness take its toll from the wife? During the 5 years prior to the field work, the wife's rate of physical illness per 100 years of risk doubled over what it had been during the period from marriage to 5 years prior to the beginning of the field work. During the 5 years before the field work began, her rate of physical illness was almost four times that of the women in the control group. The case study of the problematic year in the Gallardo family (Chapter 10) shows clearly that the husband's decompensation into schizophrenia creates multiple problems involving subsistence, health, and interpersonal relations. The impact of these problems centered on Mrs. Gallardo who believes her husband's illness is causing her own emotional disturbance. She is probably right. Could the increased rate of physical illness of the well wives married to sick men be an ominous prelude to what the future holds in store for women who confront similar problems?

Our findings indicate that the impact a disabled wife, with a galaxy of disturbing symptoms, has on the nuclear and extended family is pervasive and disruptive; her symptoms corrode the marital union, her children are trapped in a disorganized family milieu, and the extended family is fragmented. All these consequences serve to reaffirm the functional importance of the woman's role in preserving the inner coherence of the family. If the woman were afflicted with a physical handicap visible to her and to her husband instead of with a functional mental illness, would such a handicap serve to rationalize her inability to perform her role normally? The husband's response would probably be less harsh and more understanding. Would he then assume a supportive role and perform all the functions associated with the woman's role? We suggest that it is difficult, if not impossible, for the husband to bridge the role discontinuity this question raises. It implies that the husband would perform role functions inconsistent with the norms of masculinity which pervade the culture and according to which the men are socialized.

We invite further research to test, enlarge, or modify the ideas generated by this study.

APPENDIX 1

TABLE 1 Accumulative Proportion of Individuals by Age and Sex in the San Juan Metropolitan Area, as Given in the 1950 United States Census and the Sample Survey of 1957. (This Area Covers the Municipal Districts of Aguas Buenas, Bayamón, Caguas, Carolina, Cataño, Dorado, Guaynabo, Gurabo, Juncos, Loíza, Río Grande, Río Piedras, San Juan, Toa Alta, Toa Baja, Trujillo Alto.)

AGE GROUP, YEARS	MALES		FEMALES		BOTH SEXES	
	CENSUS	SAMPLE	CENSUS	SAMPLE	CENSUS	SAMPLE
Under 5	.1595	.1392	.1526	.1430	.1559	.1412
5–9	.2923	.2323	.2820	.2913	.2870	.2918
10–14	.4054	.4254	.3913	.4241	.3982	.4247
15–19	.5005	.5224	.4967	.5240	.4985	.5232
20–24	.5934	.6049	.6012	.6080	.5972	.6065
25–29	.6750	.6619	.6856	.6687	.6802	.6653
30–34	.7418	.7206	.7506	.7354	.7461	.7283
35–39	.8044	.7789	.8124	.7986	.8083	.7891
40–44	.8492	.8272	.8536	.8392	.8513	.8334
45–49	.8966	.8755	.8869	.8734	.8866	.8744
50–54	.9199	.9085	.9189	.9055	.9193	.9060
55–59	.9425	.9376	.9390	.9334	.9406	.9354
60–64	.9648	.9602	.9596	.9545	.9620	.9572
65–69	.9788	.9747	.9742	.9732	.9763	.9739
70–74	.9878	.9846	.9834	.9845	.9854	.9845
75–84	.9964	.9968	.9940	.9943	.9950	.9955
85 or more	.9992	.9991	.9992	.9992	.9990	.9991

TABLE 2 Accumulative Proportion of Individuals in Households of Different Sizes in the San Juan Metropolitan Area in the 1950 United States Census and the Sample Survey of 1957. (This Area Covers the Municipal Districts of Aguas Buenas, Bayamón, Caguas, Carolina, Cataño, Dorado, Guaynabo, Gurabo, Juncos, Loíza, Río Grande, Río Piedras, San Juan, Toa Alta, Toa Baja, Trujillo Alto.)

NO. OF PERSONS IN HOUSEHOLD	CUMULATIVE PROPORTIONS	
	CENSUS	SAMPLE
1	.0721	.0670
2	.1968	.2098
3	.3429	.3641
4	.5002	.5431
5	.6415	.6947
6	.7533	.7934
7	.8372	.8613
8	.8955	.9062
9	.9362	.9379
10 and more	.9994	.9996

APPENDIX 2

Summary of Mental Status Examination

ITEM	STATISTICAL SIGNIFICANCE	
	MALES	FEMALES
How patient meets examiner		
P. 1, I, B-2 Receptiveness (less)	$p < .05$	$p > .05$
Consciousness		
P. 3, II, C-1 Alertness (less)	$p < .01$	$p > .05$
C-5 Estrangement (more)	$p < .01$	$p < .01$
C-6 Depersonalization (more)	$p < .01$	$p < .01$
C-7a Time, sense of (less)	$p > .05$	$p < .01$
Perceptive activity		
P. 4, II, D-1 Illusions (more)	$p < .05$	$p < .01$
D-2 Hallucinations (more)	$p < .01$	$p < .01$
Thought patterns		
P. 5, III, A-1 Realistic thinking (less)	$p < .01$	$p < .01$
A-5 Phobias (more)	$p < .01$	$p > .05$
A-6 Obsessions (more)	$p > .05$	$p < .01$
A-7 Fixed ideas (more)	$p < .05$	$p < .01$
A-8 Delusions (more)	$p < .01$	$p < .01$
A-9 Paucity of ideas (more)	$p < .05$	$p > .05$
Thought processes		
P. 6, III, B-1 Speed (less)	$p < .05$	$p < .05$
B-2 Distractability (more)	$p < .05$	$p < .01$
B-3 Order and organization (less)	$p < .01$	$p < .01$
B-4 Associative trends (fewer)	$p < .01$	$p < .01$
B-6 Forgetfulness (more)	$p < .01$	$p < .01$
B-7 Blocking (more)	$p > .05$	$p < .01$
B-9 Incoherence (more)	$p < .01$	$p < .01$
B-10 Irrelevance (more)	$p < .01$	$p < .01$
B-11 Distorted thinking (more)	$p < .01$	$p < .01$
B-12a Autistic (more)	$p < .01$	$p < .01$
B-12f Concrete (more)	$p < .01$	$p < .01$
B-12g Suspicious (more)	$p < .01$	$p < .01$
B-12h Paranoid (more)	$p < .01$	$p < .01$
Powers of abstract and rational thinking		
P. 7, III, C-2 Judgment (less rational)	$p < .05$	$p < .01$

422 Appendix 2

Summary of Mental Status Examination (*Continued*)

ITEM			STATISTICAL SIGNIFICANCE	
			MALES	FEMALES
Emotions				
P. 8, IV,	A-1	Cheerful (less)	$p < .01$	$p < .05$
	A-4	Bland (more)	$p > .05$	$p < .05$
	A-5	Blunted (more)	$p < .01$	$p < .05$
	A-8	Rage (more)	$p > .05$	$p < .01$
	A-10	Fearful (more)	$p > .05$	$p < .01$
	A-12	Anxious (more)	$p < .01$	$p > .05$
	A-16	Suspicious (more)	$p < .05$	$p < .01$
Motor responses				
P. 9, V,	A-1	Spontaneity (less)	$p < .01$	$p < .01$
	A-2	Energy (less)	$p < .01$	$p < .01$
	A-3	Persistence (less)	$p < .01$	$p < .01$
	A-5a	Restlessness (more)	$p < .05$	$p < .01$
	A-5b	Agitations (more)	$p > .05$	$p < .01$
	A-5c	Impulsiveness (more)	$p < .01$	$p < .01$
	A-5e	Verbose (more)	$p > .05$	$p < .05$
P. 10, V,	A-6a	Inertia (more)	$p < .01$	$p < .01$
	A-6b	Inhibitions (more)	$p < .01$	$p < .01$
	B-1	Constructive (less)	$p < .01$	$p > .05$
	B-2	Careful (less)	$p < .05$	$p < .05$
	B-4	Helpful (less)	$p > .05$	$p < .05$
	B-5	Ineffective (more)	$p < .05$	$p < .01$
	B-6	Inefficient (more)	$p < .01$	$p < .01$
	B-9a	Manual (less)	$p < .05$	$p > .05$
Inappropriate actions				
P. 11, V,	C-2	Compulsions (more)	$p > .05$	$p < .01$
	C-7	Withdrawal (more)	$p < .01$	$p < .01$
	C-9	Peculiar habits of drinking, eating, smoking, etc.	$p > .05$	$p < .01$
	C-12	Abnormal sleeping habits	$p < .01$	$p < .01$
	C-15	Sex (abnormalities)	$p > .05$	$p < .01$
	C-16	Incongruities between emotions and actions (more)	$p < .01$	$p < .01$
	C-17	Incongruities—thought and action (more)	$p < .01$	$p < .01$

Summary of Mental Status Examination (*Continued*)

ITEM			STATISTICAL SIGNIFICANCE	
			MALES	FEMALES
Relations with other people				
P. 12, VI,	A-1	Bland (more)	$p > .05$	$p < .05$
	A-2	Rigid (more)	$p > .05$	$p < .05$
	A-3	Quiet (more)	$p > .05$	$p < .05$
	A-5	Submissive (more)	$p < .01$	$p > .05$
	A-7	Afraid (more)	$p < .01$	$p > .05$
	A-16	Demanding (more)	$p > .05$	$p < .05$
	A-17	Aggressive (more)	$p > .05$	$p < .01$
	A-18	Hostile (more)	$p > .05$	$p < .05$
Relates to self				
P. 13, VII,	A-1	Self as an individual (less realistic)	$p < .01$	$p < .01$
	A-2	Self to others (less realistic)	$p < .01$	$p < .01$
	A-3	Toward body size (less realistic)	$p < .01$	$p < .01$
	A-4	Toward strength (less realistic)	$p < .05$	$p < .01$
	A-5	Toward shape (less realistic)	$p < .01$	$p < .05$
	A-6	Toward body, organs, functions	$p < .01$	$p < .01$
	A-7	Toward mind and thinking organs	$p < .01$	$p < .01$
	A-8	Special abilities and aptitudes	$p < .01$	$p < .05$
	A-9	Self as man or woman (less real)	$p < .05$	$p < .01$
	A-10	Personal possessions (less real)	$p < .05$	$p < .05$
	A-11	Money (less real)	$p < .05$	$p < .05$
	A-12	Health (less real)	$p < .01$	$p < .01$
	A-13	Illness (less real)	$p < .05$	$p < .01$
	A-14	Ambitions (less real)	$p < .01$	$p < .01$
	A-15	Frustrations (nonrealistic)	$p < .01$	$p < .01$
	A-16	Fears (nonrealistic)	$p < .01$	$p < .01$
	A-17	Sex life (nonrealistic)	$p < .05$	$p < .01$
	A-17a	Lack of sex life (nonrealistic)	$p < .05$	$p < .01$
Toward other people				
P. 15, VII,	B-1	At home (less realistic)	$p < .01$	$p < .01$
	B-2	Work (less realistic)	$p < .01$	$p < .01$
	B-3	Church (less realistic)	$p < .01$	$p < .01$
	B-4	Community (less realistic)	$p < .01$	$p < .01$
	B-5	Strangers (less realistic)	$p < .01$	$p < .01$
	B-6	Crowds (less realistic)	$p < .01$	$p < .01$
	B-7	Individuals (less realistic)	$p < .01$	$p < .01$
	B-8	Religious (less realistic)	$p < .01$	$p < .05$

424   Appendix 2

Summary of Mental Status Examination (*Continued*)

ITEM			STATISTICAL SIGNIFICANCE	
			MALES	FEMALES
P. 15, VII,	B-9	Political parties (realistic)	$p < .05$	$p < .01$
	B-10	People of same sex (realistic)	$p < .05$	$p < .01$
	B-11	People of opposite sex (realistic)	$p < .01$	$p < .01$
	B-12	People in authority (realistic)	$p < .05$	$p < .01$
	B-13	Superiors (realistic)	$p < .05$	$p < .01$
	B-14	Peers (realistic)	$p < .01$	$p < .01$
	B-15	Subordinates (realistic)	$p < .05$	$p < .01$
Attitudes toward special situations				
P. 16, VII,	C-1	Home (less favorable)	$p < .01$	$p < .01$
	C-2	Education (less favorable)	$p < .05$	$p < .01$
	C-3	Marriage (less favorable)	$p < .01$	$p < .01$
	C-4	Children (less favorable)	$p < .01$	$p < .01$
	C-5	Responsibility (less favorable)	$p < .05$	$p < .01$
	C-6	Discipline (less favorable)	$p < .01$	$p < .01$
	C-7	Religion (less favorable)	$p < .05$	$p < .05$
	C-8	Social customs (less favorable)	$p < .05$	$p < .05$
	C-9	Morals (less favorable)	$p < .05$	$p < .05$
	C-10	Individual activities (less favorable)	$p < .01$	$p < .01$
	C-11	Group activities (less favorable)	$p < .01$	$p < .01$
	C-12	Community and state activities (less favorable)	$p < .01$	$p < .01$
	C-13	Authority (less favorable)	$p < .01$	$p < .01$
	C-14	Money (less favorable)	$p < .05$	$p < .01$
	C-15	Wealth (less favorable)	$p < .05$	$p < .01$
	C-16	Power (less favorable)	$p < .05$	$p < .05$

APPENDIX 3

TABLE 1 Replies to Question: "Do Your Hands Tremble to a Noticeable Extent?"

	OFTEN OR SOMETIMES, %	NEVER, %
A. Males		
Nonschizophrenic	49	95
Schizophrenic	51	5
$N =$	19	21
$p < .01$		
B. Females		
Nonschizophrenic	52	89
Schizophrenic	48	11
$N =$	23	17
$p < .05$		

TABLE 2 Replies to Question: "Have You Ever Noticed Your Heart Beating Very Hard?"

	OFTEN OR SOMETIMES, %	NEVER, %
A. Males		
Nonschizophrenic	61	100
Schizophrenic	39	0
$N =$	28	12
$p < .05$		
B. Females		
Nonschizophrenic	52	93
Schizophrenic	48	7
$N =$	25	15
$p < .01$		

TABLE 3 Replies to Question: "Have You Ever Had Dizzy Spells?"

	OFTEN OR SOMETIMES, %	NEVER, %
A. Males		
Nonschizophrenics	55	94
Schizophrenics	45	6
$N =$	22	18
$p < .01$		
B. Females		
Nonschizophrenics	56	92
Schizophrenics	44	8
$N =$	27	13
$p < .05$		

TABLE 4 Replies to Question: "Do You Have Shortness of Breath While Still and Not Exercising?"

	OFTEN OR SOMETIMES, %	NEVER, %
A. Males		
Nonschizophrenic	40	92
Schizophrenic	60	8
$N =$	15	25
$p < .01$		
B. Females		
Nonschizophrenic	43	94
Schizophrenic	57	6
$N =$	21	19
$p < .01$		

TABLE 5 Replies to Question: "Do You Have Cold Sweats?"

	OFTEN OR SOMETIMES, %	NEVER, %
A. Males		
Nonschizophrenic	44	95
Schizophrenic	56	5
$N =$	18	22
$p < .01$		
B. Females		
Nonschizophrenic	45	94
Schizophrenic	55	6
$N =$	22	18
$p < .01$		

TABLE 6 Replies to Question: "Have You Ever Noticed a Throbbing or Pulse in Your Neck?"

	OFTEN OR SOMETIMES, %	NEVER, %
A. Males		
Nonschizophrenic	46	91
Schizophrenic	54	9
$N =$	17	23
$p < .01$		
B. Females		
Nonschizophrenic	39	90
Schizophrenic	61	10
$N =$	18	22
$p < .01$		

TABLE 7 Replies to Question: "Does Your Chest Ever Feel Tight?"

	OFTEN OR SOMETIMES, %	NEVER, %
A. Males		
Nonschizophrenic	60	93
Schizophrenic	40	7
$N =$	25	15
$p < .05$		
B. Females		
Nonschizophrenic	52	93
Schizophrenic	48	7
$N =$	25	15
$p < .01$		

APPENDIX 4

me veo hay veces mal otras
mejor ahora lo mas que me preocupa
es causa de la señora, y me enfermo que ay dias que no tengo animo
para salir a trabajar como muy decaido
y me dan mareos apenas duermo
es penzando en tantas cosas paso hay
veces que los dias sin almorzar y vengo
a comer tarde. mi doña, hay veces que
no se apura ni por ella misma
porq. se aqueja de muchos dolores
y siempre a sido calmosa y poquita
para hacer las cosas, y yo sufro
al verla enferma imposibilitada
para todo y por todo esto yo me encuentro
enfermo porque tengo tos y no tengo
tuve al nene y se a quedado mal
de su organismo y para completar
por descuidos se a dado golpes
en la cabeza.

Index

Accidents and schizophrenia, 108–09, 159–60
Adolescent rebellion, 119, 134, 138–39
Armsen, P., 40
Aspirations, 181, 288–89, 299, 308, 390–93, 407–08
Ay Bendito! attitude, 312

Beckett, P. B. S., 4
Bowen, M., 4

Cafetín, description of, 236
Caserío, description of, 58–59
Childhood of spouses, and schizophrenia, 69–97, 405, 413
  parental controls, 85–89
  self-perceptions, 96, 100–01
  See also: Adolescent rebellion; Education; Fear; Illness, mental; Illness, physical; Parent-child relations; Socialization
Children of families, and fieldworkers, 37, 381–83, 395
  and schizophrenia, 328, 381–82, 383, 384, 393–94, 413
  death of, 161–71, 194–95, 411
  distribution of, 381
  economic burden of, 278
  emotional stability of, 212–13, 395–98
  See also: Aspirations; Discipline; Illness, physical; Parent-child relations
Clark, R. E., 6
Clausen, J. L., 4

Conformance of wife, 251, 271, 302, 318, 406
Control families, children, 395–96
  conflicts, 334–38, 350–51, 386–87
  mutual help, 180–81, 349–59
  problematic year, 176–81
  psychiatric evaluation, 175–76
  selection of, 18–19
  social control in, 294–301
  See also: Employment; Fear; Hospitalization; Marriage; Parent-child relations; Spouse relations
Courtship, and schizophrenia, 147–48
  clandestine, 137–40, 405
  entrada pattern, 136–37, 177, 405
  problems of, 136–40, 405–06
  See also: Adolescent rebellion; Sex
Cultural shock, 127

Death, and schizophrenia, 166–70, 194–95, 200
  fear of, 166, 185, 231
  of children, 166–71, 411
Dignidad, concept of, 266
Discipline, and schizophrenia, 88–89, 385–90
  as a source of conflict, 385–90
  of children, 85–89, 385–90, 407
Double schizophrenic families, children, 328, 389, 397–98
  conflict, 325, 327, 343–45, 389
  disorganization, 321–22, 415
  fantasy world of women, 273–74, 383
  hostility of women, 325, 369

431

Double schizophrenic families, mutual help, 367–70
  problematic year, 200–14
  psychiatric evaluation, 197–200
  social control, 321–33
  violence, 211, 328, 342, 368
  See also: Employment; Fear; Hospitalization; Marriage; Parent-child relations; Sex; Spouse relations
Dunham, H. W., 6

Economic problems and schizophrenia, 84, 184–85, 203–04, 279, 288–91, 362–63, 401
Economic structure, 276–85, 296–97
Education, and schizophrenia, 109–112
  attitudes toward, 63, 109–10, 391–93
  in children of families, 391–93, 407
  in families of orientation, 71–72
  in spouses, 109–10
  problems in school, 110–11
Employment, and schizophrenia, 112–14, 120, 121, 190–91, 208, 285, 286, 287–92, 301, 308, 322–23, 324, 401, 411
  job history, 112–14, 119–24, 289
  of men, 119–24, 286
  of women, 112–14, 119–24, 284, 295–96, 302–03, 304

Families, aspirations of, 288, 289, 308, 390–93, 407–08
  cohesion of, 264–65
  composition of, 82–83
  criteria for selection, 16–17
  fieldworkers' rapport with, 31, 35–36, 241, 295, 297, 382
  "ideal" roles in, 265–66, 267, 382–83, 384
  impact of schizophrenia on, 153–57, 179–80, 264–65, 413
  interpersonal relations in, 263–75
  location of, 17–19, 33–34
  mutual help in, 238, 347–59, 413–14
  of orientation, 69–84, 89–97, 404
  pseudonyms, 40–41
  representativeness of, 19–21, 402
  reversal of roles in, 303–08, 340–41, 361, 415, 416–17

Families, ruptured, 77–82
  study group defined, 8, 402–04
  See also: Children; Control families; Double schizophrenic families; Economic problems; Husband-schizophrenic families; Illness, mental; Illness, physical; Marriage; Parent-child relations; Spouse relations; Wife-schizophrenic families
Faris, R. E. L., 6
Fear, and schizophrenia, 103–05, 230–33, 341
  fieldworkers', 28–30
  in childhood, 103–05
  of death, 166, 185, 231
  of *loco* role, 216–20, 221–22, 227, 363, 412–13, 417
  of *locos*, 180, 216, 218–20, 372–73
  of sexual intercourse, 143, 341
  parental, 134
Fieldworkers, and children of families, 37, 381–82, 395
  fears of, 28–30
  freedom in interviewing, 15
  functions of, 10, 263–65
  problems of, 28–39, 239–40
  rapport with families, 31, 35–36, 241, 395, 397
  selection of, 11, 404
  training of, 395, 397
  See also: Interviewing; Schedules
Fleck, S., 4

Gerard, D. L., 4

Harding, J. S., 5
Hollingshead, A. B., 5, 6, 16
Hospitalization, for mental illness, 6, 153–54, 243
  for physical illness, 107–08, 162–63
  See also: Referral
Houston, L. G., 4
Hughes, C. C., 5
Husband-schizophrenic families, children, 306, 386, 388
  conflicts, 388
  mutual help, 360–63
  problematic year, 181–88

Husband-schizophrenic families, psychiatric evaluation, 181–83
    reduction of income, 302, 303–04, 361, 362, 371
    role reversal, 303–08, 340–41, 415
    See also: Employment; Fear; Hospitalization; Marriage; Parent-child relations; Sex; Spouse relations

Illness, mental, and rate of physical illness, 157–61
    diagnosis of, 22–23
    fear of, 180, 216–20
    explanations for, 224–30
    in children of families, 212–13
    in families of orientation, 153–57, 178–79, 225, 366, 404
    perceptions of, 153–55, 215–30, 243–54
    See also: Loco; Treatment
Illness, physical, accidents, 108–09, 123, 131, 159–60
    and schizophrenia, 108–09, 157–66
    by mental diagnosis, 107–08, 129–30
    in children of families, 165–66, 178, 191, 194–95, 200–02
    See also: Hospitalization; Treatment
Income, aspirations, 288–89
    sources of, 285–87
    See also: Economic problems; Employment; Mutual help
Inouye, E., 3
Interviewing, problems of, 28–39
    schizophrenics, 35–37, 403, 404
    See also: Fieldworkers; Schedules
Irizarry, de, A. C., 20

Jackson, D. D., 4
Jaco, E. G., 4
Jobs, *See* Employment

Kallman, F. J., 3
Kardec, A., 245, 246, 247, 254
Kay, D. W. K., 4
Kluckhohn, C., 3
Kohn, M. L., 4

Lambo, T. A., 5
Langner, T. S., 5

Leighton, A. H., 5
Leighton, D. C., 5, 6
Lidz, T., 4
Loco, attitudes toward, 15, 215, 225
    fear of identification with, 216–20, 221, 227, 263, 374, 411–13, 417
    role of, 218–21, 412–13, 417
    See also: Illness, mental
Luxenburger, H., 3

Macho, concept of, 134–36, 236, 271, 301, 333, 342, 383, 406, 415
Macklin, D. B., 5
Macmillan, A., 5, 13, 24, 42
Marriage, and schizophrenia, 147–48, 314–31, 406, 415–16
    attitudes toward, 144
    conflicts in, 333–46, 385–90, 406
    consensual, 140, 144–45, 196
    disillusionments in, 268–69, 270–73, 276–77
    expectations from, 141, 265–69
    infidelity, 74–75, 76, 78, 178, 186, 193, 195, 271, 333–46
    legal, 140, 144–46
    remarriage, 145–46
    respeto in, 266–67, 293
    satisfactions in, 268–69, 270
    stability of, 144–46
    tensions in, 143
    See also: Courtship; Families; Men; Sex
Mediums, *See* Spiritualism
Men, authority of, 296, 297–98
    freedom of, 233–34, 236, 271, 293–94, 318
    "ideal" roles, 266, 383–84
    marital dilemma, 271, 274–75
    marital dissatisfaction, 268–70
    marital expectations, 265–66
    role of, 301, 336, 371, 410–11, 415
    socialization of, 98–114, 119–20, 332–33
    See also: Macho
Michael, S. T., 5
Mobility, geographic, 125–27, 407, 418
    residential, 59, 127–29
    social, 277, 392, 407, 408
Morel, B. A., 3

Murphy, J. M., 5
Murray, H. A., 3
Mutual help, and schizophrenia, 360–77, 372–73, 413–14
  as a norm, 180–81, 238, 286–87, 370–71
  defined, 347–48
  in families, 238, 347–59, 413–14
  matriarch role in, 357–58
  wife's part in, 356–59, 362–63, 413, 417
Myers, J. K., 5

Neighborhood, acceptance of, 393–95
  See also: Aspirations
Neighbors, as a stress, 180–81, 194, 206–07, 211–12, 237, 316, 336, 394, 395, 408, 413, 417
  See also: Withdrawal

Opler, M. K., 5

Parent-child relations, 85–97, 382–84
  adolescent rebellion, 119, 134, 138–39
  and adult schizophrenia, 85–97, 383, 384
  parental controls, 85–89, 103, 134
  personality formation, 98–115
  respeto in, 85, 134, 385
  with schizophrenic fathers, 388
  with schizophrenic mothers, 383, 385, 389
  See also: Aspirations; Courtship; Discipline; Socialization
Psychiatric evaluation, of spouses, 22–23, 39, 174–76, 181–83, 188–90, 197–200
  reliability of, 23–27
  See also: Psychiatrists; Schedules
Psychiatrists, and spiritualism, 244
  attitudes toward, 243, 403
  reliability of, 23–27
  See also: Psychiatric evaluation; Treatment
Puerto Rico, history of, 44–45, 46

Rapaport, R. N., 5
Redlich, F. C., 5, 6
Referral (psychiatric), 17, 243
  See also: Hospitalization; Treatment
Reichard, S., 4
Religion, and schizophrenia, 254–56, 329
  and social class, 63
  and spiritualism, 255
  as therapy, 256
  in families, 256–58
  Mita, 257–58
Rennie, T. A. C., 5
Respeto, concept of, 85, 134, 266–67, 293, 307, 313, 385, 408
Roberts, B. H., 5
Rogler, L. H., 10, 30, 397
Role performance and schizophrenia, 293, 314, 318, 364, 371, 373, 383, 405, 409, 411, 414–15, 417–18
Role reversal in husband-schizophrenic families, 303–08, 340–41, 361, 415, 416–17
Rosenthal, D., 4
Roth, B., 3
Roth, M., 4

San Juan, growth, 33, 45, 46
  physical description, 45–46, 49
  population, by class, 46–47
    by education, 48–49
    by income, 51
    by marital status, 52
    by occupation, 46–48
    by residence, 49–50
Sanua, V. D., 4
Schedules, administration of, 14–15, 18
  analysis of, 21, 39–41, 59, 264, 288–89, 402–03
  assessment, 41
  Conceptions of Mental Health, 13
  development of, 11–12
  Family Life, 13, 14
  H. O. S., 12–13, 23–27
  Life History, 13
  Mental Status Examination, 12, 14, 22, 23, 26
  Problematic Areas, 14, 173–75
  Screening, 12, 14, 18

Schedules, Spiritualism in Everyday Life, 7–8, 244
  See also: Fieldworkers; Interviewing
Schizophrenia, and adolescent experiences, 112–32, 405
  and courtship patterns, 147–48
  and cultural shock, 127
  and death of child, 166–70, 194–95, 200, 411
  and early childhood experiences, 60–97, 98–114, 404–05
  and economic problems, 84, 184–85, 203–04, 208, 287, 288–91, 309, 362
  and education, 109–12
  and employment, 112–15, 120, 121, 190–91, 208, 285, 287–92, 301, 308, 322–23, 401
  and family cohesion, 77–82, 263–65
  and fantasy world of women, 273–74, 383
  and geographic mobility, 125–27, 407
  and hostility of women, 325–69, 415
  and job history, 121–24, 361
  and marriage, 147–48, 314–31, 406, 415–16
  and mutual help, 360–77, 413–14
  and need to confide, 36, 240–41, 404
  and nightmares, 104–05, 405
  and physical illness, 107, 157–61, 417–18
  and religion, 254–56, 329
  and residential stability, 127–29
  and role obligations, 270, 293, 309–11, 314–15, 413, 414–15
  and social environment, 6–9, 401, 405, 409–18
  and spiritualism, 247–48, 254, 412
  impact on children, 328, 383, 413
  impact on spouses, 187, 209, 212–13, 302, 317, 328, 413, 417–18
  in family of orientation, 154–57, 179–80, 404
  perceptions of, 224–31, 302, 315–21
  spouses' concept of, 237, 284, 309, 314, 315, 316, 317–18, 320, 339–42
  theories of, 3–4

Schizophrenia, withdrawal in, 221, 223–24, 301, 339, 342, 371, 411–12
  See also: Illness, mental; *Loco*; Psychiatric evaluation; Role performance; Sex; Symptoms
Schroeder, C. W., 6
Sex, and schizophrenic men, 185–86, 338–41, 343–45, 346
  and schizophrenic women, 341–45
  conflicts about, 332–45
  first experiences, 141–44, 177–78, 406
  social concepts of, 133–36, 178, 333–35, 405
  See also: Courtship; *Macho*; Marriage; Spouse relations
Slums, description of, 53–58, 349, 360–61, 364, 366, 367
Social classes, acceptance of, 60
  class V, description, 51, 52–66
  interclass relations, 34, 63–64, 404
  perceptions of, 14–15, 60–65, 390–91
  structure of, 46–51
Socialization, and personality formation, 95–115, 133, 408
  of boys, 134–36, 332, 405
  of girls, 133–34, 405
  See also: Childhood of spouses; Children of families, Parent-child relations
Spiritualism, and doctors, 249, 251–52
  and psychiatry, 244, 253–54
  and religion, 255
  and schizophrenia, 247, 248, 254, 412
  as therapy, 246, 253–54
  belief in, 31–32, 63, 193, 245–54
  description of session, 246–47
  ideology, 244, 246, 249–50
  mediums, 244, 246, 247, 249, 251
  schedule on, 13–14
Spouse relations, 263–75, 314–21, 323–25, 409
  conformance in, 251, 271, 302, 318, 406
  male freedom, 233–34, 236, 271
  respeto in, 266–67, 293
  restriction of women, 233–35, 273, 293–94, 334–56

Spouse relations,
  See also: Control families; Double schizophrenic families; Husband-schizophrenic families; *Macho;* Marriage; Men; Wife-schizophrenic families; Women
Srole, L., 5, 6
Sterilization, and schizophrenia, 160
  of men, 300
  of women, 162–63
Stress and schizophrenia, 183, 187–88, 196–97, 213–14, 405
Symptoms (schizophrenic), attempts to control, 240, 301
  explanations of, 225–29
  onset, 186–87, 197, 208, 227, 362, 411

Tillman, C., 4
Treatment, for mental illness, 6, 154, 229, 243–44, 306, 363
  for physical illness, 107–09, 354
  perceptions of, 221
  through spiritualism, 246, 253–54
  See also: Hospitalization; Referral

Wife-schizophrenic families, children, 389–90
  conflicts, 341–43, 375, 388
  fantasy world of women, 273–74, 383
  mutual help, 363–67, 373
  problematic year, 190–97
  social control, 314–21
  violence, 318–19, 342, 395
  See also: Employment; Fear; Hospitalization; Marriage; Parent-child relations; Sex
Withdrawal (schizophrenic), 221, 223–41, 301, 339, 342, 371, 412
Women, and mutual help, 356–59, 362–63, 413, 417
  conformance of, 251, 271, 302, 318, 406
  employment of, 112–14, 119–24, 284, 295–96, 302–03, 304
  "ideal" roles, 265–66, 282–83
  obligations of, 270, 314–15, 334, 382–83, 410
  restriction of, 233–35, 273, 293–94, 334, 356
Wynne, L. C., 4